AF443394

COMBATING THE THREAT OF PANDEMIC INFLUENZA

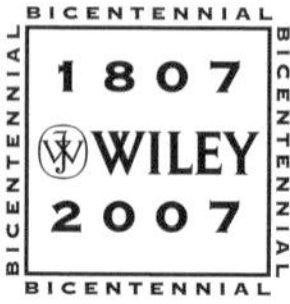

THE WILEY BICENTENNIAL–KNOWLEDGE FOR GENERATIONS

Each generation has its unique needs and aspirations. When Charles Wiley first opened his small printing shop in lower Manhattan in 1807, it was a generation of boundless potential searching for an identity. And we were there, helping to define a new American literary tradition. Over half a century later, in the midst of the Second Industrial Revolution, it was a generation focused on building the future. Once again, we were there, supplying the critical scientific, technical, and engineering knowledge that helped frame the world. Throughout the 20th Century, and into the new millennium, nations began to reach out beyond their own borders and a new international community was born. Wiley was there, expanding its operations around the world to enable a global exchange of ideas, opinions, and know-how.

For 200 years, Wiley has been an integral part of each generation's journey, enabling the flow of information and understanding necessary to meet their needs and fulfill their aspirations. Today, bold new technologies are changing the way we live and learn. Wiley will be there, providing you the must-have knowledge you need to imagine new worlds, new possibilities, and new opportunities.

Generations come and go, but you can always count on Wiley to provide you the knowledge you need, when and where you need it!

WILLIAM J. PESCE
PRESIDENT AND CHIEF EXECUTIVE OFFICER

PETER BOOTH WILEY
CHAIRMAN OF THE BOARD

COMBATING THE THREAT OF PANDEMIC INFLUENZA

Drug Discovery Approaches

Edited by

PAUL F. TORRENCE
Northern Arizona University
Department of Chemistry and Biochemistry
Flagstaff, Arizona

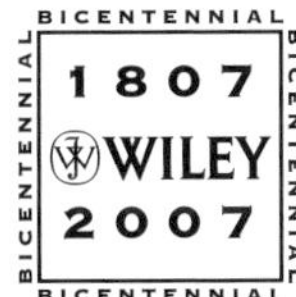

WILEY-INTERSCIENCE
A JOHN WILEY & SONS, INC., PUBLICATION

Library of Congress Cataloging-in-Publication Data:

Combating the threat of pandemic influenza : drug discovery approaches / edited by Paul F. Torrence.
     p. ; cm.
  Includes bibliographical references and index.
  ISBN 978-0-470-11879-5 (cloth)
  1. Antiviral agents. 2. Influenza—Chemotherapy. I. Torrence, Paul F.
  [DNLM: 1. Influenza, Human—drug therapy. 2. Influenza, Human—prevention & control. 3. Antiviral Agents—therapeutic use. 4. Disease Outbreaks—prevention & control. 5. Drug Design. 6. Influenza Vaccines—therapeutic use. WC 515 C729 2008]
  RM411.C66 2008
  616.2′03061—dc22

2007011326

CONTENTS

CONTRIBUTORS

Laura M. Aschenbrenner, NexBio, Inc., San Diego, CA 92121

Ben Berkhout, Laboratory of Experimental Virology, Center for Infection and Immunity Amsterdam (CINIMA), Academic Medical Center of the University of Amsterdam, 1105 AZ Amsterdam, The Netherlands

Nicolai V. Bovin, Shemyakin Institute of Bioorganic Chemistry RAS, 117997, Moscow, Russia

Mary E. Christopher, Chemical and Biological Defence Section, Defence R&D Canada—Suffield, Ralston, Alberta T1A 8K6, Canada

Murray Cairns, School of Biomedical Sciences, Faculty of Health, University of Newcastle, NSW 2308, Australia

Roderic M. K. Dale, Oligos Etc. Inc., Wilsonville, OR 97070

Erik De Clercq, Rega Institute for Medical Research, Katholieke Universiteit Leuven, B-3000 Leuven, Belgium

Heather Ezelle, Marlene and Stewart Greenebaum Cancer Center, University of Maryland, Baltimore School of Medicine, Baltimore, MD

Fang Fang, NexBio, Inc., San Diego, CA 92121

Alexandra S. Gambaryan, Shemyakin Institute of Bioorganic Chemistry RAS, 117997, Moscow, Russia

George F. Gao, Department of Molecular Immunology and Molecular Virology, Institute of Microbiology, Chinese Academy of Sciences, Datunlu, Beijing 100101, People's Republic of China

Joost Haasnoot, Laboratory of Experimental Virology, Department of Medical Microbiology, Center for Infection and Immunity Amsterdam (CINIMA), Academic Medical Center of the University of Amsterdam, 1105 AZ Amsterdam, The Netherlands

Corwin Hansch, Department of Chemistry, Pomona College, Claremont, CA 91711

Minoru Hashimoto, Riken Vitamin Co., Ltd., Chiyoda-ku, Tokyo 101-8370, Japan

Bret A. Hassel, Marlene and Stewart Greenebaum Cancer Center and Department of Microbiology and Immunology, University of Maryland, Baltimore School of Medicine, Baltimore, MD 21201

Kyoko Hayashi, Graduate School of Medicine and Pharmaceutical Sciences, University of Toyama, 2630 Sugitani, Toyama 930-0194, Japan

Toshimitsu Hayashi, Graduate School of Medicine and Pharmaceutical Sciences, University of Toyama, 2630 Sugitani, Toyama 930-0194, Japan

Kenji Kanekiyo, Graduate School of Medicine and Pharmaceutical Sciences, University of Toyama, 2630 Sugitani, Toyama 930-0194, Japan

Jung-Bum Lee, Graduate School of Medicine and Pharmaceutical Sciences, University of Toyama, 2630 Sugitani, Toyama 930-0194, Japan

Takahisa Nakano, Riken Vitamin Co., Ltd., 32-9-28 Misaki-cho, Chiyoda-ku, Tokyo 101-8370, Japan

Diana L. Noah, Southern Research Institute, Drug Discovery Division, Birmingham, AL 35205

James W. Noah, Drug Discovery Division, Southern Research Institute, Birmingham, AL 35205

Yuko Ohta, Graduate School of Medicine and Pharmaceutical Sciences, University of Toyama, 2630 Sugitani, Toyama 930-0194, Japan

Nicole Pelletier, NexBio, Inc., San Diego, CA 92121

Andres M. Salazar, Oncovir Inc., Washington, DC 20008

Shiro Shigeta, Fukushima Medical University and Bureau of Prefectural Hospitals of Fukushima, Fukushima 960-8043, Japan

L.-Q. Sun, Oligos Etc. Inc., Wilsonville, OR 97070

Jonathan P. Wong, Chemical and Biological Defence Section, Defence R&D Canada—Suffield, Ralston, Alberta T1A 8K6, Canada

Rajeshwar P. Verma, Department of Chemistry, Pomona College, Claremont, CA 91711

E. Lucile White, Drug Discovery Division, Southern Research Institute, Birmingham, AL 35205

Mang Yu, NexBio, Inc., San Diego, CA 92121

PREFACE

It seems impossible not to see or hear of the threat of avian influenza in the printed media or the nightly news. The avian influenza A (H5N1) epizootic that is occurring in Asia and in parts of Europe, the Near East, and Africa will not likely diminish soon. Thus far, there is no evidence to suggest genetic recombination between avian influenza A virus and human genes. Nonetheless, since there is little preexisting natural immunity to H5N1 infection in human populations, if H5N1 viruses become able to maintain efficient and sustained transmission among humans, an influenza pandemic could result. High rates of morbidity and mortality could result along with staggering economic and societal disruption.[1-4]

While vaccines will likely be the most effective at reducing morbidity and mortality, they may be available in the beginning of a pandemic because of production capacity.[5] Therefore, antivirals, such as neuraminidase inhibitors, would be expected to provide pharmaceutical intervention until sufficient vaccine can be produced.[6-8] This places a huge onus on antiviral chemotherapy, especially when the phenomenon of emerging resistance is considered.[9] Of great significance is the finding that H5N1 viruses from humans in Thailand and Vietnam show resistance to amantadine and rimantadine, Therefore, novel approaches of all kinds to effective therapeutics for influenza should be sought. The contributions in this volume provide some insight into such possibilities.

In Chapter 1, De Clercq provides an overview of the current state of antiviral therapeutics for influenza. Covered are: M2 ion-channel inhibitors such as amantadine, rimantadine, and new adamantanamine congeners; interferon and interferon inducers; neuraminidase inhibitors such as the well-known zanamivir and oseltamivir as well as more recent compounds such as peramivir and other cyclopentane or pyrrolidine derivatives and dimeric zanamivir derivatives; the IMP dehydrogenase inhibitors ribavirin and viramidine; RNA polymerase inhibitors such as 2′-deoxy-2′-fluoroguanosine and the newer thiadiazolo[2,3-a]pyrimidine and pyrimidinyl acylthiourea. In addition, the key issues of drug combinations and resisitance devlopment are treated.

The vital matter of high-throughput screening (HTS) to aid in the identification of new leads for influenza antivirals is dealt with by Noah et al. in Chapter 2. Described is the potential of each influenza component as an assay target, along with the current state of influenza assays that are adaptable or have already been adapted to HTS formats for diagnostic strain characterization, vaccine evaluation, and identification of potential antivirals.

Interferon and interferon inducers have been around for some time and may prove to be of use as interferon antivirals, but it may well be the targets revealed through mechanisms of their antiviral activity that will provide clues for alternative therapeutics. In Chapter 3, Ezelle and Hassel review the ever-expanding knowledge base of interferon actions.

In Chapter 4, Shigeta describes his laboratory's experiences in mass-screening trial of potential anti-myxovirus agents including both synthetic and natural substances, Several broad-spectrum anti-myxovirus agents have been found in these studies, and some of these compounds exceeded ribavirin in potency and selectivity *in vitro* and some displayed activity *in vivo*.

Wong and colleagues look at nucleic acid-based agents (with the exception of RNAi interference) as antiviral agents in Chapter 5, whereas Haasnoot and Berkhout review the activity and potential of RNA interference against influenza and other respiratory viruses in Chapter 6.

Hayashi and co-workers review their research on fucoidan, a sulfated polysaccharide isolated from an edible alga *Undaria pinnatifida*, as an inhibitor of influenza A virus replication in Chapter 7. This fucoidan shows *in vitro* antiviral activity and synergistic antiviral action in combination with oseltamivir.

Carbohydrate chains of mammalian host cells are known to be receptors for influenza virus and many other viruses and bacteria. In Chapter 8, Bovin and Gambaryan presented the rational design of an anti-adhesion drug for influenza. This includes self-assembling glyco-peptides and symmetric star-like molecules.

Verma and Hansch apply quantitative structure–activity relationships (QSAR) in the search for new neuraminidase inhibitors as anti-influenza drugs in Chapter 9. From data gathered on known specific influenza A and B neuraminidase inhibitors, the authors have developed two QSAR models that may be used to narrow the synthetic challenges required to develop new inhibitors.

In Chapter 10, Gao relates recent progress in the development of anti-virus fusion peptides by addressing the important hepted repeat (HR) polypeptides in some notorious viruses, such as HIV, Newcastle disease virus (NDV), and influenza virus, which are all Class I enveloped viruses.

Finally, in Chapter 11, Aschenbrenner and colleagues describe several new approaches under development at NexBio, Inc. These include a chemical entity that inactivates the virus receptor and another that inhibits the viral RNA polymerase.

REFERENCES

1. Ferguson, N. M.; Cummings, D. A.; Fraser, C.; Cajka, J. C.; Cooley, P. C.; Burke, D. S. Strategies for mitigating an influenza pandemic. *Nature.* **2006**, *442*(7101), 448–452.

2. Donis, R. O. Avian influenza: An omnipresent pandemic threat. *Pediatr. Infect. Dis. J.* **2005**, *24*(11 Suppl.), S208–S216, discussion S215.

3. Duley, M. G. The next pandemic: Anticipating an overwhelmed health care system. *Yale J. Biol. Med.* **2005**, *78*(5), 355–362.

4. Gust, I. D.; Hampson, A. W.; Lavanchy, D. Planning for the next pandemic of influenza. *Rev. Med. Virol.* **2001**, *11*(1), 59–70.

5. Arras, J. D. Rationing vaccine during an avian influenza pandemic: Why it won't be easy. *Yale J. Biol. Med.* **2005**, *78*(5), 287–300.

6. Oshitani, H. Potential benefits and limitations of various strategies to mitigate the impact of an influenza pandemic. *J. Infect. Chemother.* **2006**, *12*(4), 167–171.

7. Monto, A. S. Vaccines and antiviral drugs in pandemic preparedness. *Emerg. Infect. Dis.* **2006**, *12*(1), 55–60.

8. Cox, M. M. Pandemic influenza: Overview of vaccines and antiviral drugs. *Yale J. Biol. Med.* **2005**, *78*(5), 321–328.

9. Romanova, J. The fight against new types of influenza virus. *Biotechnol. J.* **2006**, *1*(12), 1381–1392.

PAUL F. TORRENCE

Flagstaff, AZ

1

EXISTING INFLUENZA ANTIVIRALS: THEIR MECHANISMS OF ACTION AND POTENTIAL IN THE FACE OF AVIAN INFLUENZA*

ERIK DE CLERCQ

Rega Institute for Medical Research, Katholieke Universiteit Leuven, B-3000 Leuven, Belgium

INTRODUCTION

The outbreaks of avian influenza A (H5N1) in Southeast Asia[2] (with several clusters recently identified in Indonesia[3]), the expanding geographic distribution of this epizootic virus (with well-documented cases in Eastern Turkey in 2006[4]), and the ability of influenza A to transfer to humans and cause severe infection have aroused serious concerns on the control measures that should be undertaken if a pandemic with influenza A, whether avian or human, would strike. In the wake of such pandemic, several preventive and therapeutic strategies have been formulated, among which are the stockpiling of antiviral drugs[2,5] and in particular the neuraminidase inhibitors oseltamivir (Tamiflu™) and zanamivir (Relenza™).

*This chapter represents an adjusted and updated version of De Clercq, E. Antiviral agents active against influenza viruses, *Nature Rev. Drug Discovery* **5**:1015–1025 (2006).[1]

Combating the Threat of Pandemic Influenza: Drug Discovery Approaches,
Edited by Paul F. Torrence
Copyright © 2007 by John Wiley & Sons, Inc.

Many governments are now stockpiling large quantities of oseltamivir, providing an expanding and durable market for the drug.[6] Public and media interest in avian influenza has sparked demand for oseltamivir in the private sector, leading to increases in prescriptions amid fears of a shortage.[6] Roche has announced plans to dramatically increase production by as much as 8- to 10-fold to meet these demands. Other companies are now considering to resurrect their antiviral programs to take advantage of the increased interest generated by the possibility of a pandemic.[6] Given the considerable challenges to the rapid development of an effective vaccine against influenza A (H5N1) antiviral agents will play an important role as a first-line defense if a new pandemic strikes.[7] However, the large-scale use of drugs for chemoprophylaxis and chemotherapy imposes new challenges—that is, those of the selection and ensuing transmission of drug-resistant virus strains.[7]

There are, in principle, two mechanisms by which pandemic influenza may originate (i) by direct transmission (of a mutated virus?) from animal (bird) to man, as happened in 1918 with the "Spanish influenza" (H1N1), "the mother of all pandemics," [8] or (ii) through reassortment of an avian with a human influenza virus, as occurred in 1957 with the "Asian influenza" (H2N2) and, again, in 1968 with the "Hong Kong influenza" (H3N2)[9] (Fig. 1.1).[10] Whether a new influenza pandemic may arise through (i) antigenic "drift" from an avian influenza or (ii) antigenic "shift" by recombination of an avian and human influenza virus can only be speculated upon. Whereas this question is of crucial importance for future vaccine development, it basically should have little bearing on antiviral drug design, because the antiviral drug targets, as depicted in Fig. 1.2, should be applicable to all influenza A virus variants.[11]

M2 ION-CHANNEL INHIBITORS: AMANTADINE, RIMANTADINE, AND NEW ADAMANTANAMINE DERIVATIVES

The first synthetic compound ever shown to inhibit influenza virus replication was amantadine.[12] As indicated in Fig. 1.2 amantadine blocks, within the endosomes, the migration of H^+ ions (protons) into the interior of the virus particles (virions), a process that is needed for the uncoating to occur. The H^+ ions are imported through the M2 (matrix 2) channels.[13] The transmembrane domain of the M2 protein, with the amino acid residues facing the ion-conducting pore,[14] is shown in Fig. 1.3. Amantadine has been postulated to plug up the interior

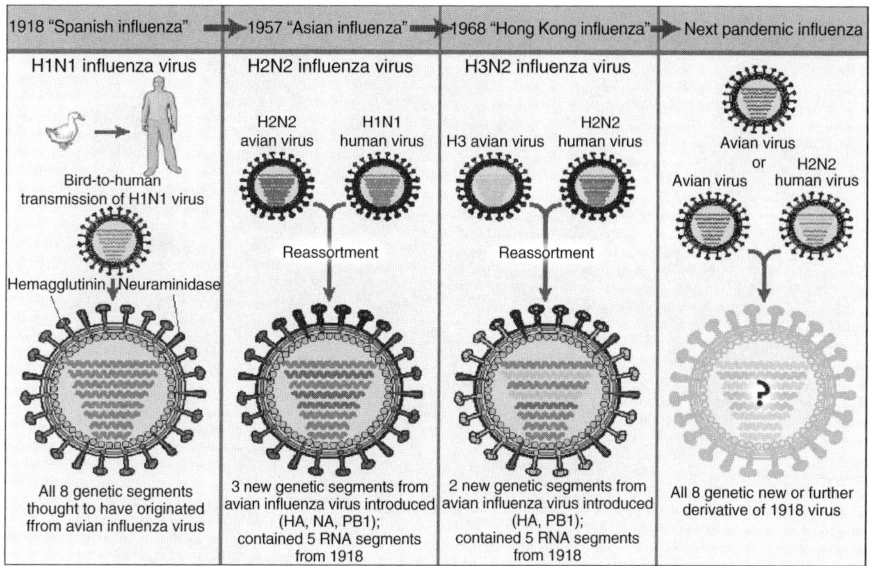

Fig. 1.1. The two mechanisms whereby pandemic influenza originates. In 1918, the "Spanish influenza" H1N1 virus closely related to an avian virus adapted to replicate efficiently in humans. In 1957 and 1968, reassortment events led to, respectively, the "Asian influenza" H2N2 virus and the "Hong Kong influenza" H3N2 virus. The "Asian influenza" H2N2 virus acquired three genetic segments from an avian species [a hemagglutinin, a neuraminidase, and a polymerase (PB1) gene]. The "Hong Kong influenza" H3N2 virus acquired two genetic segments from an avian species (hemagglutinin and PB1). Future pandemic strains could arise through either mechanism.[10] (Taken from Belshe.[10]) See color insert.

channel within the tetrameric M2 helix bundle.[15] The adamantan(amin)e derivatives amantadine and rimantadine (Fig. 1.4) have for a considerable time been available for both the prophylaxis and therapy of influenza A virus infections, but their use has been limited essentially because of the rapid emergence of virus-drug resistance, the ready transmissibility of the drug-resistant viruses.

In addition to amantadine and rimantadine, a variety of new adamantanamine derivatives have been accredited with marked activity against influenza A (H2N2 and/or H3N2): spiro[cyclopropane-1,2′-adamantan]-2-amine,[16] spiro[pyrrolidine-2,2′-adamantane],[16] spiro[piperidine-2,2′-adamantane],[17] 2-(2-adamantyl)piperidine,[18] 3-(2-adamantyl)pyrrolidine,[19] rimantadine 2-isomers,[20] 2-(1-adamantyl)piperidine,[21] 2-(1-adamantyl)pyrrolidine,[21] and 2-(1-adamantyl)-2-methyl-pyrrolidine[22] (Fig. 1.4). Whether any of these new adamantyl derivatives may offer any advantage—in terms of potency, selectivity, safety, or resistance

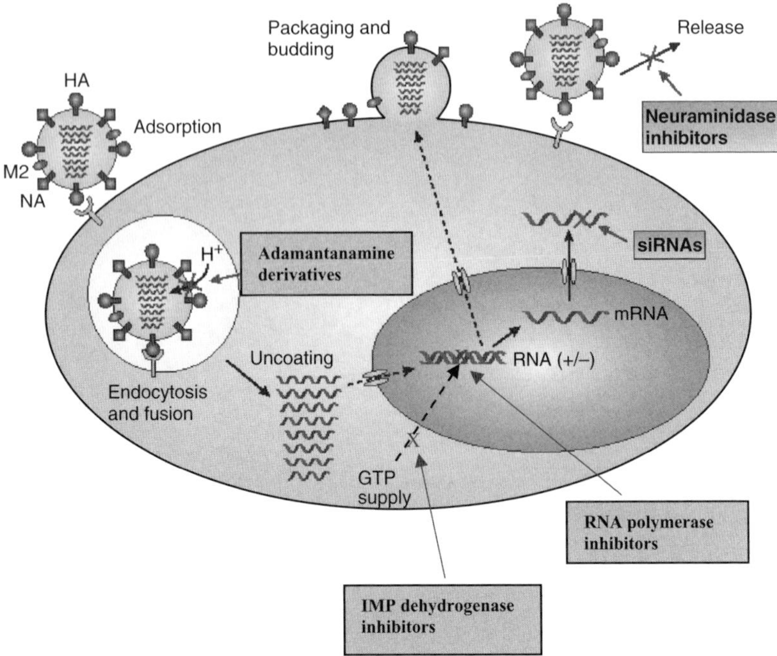

Fig. 1.2. Inhibition of influenza virus replication cycle by antivirals. After binding to sialic acid receptors, influenza virions are internalized by receptor-mediated endocytosis. The low pH in the endosome triggers the fusion of viral and endosomal membranes, and the influx of H^+ ions through the M2 channel releases the viral RNA genes in the cytoplasm. Adamantanamine derivatives block this uncoating step. RNA replication/ transcription occurs in the nucleus. This process can be blocked by inhibitors of IMP dehydrogenase (a cellular enzyme) or viral RNA polymerase. The stability of the viral mRNA and its translation to viral protein may be prevented by siRNAs. Packaging and budding of virions occur at the cytoplasmic membrane. Neuraminidase inhibitors block the release of the newly formed virions from the infected cells. (Taken from Palese,[11] with modifications.[1]) See color insert.

profile—over the parent compounds amantadine and rimantadine needs to be further explored.

RESISTANCE TO THE M2 ION-CHANNEL INHIBITORS AMANTADINE AND RIMANTADINE

Resistance to amantadine and rimantadine develops rapidly as a result of single amino acid substitutions 26, 27, 30, 31, or 34 within the transmembrane domain of the M2 protein.[23] In particular, the Ser → Asn mutation at position 31 (S31N) engenders high-level resistance to

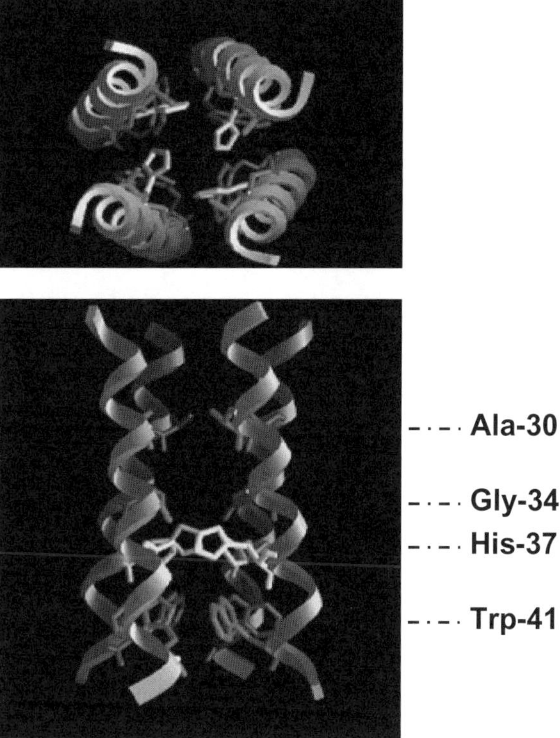

Fig. 1.3. Model of the proposed transmembrane domain of the M2 protein, showing top view as seen from the extracellular side and a cross section in the plane of the lipid layer. Residues that were identified as facing the ion-conducting aqueous pore are indicated. (Taken from Shuck et al.[14]) See color insert.

adamantan(amin)es (Fig. 1.5).[24] The incidence of adamantan(amin)e (M2-inhibitor) resistance among human influenza A (H3N2) virus in the United States has increased from less than 2% until 2004 to 14.5% for the period October 2004–March 2005 to 92.3% for the period October–December 2005.[24] The incidence of adamantane resistance among influenza A (H3N2) viruses isolated in the United States[25] and worldwide[26] has been a cause for concern. More than 98% of the adamantane-resistant isolates identified worldwide between 1995 and 2005 contain the same S31N substitution.[26]

The rate of adamant(amin)e resistance began to increase in Asia in the 1997–1998 influenza season and increased markedly in China to 57.5% in 2002–2003 and 73.8% in 2003–2004.[26] Misuse of the adamant(amin)es most likely contributed to this rapid increase in resistance. In China, Russia, and some other countries, amantadine and

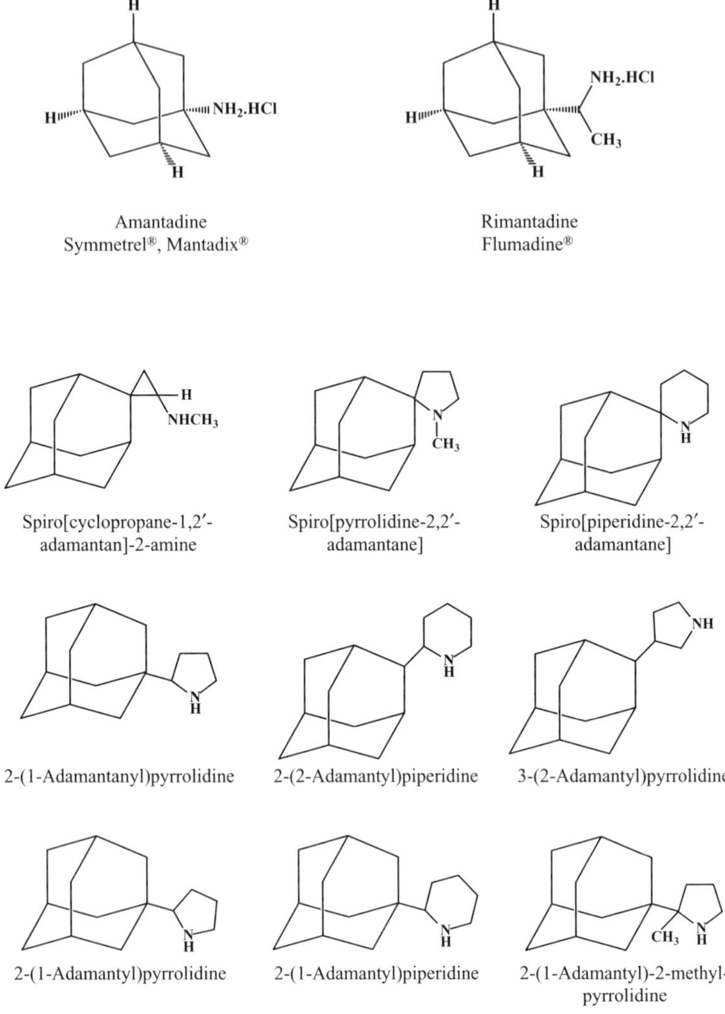

Fig. 1.4. The adamantane (or adamantanamine) derivatives amantadine and rimantadine and various new adamantanamine derivatives. Amantadine, rimantadine, and adamantanamine derivatives share a number of common structural features, which relate to their eventual mode of action—that is, blockage of the M2 channel—responsible for transporting H^+ ions (protons) into the interior of the virions and initiating the viral uncoating process (see legend to Fig. 1.2). Several new adamantamine derivatives were found to be more active than amantadine: i.e. 230-fold (spiro[pyrrolidine-2,2′-adamantane), 101-fold (spiro[cyclopropane-1,2′-adamantan]-2-amine), and 4.3-fold (3-[2-adamantyl]pyrrolidine).[22]

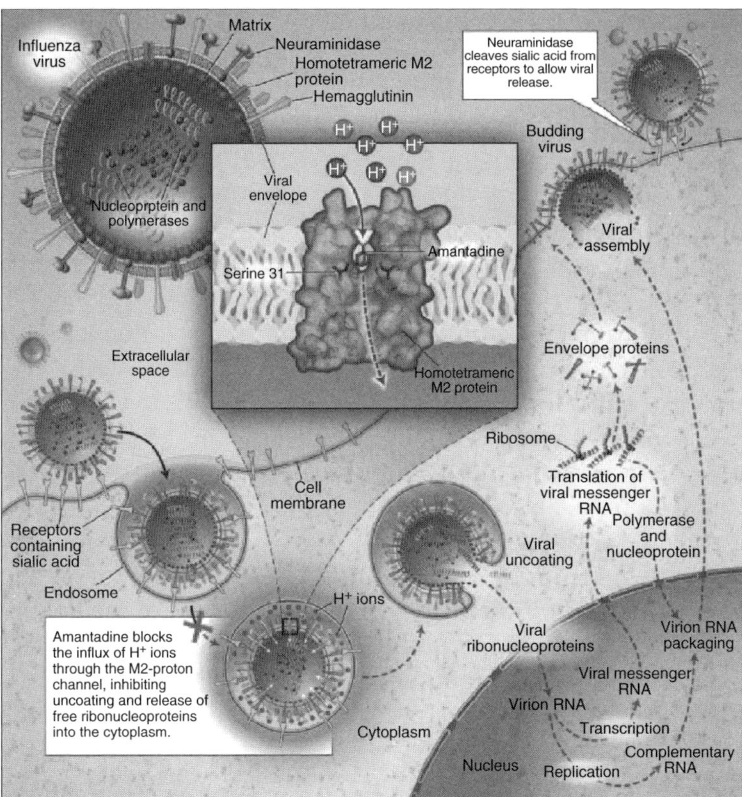

Fig. 1.5. Mechanism of action of and development of resistance to M2 inhibitors. In the absence of amantadine, the proton channel mediates an influex of H⁺ ions into the infecting virion early in the viral replication cycle, which facilitates the dissociation of the ribonucleoproteins from the virion interior and allows them to be released into the cytoplasm and transported into the cell nucleus. In highly pathogenic avian viruses (H5 and H7), the M2-proton channel protects the hemagglutinin from acid-induced inactivation in the trans-Golgi network during transport to the cell surface. In the presence of amantadine, the channel is blocked and replication is inhibited. The serine at position 31 lies partially in the protein–protein interface and partially in the channel (see inset). Replacement of serine by a larger asparagine leads to the loss of amantadine binding and the restoration of channel function. Depending on the particular amino acid, other mutations at position 26, 27, 30, or 34 may inhibit amantadine binding or allow binding without the loss of ion-channel function. [Taken from Hayden.[24] Inset courtesy of Rupert Russell, Phillip Spearpoint, and Alan Hay (National Institute for Medical Research, London).] See color insert.

rimantadine are both available without a prescription and are included in over-the-counter "antiflu" and "cold" preparations at a range of doses.[27] In North America, the increase in resistance began about 5 years after the initial increase in Asia to reach the current 92%.[25] In January 2006, the Centers for Disease Control (CDC) issued a Health Alert and recommended that neither amantadine nor rimantadine should be used for the treatment or prophylaxis of influenza A infections in the United States for the remainder of the 2005–2006 influenza season.[27]

The distribution of amantadine-resistant avian influenza H5N1 in Asia has been examined.[28] More than 95% of the H5N1 viruses isolated in Vietnam and Thailand contained resistance mutations, as compared to 6.3% in Indonesia and 8.9% in China. The dual mutation Leu26Ile and Ser31Asn was found almost exclusively in all resistant isolates from Vietnam, Thailand, and Cambodia.[28]

The startling increase in the incidence of adamantan(amin)e resistance in the United States[25] has obviously been looking for an explanation, one (still hypothetical) being the wide-scale use of the amantadine derivative memantine (3,5-dimethyl-L-adamantanamine). Memantine, which interacts with the N-methyl-D-aspartate (NMDA) receptor,[29] has been launched in March 2004 for the treatment of Alzheimer's disease, accounting for 26% of all prescriptions for this disease by March 31, 2005. The introduction of memantine may, according to this provocative hypothesis,[29] have inadvertently led to the inability of amantadine to be used in the prophylaxis or therapy of influenza A.

NEURAMINIDASE INHIBITORS: ZANAMIVIR AND OSELTAMIVIR

Whereas the viral hemagglutinin (H) is needed for the virus to interact with the receptor bearing the N-acetylneuraminic acid (NANA, sialic acid), the viral neuraminidase (N) that cleaves off NANA enables the progeny virions to leave the infected cells and to spread to other host cells. By blocking the release of these newly formed virus particles, neuraminidase inhibitors should prevent further spread of the virus[30,31] (Fig. 1.6). The neuraminidase may also play a role early in influenza infection of the human airway epithelium.[32] The viral neuraminidase cleaves NANA (sialic acid or SA) from the cell surface glycoprotein at a specific bond [SAα2,3Gal (sialic acid linked to galactose by an α-2,3 linkage) or SAα2,6Gal (sialic acid linked to galactose by an α-2,6 linkage)] (Fig. 1.7).

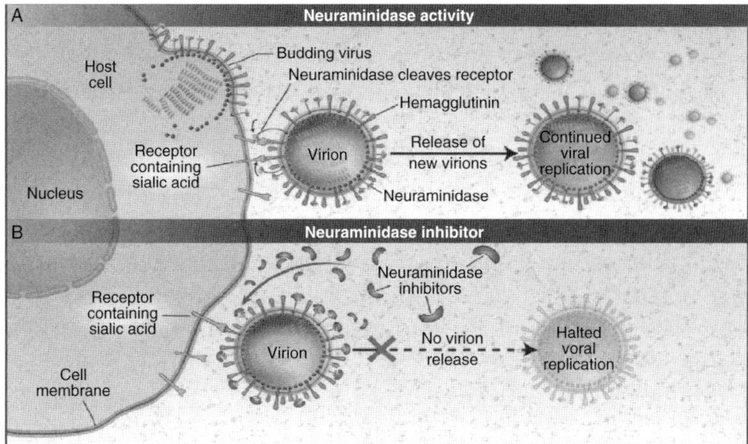

Fig. 1.6. Mechanism of action of neuraminidase inhibitors. Neuraminidase inhibitors, such as zanamivir and oseltamivir (see Fig. 1.8), interfere with the release of progeny influenza virions from the surface of infected host cells. In doing so, the neuraminidase inhibitors prevent virus infection of new host cells and thereby halt the spread of infection in the respiratory tract. The neuraminidase cleaves off sialic acid (*N*-acetylneuraminic acid) from the cell receptor for influenza virus (see Fig. 1.7), so that the newly formed virus particles can be released from the cells. Neuraminidase inhibitors prevent this process. (Taken from Moscona.[31]) See color insert.

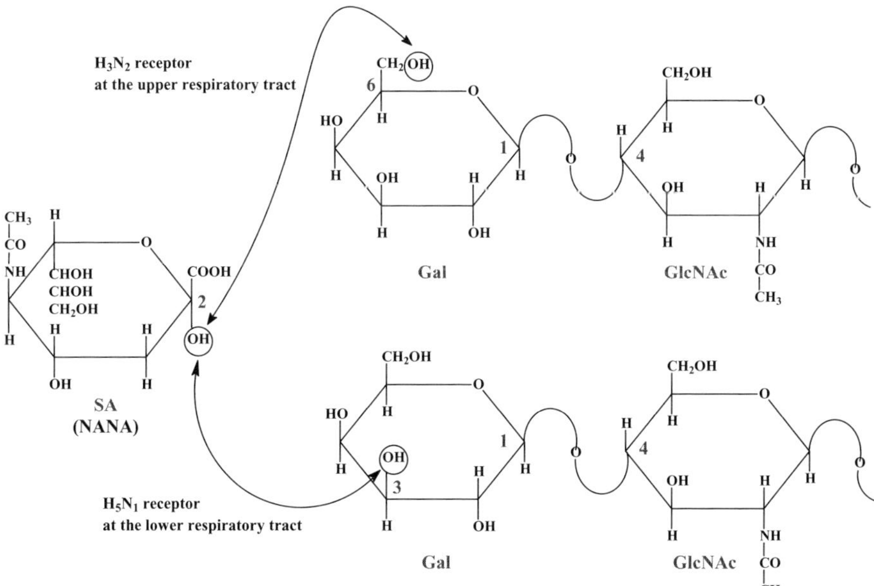

Fig. 1.7. Sialic acid (SA) [also known as *N*-acetylneuraminic acid (NANA)] linked to galactose (Gal) by an α2–3 linkage (SAα2–3Gal) or α2–6 linkage (SAα2–6Gal). Galactose is linked to *N*-acetylglucosamine (GlcNAc through a β1–4 linkage).

Avian (H5N1) influenza and human (H3N2, H1N1) influenza viruses seem to target different receptors of the human respiratory tract: Whereas human-derived viruses preferentially recognize SAα2,6Gal located on epithelial cells of the nasal mucosa, paranasal sinuses, pharynx, trachea, and bronchi, avian viruses would preferentially recognize SAα2,3Gal located more deeply in the respiratory tract, at the alveolar cell wall and junction between the respiratory bronchiole and alveolus.[33] The avian influenza H5N1 virus may cause severe lower respiratory tract (LRT) disease in humans because it attaches predominantly to type II pneumocytes, alveolar macrophages, and nonciliated bronchiolar cells of the human LRT.[34] In terms of the effectiveness of neuraminidase inhibitors, it would not, in theory, matter whether NANA is bound via an α-2,3 or α-2,6 linkage, because the neuraminidase inhibitors act as transition state analogues[35] of NANA, irrespective on how it is bound to the penultimate galactose unit.

The first neuraminidase inhibitors designed according to the "transition state analogue" principle were DANA and FANA. They served as the lead compounds for the development of the neuraminidase inhibitors that were eventually marketed for the treatment (and prophylaxis) of influenza A and B virus infections: zanamivir (Relenza®, 4-guanidino-Neu5Ac2en, GG167)[36] and oseltamivir (Tamiflu®, GS4071 ethyl ester, GS4104, Ro64-0796)[37] (Fig. 1.8). Both compounds have been found to be highly potent inhibitors ($IC_{50} \leq 1\,ng/ml$) of the influenza neuraminidase, to inhibit influenza A and B virus replication *in vitro* and *in vivo* (mice, ferrets), to be well-tolerated, and to be both prophylactically (significant reduction in number of ill subjects) and therapeutically (significant reduction in duration of illness) effective against influenza A/B virus infection in humans. A crucial difference between zanamivir and oseltamivir, however, is that zanamivir has to be administered by inhalation (10 mg bid), whereas oseltamivir can be administered orally (75 or 150 mg b.i.d.).

The benefits to be expected from the neuraminidase inhibitors are that they may be expected to reduce illness duration by 1–3 days, to reduce the risk of virus transmission to household or health-care contacts, to reduce the number and severity of complications (sinusitis, bronchitis), to reduce the use of antibiotics and to prevent seasonal influenza virus infection. As shown in particular for oseltamivir, the earlier the administration of oseltamivir, the shorter the duration of fever, the greater the alleviation of symptoms and the faster the return to baseline activity and health scores.[38] Oseltamivir treatment of influenza illness reduces lower respiratory tract complications (LRTCs), particularly bronchitis and pneumonia, concomitantly with a reduction

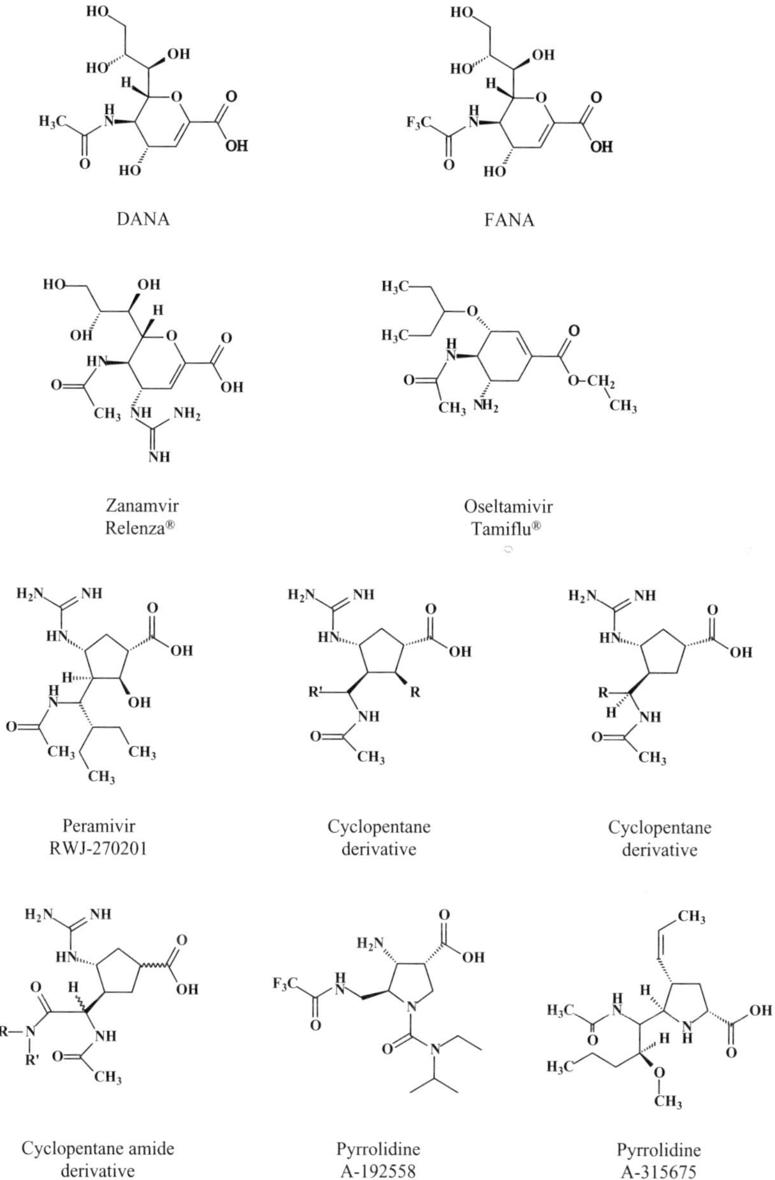

Fig. 1.8. DANA, FANA, eanamivir (Relenza®, 4-guanidino-Neu5Ac2en, GG167), oseltamivir (Tamiflu®, GS4071 ethyl ester, GS4104, Ro64-0796), peramivir (RWJ-270201), and cyclopentane and pyrrolidine derivatives.

in antibiotic use and need for hospitalization.[39] Also, post-exposure prophylaxis with oseltamivir, 75 mg once daily for 7 days, was found to protect close contacts of influenza-infected persons against influenza illness and prevented spread within households.[40] Post-exposure prophylaxis with oseltamivir can be considered an effective option for preventing the transmission of influenza within households.[41] It should be recognized, however, that oseltamivir is less effective against influenza B than against influenza A—that is, with regard to duration of fever and virus persistence.[42]

The neuraminidase inhibitors (i.e., GS4071) have been positioned in the active center of the neuraminidase (Fig. 1.9).[37,43] The structure of

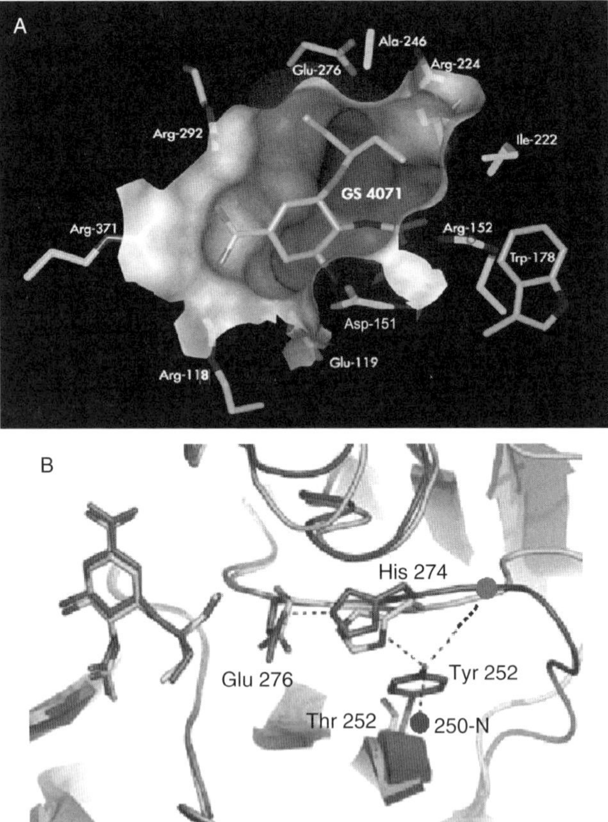

Fig. 1.9. GS4071 within the active site of the influenza A viral neuraminidase. Locations of oseltamivir-resistance mutations (i.e., H274Y) showing that the tyrosine at position 252 is involved in a network of hydrogen bonds in group-1 (H5N1 and H1N1) neuraminidases.[44] (Figure 1.9A was taken from Kim et al.[37] and De Clercq,[43] and Fig. 1.9B was taken from Russell et al.[44]) See color insert.

the influenza A virus neuraminidase has recently been resolved in two groups (group 1 contains the subtypes N1 (as in H5N1), N4, N5, and N8, and group 2 contains the subtypes N2 (as in H3N2), N3, N6, N7, and N9).[44] The crystal structures of the N1, N4, and N8 neuraminidases reported by Russell et al.,[44] surprisingly reveal that the active site of these group 1 enzymes have a different three-dimensional structure from that of group-2 enzymes.[45] The differences lie in a loop of amino acids known as the 150-loop. Group-1 neuraminidases contain a cavity adjacent to their active site that closes on ligand binding (Fig. 1.10).[44] When an inhibitor binds to group-1 subtypes, the 150-loop adopts a conformation similar to that of group-2 neuraminidases.[45] The cavity near the active site that is exposed by the open conformation of the 150-loop might be exploited in further drug design.[45]

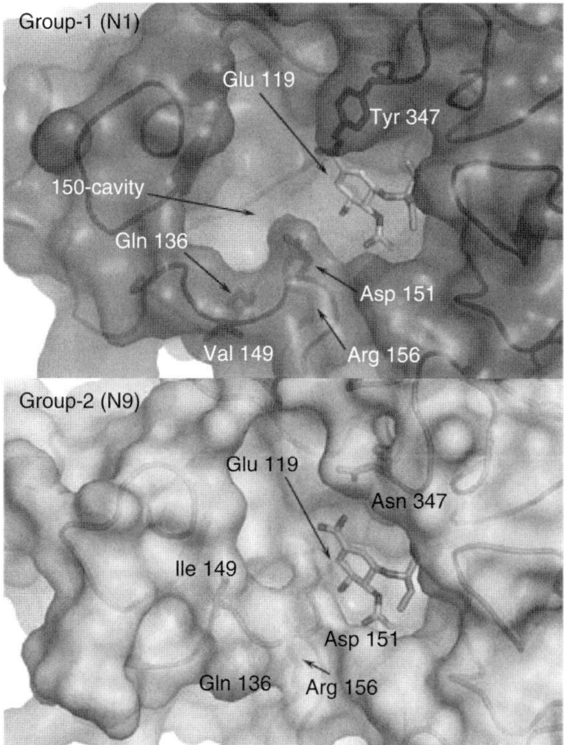

Fig. 1.10. Molecular surfaces of group-1 (N1) and group-2 (N9) neuraminidases with bound oseltamivir showing the 150-cavity in the group-1 (N1) structure that arises because of the distinct conformation of the 150-loop. (Taken from Russell et al.[44]) See color insert.

RESISTANCE TO NEURAMINIDASE INHIBITORS ZANAMIVIR AND OSELTAMIVIR

The neuraminidase inhibitors zanamivir and oseltamivir make contact, through their carboxylic acid group, with the neuraminidase amino acid residue arginine in position 292 and, through their basic amine (oseltamivir) or guanidinium (zanamivir) group, with the neuraminidase amino acid residue glutamic acid in position 119. Hence, it is not surprising that at these positions (R292K, E119G), mutations may arise that engender resistance to both zanamivir and oseltamivir.[46] The R292K mutation causes high-level resistance to oseltamivir but only low-level (5- to 30-fold) resistance to zanamivir.

In a comprehensive study of over 1000 clinical influenza isolates recovered from 1996 to 1999, there was no evidence of naturally occurring resistance to either oseltamivir or zanamivir in any of the isolates.[47] During the subsequent 3 years (1999–2002) the frequency of variants with decreased sensitivity to the neuraminidase inhibitors did not increase significantly (the percent variants with a >10-fold decrease in susceptibility to oseltamivir was 0.41% in 2002, as compared to 0.33% in 2000).[48] However, in children treated for influenza with oseltamivir, Kiso et al.[49] found neuraminidase mutations in viruses from nine patients (18%), six of whom had mutations at position 292 (R292K) and two at position 119 (E119V). It has been postulated that zanamvir-resistant influenza H3N2 viruses may not readily arise *in vivo* due to their poor viability (reduced fitness).[50]

Recombinant viruses containing either the wild-type neuraminidase or a single amino acid change at residue 119 (E119V) or 292 (R292K) were generated in the influenza A (H3N2) influenza virus background by reverse genetics: Both mutants showed decreased sensitivity to oseltamivir, and the R292K virus showed cross-resistance to zanamivir. The R292K mutation was associated with compromised viral growth and transmissibility (in accordance with earlier studies[51,52]), whereas the growth and transmissibility of the E119V virus was comparable to those of wild-type virus.[53]

Of note, influenza virus A (H3N2) carrying the R292K mutation in the neuraminidase gene did not transmit to ferrets under conditions the wild-type virus was readily transmitted.[51] However, other mutant viruses of influenza A (H3N2) (i.e., E119V and H274Y, both engendering resistance to oseltamivir) were found to be readily transmissible in ferrets, although the H274Y mutant required a 100-fold higher dose for infection and was transmitted more slowly than the wild type.[52]

It has been hypothesized that neuraminidase inhibitors could, in theory, inhibit the 1918 pandemic virus.[54] In fact, recombinant viruses possessing the 1918 neuraminidase, or both the 1918 neuraminidase and 1918 hemagglutinin, were shown to be effectively inhibited, both *in vitro* and *in vivo* (mice) by the neuraminidase inhibitors zanamivir and oseltamivir; and a recombinant virus possessing the 1918 M2 ion channel could be effectively inhibited by amantadine and rimantadine. This means that current antiviral strategies would be effective in curbing a reemerging 1918 or 1918-like influenza (H1N1) virus.[55]

Particular vigilance is warranted for drug-resistant influenza virus in immunocompromised patients, which may harbor, and shed, multi-drug-resistant influenza A (H3N2) for a prolonged time (1 year), as has been demonstrated for H3N2 influenza A H3N2 carrying the neuraminidase E119V mutation.[56,57]

The conserved amino acid residues that interact with neuraminidase inhibitors are under selective pressure, but only a few have been linked to resistance. In the A/Wuhan/359 (H3N2) recombinant virus background, seven charged neuraminidase residues (R118, R371, E227, R152, R224, E276, and D151) were characterized that directly interact with the neuraminidase inhibitors but have not been reported to confer resistance to neuraminidase inhibitors.[58] Of the mutations that may arise at these positions, only the E276D mutation was predicted to likely emerge under selective pressure.[58] Other mutations, in addition to those that are currently associated with influenza resistance to zanamivir and oseltamivir (E119G, R152K, H274Y, and R292K), are so-called "outlier" mutations (i.e., A18S, L23F, C42F, R143V, E199K, S332F, and K431N): these "outlier" mutations have not been associated with resistance to neuraminidase inhibitors.[59]

Resistance of influenza H5N1 to oseltamivir due to the H274Y mutation in the N gene has been described:[60] The patient from whom the oseltamivir-resistant H5N1 strain was isolated recovered from the disease, and the virus was found to be less pathogenic in ferrets than the parent strain and did not show cross-resistance to zanamivir. Although the H274Y mutation in influenza A H1N1 neuraminidase had been previously reported,[61,62] its occurrence in influenza A (H5N1) infection raised concern because it was associated with death in two of the eight influenza A (H5N1) virus-infected patients.[63] Whether there was a causal relationship between the emergence of the H274Y mutation and the lethal outcome could not be ascertained, however.[63]

The efficacy of oseltamivir in the treatment of H5N1 infection in humans could, because of its anecdotal use, not been unequivocally demonstrated. Yet, it should be pointed out that oseltamivir has been shown to protect ferrets against lethal influenza H5N1 infection: Treatment with oseltamivir at 5 mg/kg/day for 5 days twice daily (orally) resulted in complete inhibition of virus replication in the lungs and small intestine on day 5 p.i. and, consequently, prevented mortality.[64] Similarly, oseltamivir has proven efficacious in the treatment of mice infected with the highly pathogenic H5N1 A/Vietnam/1203/04 influenza virus strain, although prolonged and higher-dose oseltamivir regimens were required for achieving the most beneficial antiviral effect.[65]

Recent data have demonstrated that the sensitivities of the neuraminidase of H5N1 viruses isolated in 2004 and 2005 to oseltamivir are about 10-fold higher than those of earlier H5N1 viruses.[66] Although the clinical relevance of a 10-fold increase in sensitivity of neuraminidase to oseltamivir needs to be investigated further, the possibility that sensitivity to neuraminidase inhibitors could increase (or possibly decrease) significantly, even in the absence of treatment, underscores the need for continuous evaluation especially for influenza viruses with pandemic potential.[66]

NEURAMINIDASE INHIBITORS: PERAMIVIR AND OTHER CYCLOPENTANE OR PYRROLIDINE DERIVATIVES AND DIMERIC ZANAMIVIR DERIVATIVES

Whereas oseltamivir can be described as a cyclohexenyl derivative, there are a number of cyclopentane and pyrrolidine derivatives that have been described as neuraminidase inhibitors: peramivir (RWJ-270201, BCX-1182)[67–69] and other cyclopentane[69,70] and cyclopentane amide[71] derivatives as well as a variety of pyrrolidine derivatives, including A-192558,[72] A-315675,[73–75] and other pyrrolidines[76] (Fig. 1.8). Also, 2,3-disubstituted tetrahydrofuran-5-carboxylic acid derivatives have been described as influenza neuraminidase inhibitors, albeit with reduced inhibitory potency as compared to the corresponding pyrrolidine analogues.[77]

Peramivir (RWJ-270201) and A-315675 represent novel neuraminidase inhibitors that were shown to retain activity against various zanamivir- and oseltamivir-resistant influenza A and B viruses:[78] Specifically, a new oseltamivir-resistant influenza B variant carrying the D198N substitution at the viral neuraminidase was found to retain susceptibility to peramivir and A-315675. Also, the neuraminidase E119V mutant displaying 6000-fold lower susceptibility to oseltamivir and 175-fold lower susceptibility to zanamivir than did wild-type virus still retained full susceptibility to A-315675.[79]

Taken together the different studies performed with influenza A (H3N2) virus mutants,[49–53,78,79] it appears that neuraminidase inhibitors may select for mutations at a number of positions (E119V, R152K, D198N, H274Y, and R292K) that do only partially overlap,[80] that is, only partially engender cross-resistance.

In vivo, peramivir (BCX-1812, RWJ-270201) was found to strongly suppress influenza A (H1N1) infection in mice upon a single intramuscular injection (10 mg/kg). This was ascribed to a tight binding of peramivir to the neuraminidase.[81] Complete protection against lethality was afforded by peramivir given once daily for five days after influenza A virus infection in a murine model.[82] Similarly, a single intramuscular/ intravenous injection of peramivir, 1 hour pre-virus exposure, offered protection against influenza A (H5N1) in mice.[83] When given orally to humans, however, peramivir did not offer robust protection against human influenza A virus infection, which was attributed to the very low oral bioavailability (<5%) of peramivir;[84] further studies with parenteral formulations of peramivir are, therefore, warranted.

Dimeric derivatives of zanamivir with linking groups of 14–18 atoms in length were found to be 100-fold more potent inhibitors of influenza virus replication *in vitro* and *in vivo* than zanamivir.[85,86] These compounds exhibited long-lasting antiviral activity due to extremely long resistance times in the lungs, thus allowing a once-weekly dosing regimen. This raises the prospect for a new type of anti-influenza drug that could be administered as a single dose in the treatment of influenza, or just once a week in the prevention of infection.[86]

IMP DEHYDROGENASE INHIBITORS: RIBAVIRIN AND VIRAMIDINE

Ribavirin has long been recognized as a broad-spectrum antiviral agent with particularly distinct activity against orthomyxo (i.e., influenza) and paramyxo (i.e., measles, respiratory syncytial) viruses.[87] Respiratory syncytial virus (RSV) infection is the only (−)RNA virus infection for which aerosolized ribavirin has been formally approved. Oral ribavirin is also used, in combination with parenteral pegylated α-interferon, in the treatment of chronic hepatitis C virus (HCV) infection. The intravenous form of ribavirin has been registered for the treatment of hemorrhagic fever with renal syndrome (HFRS). In addition to ribavirin, viramidine, which can actually be considered as the amidine prodrug of ribavirin (Fig. 1.11), has been accredited with marked potential as an anti-influenza drug.[88] Of interest, ribavirin has not been shown to generate virus-drug resistance, and resistance of influenza virus replication to ribavirin has not been reported to date. Obviously, this lack of drug

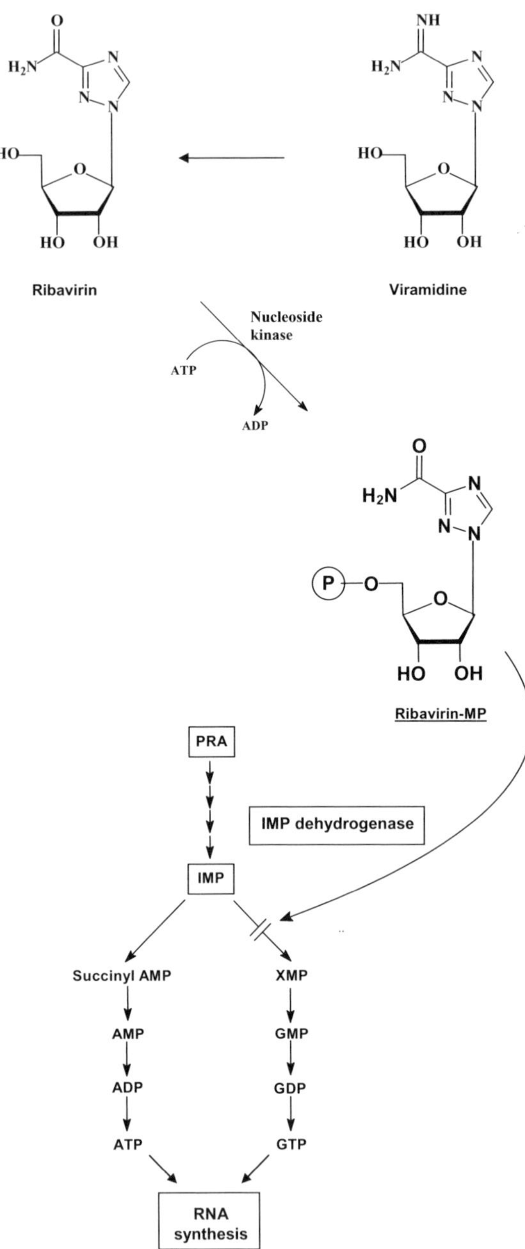

Fig. 1.11. Ribavirin and viramidine, with IMP dehydrogenase being the target enzyme for ribavirin 5′-monophosphate. Viramidine acts as a prodrug (precursor) of ribavirin, which is converted intracellularly to its 5′-monophosphate derivative, ribavirin-MP. The latter inhibits IMP dehydrogenase, a crucial enzyme in the biosynthesis of RNA, including viral RNA. The IMP dehydrogenase is responsible for the conversion of IMP (inosine 5′-monophosphate) to XMP (xanthosine 5′-monophosphate), which, in turn, is further converted to GMP (guanosine 5′-monophosphate), GDP (guanosine 5′-diphosphate), and GTP (guanosine 5′-triphosphate). The latter serves as substrate, together with ATP, UTP, and CTP, in the synthesis of RNA.

resistance development is due to the fact that ribavirin's main target of antiviral action (as demonstrated for paramyxo- and flaviviruses[89]) is a cellular enzyme, the inosine 5′-monophosphate (IMP) dehydrogenase (responsible for the conversion of IMP to XMP), a key enzyme involved in the biosynthesis of GTP and viral RNA synthesis (Fig. 1.11).

Ribavirin is active against both human and avian (H5N1) influenza viruses within the 50% effective concentration (EC_{50}) range of 6–22 μM.[88] Of the three routes (oral, aerosolized, intravenous) by which ribavirin could be administered in the treatment of avian/human influenza, the intravenous should be the preferred route when it comes to therapy of an acute influenza virus infection. Oral ribavirin did not offer the expected clinical or virological efficacy in earlier studies with influenza A (H1N1).[90] Ribavirin aerosol has been used successfully (based on reduction of virus shedding and clinical symptoms) in the treatment of influenza virus infections in college students.[91] Intravenous ribavirin (producing mean plasma concentration at 20–60 μM) was associated with symptomatic improvements and elimination of influenza virus from nasopharyngeal swabbings and tracheal aspirates.[92]

Intravenous ribavirin has been further investigated, with success, in the treatment of Lassa fever[93] and HFRS.[94] Both studies demonstrated significant benefits of ribavirin in terms of survival and reduction of disease severity. The dosing regimen for intravenous ribavirin consists of a loading dose of 2 g of ribavirin followed by 1 g every 6 hr for 4 days. During the next 5 days, a maintenance dose of 0.5 g should be administered every 8 hr. This should generate the effective concentrations needed for achieving suppression of (human and avian) influenza virus replication. Dose-limiting toxicity would be hemolytic anemia, which should be reversible upon cessation of therapy.

SHORT INTERFERING RNAS AND PHOSPHOROTHIOATE OLIGONUCLEOTIDES

Short interfering RNAs (siRNAs) specific for conserved regions of influenza virus genes were found to reduce virus production in the lungs of infected mice, when the siRNAs were given intravenously (i.v.) in complexes with a polycation carrier either before or after initiating virus infection.[95] Delivery of siRNAs specific for highly conserved regions of the nucleoprotein or acidic polymerase significantly reduced lung virus titers in influenza A virus-infected mice and protected the animals from lethal challenge. This protection was specific and not mediated by an antiviral interferon response. The influenza-specific siRNA treatment was broadly effective and protected animals against lethal challenge with highly pathogenic avian influenza A viruses of the H5 and H7 subtypes.[96] That specific siRNA would be effective against influenza could be readily predicted from equally effective results obtained with other specific siRNAs—that is, against the SARS (severe acute respiratory syndrome) coronavirus in comparable situations.[97]

Phosphorothioate oligonucleotides (PS-ONs) (i.e., REP, a 40-mer PS-ON) offer potential, when administered as aerosol in the prophylaxis and therapy of influenza infection.[98] Similarly, antisense phosphorodiamidate morpholino oligomers (ARP-PMOs) could be further pursued for their potential in the treatment of H5N1 influenza A virus infections.[99] Similarly, peptide-conjugated phosphorodiamidate morpholino oligomers (P-PMO), designed to base-pair with influenza viral RNA sequences that are highly conserved across viral subtypes, proved highly efficacious in reducing the viral titer in a dose-responsive and sequence-specific manner in influenza A virus-infected cells.[100]

INFLUENZA VIRUS RNA POLYMERASE INHIBITORS

The influenza viral RNA polymerase consists of a complex of three virus-encoded polypeptides (PB1, PB2, and PA), which, in addition to the RNA replicative activity, also contains an endonuclease activity so as to ensure "cap snatching" for initiating the transcription and subsequent translation process.[101] The polymerase complex genes[102] contribute to the high virulence of the human H5N1 influenza virus isolate A/Vietnam/1203/04. This observation underscores the importance of novel antivirals targeting the polymerase for further development for the therapy and prophylaxis of human and avian influenza virus infections.

Few compounds have been reported to be operating at either the RNA replicase (RNA polymerase) or endonuclease level. In analogy with the inhibitors that have been identified to inhibit the reverse transcriptase (RNA-dependent DNA polymerase) of HIV or RNA replicase (RNA-dependent RNA polymerase) of HCV, influenza RNA replicase inhibitors could be divided into two classes: nucleoside and non-nucleoside type of inhibitors. Examples of the nucleoside type of inhibitors are 2′-deoxy-2′-fluoroguanosine (FdG)[103,104] and T-705[105–107] (Fig. 1.12).

T-705 is a substituted pyrazine that has been found to exhibit potent anti-influenza virus activity *in vitro* and *in vivo*. According to a com-

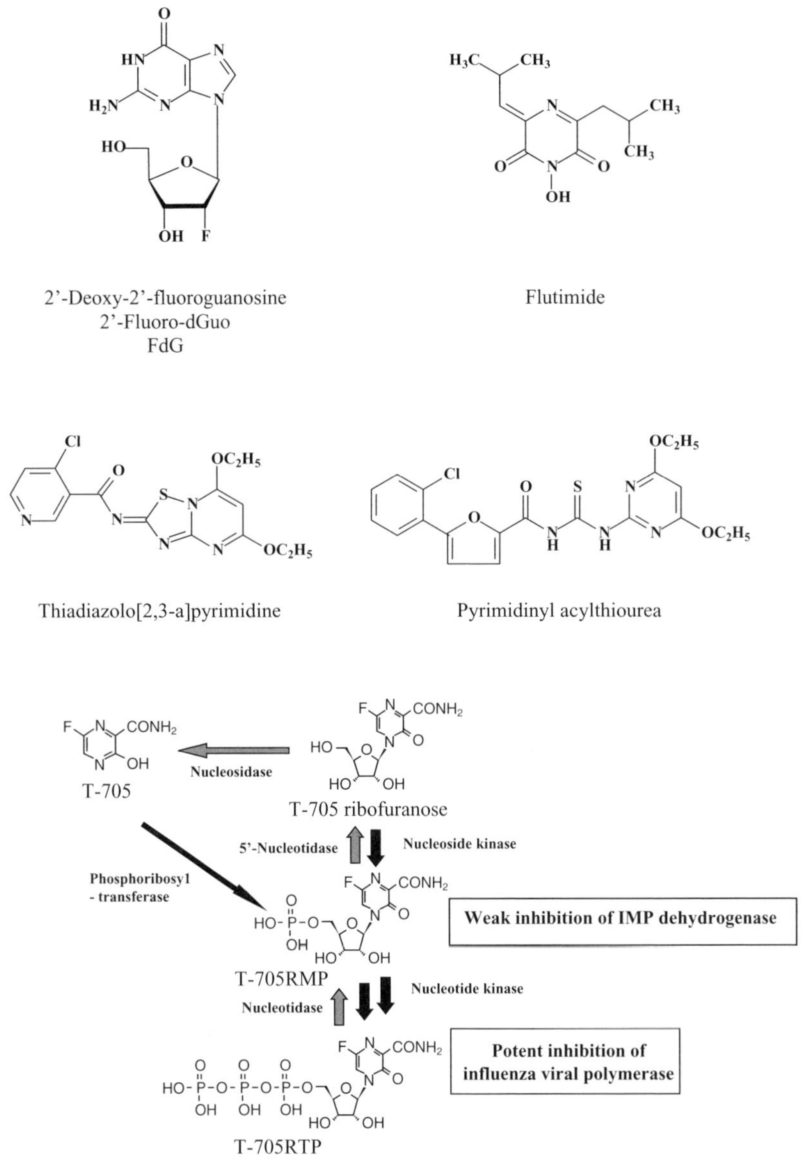

2'-Deoxy-2'-fluoroguanosine
2'-Fluoro-dGuo
FdG

Flutimide

Thiadiazolo[2,3-a]pyrimidine

Pyrimidinyl acylthiourea

T-705

Nucleosidase

T-705 ribofuranose

5'-Nucleotidase

Nucleoside kinase

Phosphoribosyl - transferase

Weak inhibition of IMP dehydrogenase

T-705RMP

Nucleotidase

Nucleotide kinase

Potent inhibition of
influenza viral polymerase

T-705RTP

Fig. 1.12. FdG, Flutimide, thiadiazolo[2,3-*a*]pyrimidine, pyrimidinyl acylthiourea, and T-705, with the postulated mode of action of T-705, according to Furuta et al.[107]

parative study, T-705 would even be more potent than oseltamivir when increasing the multiplicity of infection (*in vitro*) or using a higher virus challenge dose (*in vivo*).[106] It has been postulated that T-705 would be converted intracellularly to its ribonucleotide, T-705 4-ribofuranosyl-5'-monophosphate (T-705 RMP), through a phosphoribosyl transferase, and, upon further phosphorylation to its 5′-triphosphate (Fig. 1.12), T-705 RTP would then inhibit influenza virus RNA polymerase in a GTP-competitive manner.[107] Unlike ribavirin 5′-monophosphate, T-705 RMP did not significantly inhibit IMP dehydrogenase, indicating that it owes its anti-influenza virus activity mainly, if not exclusively, to an inhibition of the influenza virus RNA polymerase.

In addition to the RNA polymerase, the "cap snatching" or "cap scavenging" endonuclease activity associated with the PB1-PB2-PA complex could be considered as an attractive target for influenza virus inhibitors: It can be inhibited by 4-substituted 2,4-dioxobutanoic acid derivatives[108] and N-hydroxamic acid/N-hydroxy-imide derivatives.[109] Likewise, flutimide, a 2,6-diketopiperazine (Fig. 1.12), identified in extracts of the fungal species *Delitschia confertaspora*, has been demonstrated to specifically inhibit the cap-dependent endonuclease activity associated with influenza viral RNA polymerase and to inhibit the replication of influenza A and B virus in cell culture.[110] Both the viral RNA polymerase and endonuclease should be further explored as targets for the development of anti-influenza agents.

Recently, a new class of potent influenza virus inhibitors (EC$_{50}$ for virus replication: 0.08–0.09 µM), as represented by thiadiazolo[2,3-*a*]pyrimidine and pyrimidinyl acylthiourea (Fig. 1.12), has been reported.[111] Although the mechanism of action of this highly potent and selective inhibitors of influenza virus remains to be established, they represent a highly interesting lead worth pursuing. A series of novel bisheterocycle tandem derivatives consisting of methyloxazole and thiazole may also serve as leads for further optimization, although the lead compounds exhibited only modest activity against influenza A virus.[112]

INTERFERON (INDUCERS)

Interferon was originally discovered, exactly 50 years ago, with influenza virus as inducer.[113] In some earlier studies, interferon, instilled by the intranasal route, did not offer much protection in the prophylaxis of influenza A virus infections.[114,115] Meanwhile, interferon has come a long way, and pegylated α-interferon (injected parenterally), in combination with (oral) ribavirin, has become the standard therapy for chronic hepatitis C virus (HCV) infections. This means that with this combination, extensive experience has been accumulated,[116] which could be readily implemented in the prophylaxis and therapy of human and avian influenza virus infections in humans. In the prophylaxis/ therapy of influenza virus infections, the duration of treatment would be much shorter than that for hepatitis C, which would obviously reflect on the convenience (cost/benefit) and side effects that are inherently linked to the use of interferon and ribavirin.

In addition to interferon, interferon inducers such as poly(I)·poly(C), discovered some 40 years ago,[117] may also play a role in the control of influenza virus infections. Prophylaxis using liposome-encapsulated double-stranded RNA [poly(I)·poly(C)] provided complete and long-lasting protection against influenza A virus infection.[118] Furthermore, poly(I)·poly(C), when combined with (intranasal) vaccination, conferred complete protection against influenza virus infection, which may have been mediated by an upregulated expression of Toll-like receptor 3 and α/β interferons as well as Th1- and Th2-related cytokines.[119] It is unclear whether the use of exogenous interferon, or the induction of endogenous interferon by poly(I)·poly(C) or other double-stranded RNAs, may help in the prophylaxis or therapy of avian or human influenza virus infections, but in view of the "renaissance" of interferon, as witnessed in the treatment of HCV infection, the potential of interferon in control measures against influenza may well deserve to be revisited.

ANTIVIRAL DRUG COMBINATIONS

From the drug combination regimens utilized in the treatment of *Mycobacterium tuberculosis* and human immunodeficiency virus (HIV) infections (AIDS), we have learned that such drug combinations (i) achieve greater benefit than each compound given individually, (ii) reduce the likelihood of drug resistance development, and (iii) may allow us to decrease the individual drug doses, thereby diminishing adverse side effects. The concept of using two or more antivirals for influenza to enhance antiviral efficacy and possibly reduce resistance emergence is several decades old,[120–123] and it was first demonstrated for the combination of interferon with amantadine.[121] Many more drug combinations are possible, even if limited only to those compounds that are available (marketed) today: neuraminidase inhibitors (oseltamivir and zanamivir), adamantanamines (amantadine and rimantadine), ribavirin, and (pegylated) interferon (Fig. 1.13).

In the therapy (or prophylaxis) of influenza virus infections, the combination of (pegylated) interferon and ribavirin could be further complemented with amantadine (or rimantadine). This triple-drug combination has shown efficacy in the treatment of chronic HCV infection,[124] and it may also be worth pursuing in the treatment (or

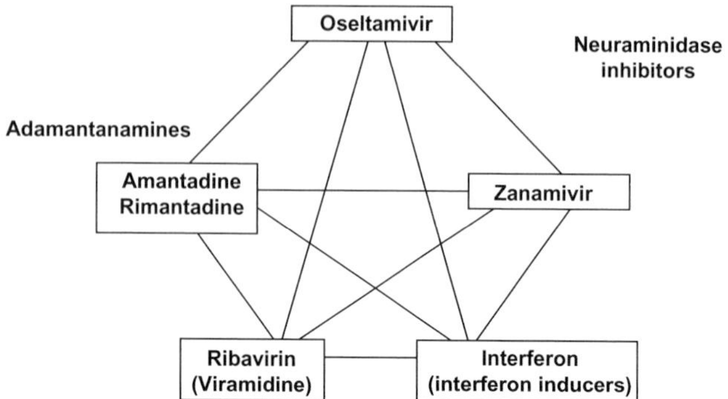

Fig. 1.13. Drug combination possibilities among neuraminidase inhibitors (oseltamivir and zanamivir), adamantanamines (amantadine or rimantadine), ribavirin (or viramidine), and interferon (or interferon inducers).

prophylaxis) of influenza. The three drugs are, individually, all active against influenza virus replication *in vitro* and act through different mechanisms, which implies that, when combined, they may achieve an additive or even synergistic action while reducing the risk of emergence of drug-resistant virus variants. As early as 1984, Hayden et al.[125] pointed to the additive synergistic action between interferon-α2, rimantadine, and ribavirin.

Also combinations of (pegylated) interferon with neuraminidase inhibitors (zanamivir, oseltamivir, peramivir) may be considered, and thus might be combinations of ribavirin (or viramidine) with the neuraminidase inhibitors, although in a recent study with a lethal influenza A (H1N1) infection model in mice, Smee et al.[126] found that the combination of oseltamivir with ribavirin did not score better than ribavirin alone. On the other hand, combination of oseltamivir with amantadine appeared to effect a significantly greater antiviral activity against influenza A (H1N1, H3N2, and H5N1) while reducing the emergence of drug-resistant influenza A variants.[127]

Combinations of the adamantan(amin)es (i.e., amantadine or rimantadine) with the neuraminidase inhibitors (zanamivir or oseltamivir) should, therefore, receive due attention. *In vitro*, rimantadine was found to act synergistically with zanamivir, oseltamivir, or peramivir in reducing the extracellular yield of influenza A (H3N2) virus.[128] *In vivo*, oseltamivir at 10 mg/kg/day and amantadine at 15 mg/kg/day provided similar protection against influenza A (H5N1)-associated death risk in mice; but when both were combined, they provided an incremental protection against lethality as combined to both compounds given as single-agent chemotherapy.[129] The only controlled study in humans was a comparison of rimantadine alone versus rimantadine plus inhaled zanamivir in hospitalized (adult) patients with serious influenza;[130] although preliminary, this study pointed to a higher clinical benefit for the combination of zanamivir with rimantadine.

RECOMMENDATIONS

Among the antivirals, the neuraminidase inhibitors oseltamivir and zanamivir are the most likely to be considered for use against an avian influenza H5N1 pandemic, with oseltamivir being the preferable option of the two neuraminidase inhibitors because it is less expensive and administered orally (whereas zanamivir is administered by inhalation).[131] The stockpiling of an appropriate antiviral agent such as oseltamivir is currently the most crucial single defense to be utilized against influenza H5N1.[132]

Zanamivir remains an attractive antiviral drug for combination with oseltamivir because of a non-overlapping resistance pattern, but then the route of administration will need to be reconsidered, since, if administered by inhalation, it does not reach the sites (lower respiratory tract and extrapulmonary) where avian influenza H5N1 replicates.[133]

Some authors have questioned the effectiveness of neuraminidase inhibitors in interrupting viral spread and argued that their use in a serious epidemic or pandemic should not be considered without concomitant public-health measures such as barriers, distance, and personal hygiene.[134] The same authors also argued against the use of amantadine and rimantadine.[134] Yet, in severe influenza A virus infections, amantadine may be lifesaving,[135] due to the fact that, independently of its antiviral properties (and thus unaffected by antiviral resistance), it may increase distal airway function and thus improve oxygenation.[136]

Finally, when considering the use of antivirals in the prevention and/or treatment of influenza, particular attention should be paid to high-risk groups: children, pregnant women, immunocompromised hosts, and nursing home residents.[137]

CONCLUSIONS

Several drugs are available that could be used, either alone or in combination, in the treatment (or prophylaxis) of a pandemic influenza virus infection, whether avian or human. These include adamantan(amin)e derivatives (i.e., amantadine, rimantadine), neuraminidase inhibitors (i.e., zanamivir, oseltamivir), ribavirin, and interferon. In the meantime, attempts should be intensified to further design and develop new antivirals whether based on known molecular targets, such as the neuraminidase and M2 ion channel, or on yet relatively unexplored targets such as the viral RNA polymerase. The latter could, in principle, be targeted by both nucleoside and non-nucleoside inhibitor types, an approach that has proven most successful in the cases of the HIV reverse transcriptase and HCV RNA polymerase.

ACKNOWLEDGMENTS

I thank Christiane Callebaut for her invaluable editorial assistance.

REFERENCES

1. De Clercq, E. Antiviral agents active against influenza A viruses. *Nature Rev. Drug Discov.* **2006**, *5*, 1015–1025.

2. Ferguson, N. M.; Cummings, D. A.; Cauchemez, S.; Fraser, C.; Riley, S.; Meeyai, A.; Iamsirithaworn, S.; Burke, D. S. Strategies for containing an emerging influenza pandemic in Southeast Asia. *Nature* **2005**, *437*, 209–214.

3. Kandun, I. N.; Wibisono, H.; Sedyaningsih, E. R.; Yusharmen, D. P. H.; Hadisoedarsuno, W.; Purba, W.; Santoso, H.; Septiawati, C.; Tresnaningsih, E.; Heriyanto, B.; Yuwono, D.; Harun, S.; Soeroso, S.; Giriputra, S.; Blair, P. J.; Jeremijenko, A.; Kosasih, H.; Putnam, S. D.; Samaan, G.; Silitonga, M.; Chan, K. H.; Poon, L. L.; Lim, W.; Klimov, A.; Lindstrom, S.; Guan, Y.; Donis, R.; Katz, J.; Cox, N.; Peiris, M.; Uyeki, T. M. Three Indonesian clusters of H5N1 virus infection in 2005. *N. Engl. J. Med.* **2006**, *355*, 2186–2194.

4. Oner, A. F.; Bay, A.; Arslan, S.; Akdeniz, H.; Sahin, H. A.; Cesur, Y.; Epcacan, S.; Yilmaz, N.; Deger, I.; Kizilyidiz, B.; Karsen, H.; Ceyhan, M. Avian influenza A (H5N1) infection in Eastern Turkey in 2006. *N. Engl. J. Med.* **2006**, *355*, 2179–2185.

5. Ferguson, N. M.; Cummings, D. A.; Fraser, C.; Cajka, J. C.; Cooley, P. C.; Burke, D. S. Strategies for mitigating an influenza pandemic. *Nature* **2006**, *442*, 448–452.

6. McCullens, J. A. The clinical need for new antiviral drugs directed against influenza virus. *J. Infect. Dis.* **2006**, *193*, 751–753.

7. Regoes, R. R.; Bonhoeffer, S. Emergence of drug-resistant influenza virus: Population dynamical considerations. *Science* **2006**, *312*, 389–391.

8. Taubenberger, J. K.; Morens, D. M. Influenza: The mother of all pandemics. *Emerging Infect. Dis.* **2006**, *12*, 15–22.

9. Kilbourne, E. D. Influenza pandemics of the 20th century. *Emerging Infect. Dis.* **2006**, *12*, 9–14.

10. Belshe, R. B. The origins of pandemic influenza—Lessons from the 1918 virus. *N. Engl. J. Med.* **2005**, *353*, 2209–2211.

11. Palese, P. Influenza: Old and new threats. *Nature Med.* **2004**, *10*, S82–S87.

12. Davies, W. L.; Grunert, R. R.; Haff, R. F.; McGahen, J. W.; Neumayer, E. M.; Paulshock, M.; Watts, J. C.; Wood, T. R.; Hermann, E. C.; Hoffmann, C. E. Antiviral activity of 1-adamantanamine (amantadine). *Science* **1964**, *144*, 862–863.

13. Horimoto, T.; Kawaoka, Y. Influenza: Lessons from past pandemics, warnings from current incidents. *Nature Rev. Microbiol.* **2005**, *3*, 591–600.

14. Shuck, K.; Lamb, R. A.; Pinto, L. H. Analysis of the pore structure of the influenza A virus M_2 ion channel by the substituted-cysteine accessibility method. *J. Virol.* **2000**, *74*, 7755–7761.

15. Sansom, M. S.; Kerr, I. D. Influenza virus M2 protein: A molecular modelling study of the ion channel. *Protein Eng.* **1993**, *6*, 65–74.

16. Kolocouris, N.; Foscolos, G. B.; Kolocouris, A.; Marakos, P.; Pouli, N.; Fytas, G.; Ikeda, S.; De Clercq, E. Synthesis and antiviral activity evaluation of some aminoadamantane derivatives. *J. Med. Chem.* **1994**, *37*, 2896–2902.

17. Kolocouris, N.; Kolocouris, A.; Foscolos, G. B.; Fytas, G.; Neyts, J.; Padalko, E.; Balzarini, J.; Snoeck, R.; Andrei, G.; De Clercq, E. Synthesis and antiviral activity evaluation of some new aminoadamantane derivatives. 2. *J. Med. Chem.* **1996**, *39*, 3307–3318.

18. Kolocouris, N.; Tataridis, D.; Fytas, G.; Mavromoustakos, T.; Foscolos, G. B.; Kolocouris, N.; De Clercq, E. Synthesis of 2-(2-adamantyl)piperidines and structure anti-influenza virus A activity relationship study using a combination of NMR spectroscopy and molecular modeling. *Bioorg. Med. Chem. Lett.* **1999**, *9*, 3465–3470.

19. Stamatiou, G.; Kolocouris, A.; Kolocouris, N.; Fytas, G.; Foscolos, G. B.; Neyts, J.; De Clercq, E. Novel 3-(2-adamantyl)pyrrolidines with potent activity against influenza A virus—Identification of aminoadamantane derivatives bearing two pharmacophoric amine groups. *Bioorg. Med. Chem. Lett.* **2001**, *11*, 2137–2142.

20. Zoidis, G.; Kolocouris, N.; Foscolos, G. B.; Kolocouris, A.; Fytas, G.; Karayanis, P.; Padalko, E.; Neyts, J.; De Clercq, E. Are the 2-isomers of the drug rimantadine active anti-influenza A agents? *Antiviral Chem. Chemother.* **2003**, *14*, 153–164.

21. Stamatiou, G.; Foscolos, G. B.; Fytas, G.; Kolocouris, A.; Kolocouris, N.; Pannecouque, C.; Witvrouw, M.; Padalko, E.; Neyts, J.; De Clercq, E. Heterocyclic rimantadine analogues with antiviral activity. *Bioorg. Med. Chem.* **2003**, *11*, 5485–5492.

22. Zoidis, G.; Fytas, C.; Papanastasiou, I.; Foscolos, G. B.; Fytas, G.; Padalko, E.; De Clercq, E.; Naesens, L.; Neyts, J.; Kolocouris, N. Heterocyclic rimantadine analogues with antiviral activity. *Bioorg. Med. Chem.* **2006**, *14*, 3341–3348.

23. Belshe, R. B.; Smith, M. H.; Hall, C. B.; Betts, R.; Hay, A. J. Genetic basis of resistance to rimantadine emerging during treatment of influenza virus infection. *J. Virol.* **1988**, *62*, 1508–1512.

24. Hayden, F. G. Antiviral resistance in influenza viruses—Implications for management and pandemic response. *N. Engl. J. Med.* **2006**, *354*, 785–788.

25. Bright, R. A.; Shay, D. K.; Shu, B.; Cox, N. J.; Klimov, A. I. Adamantane resistance among influenza A viruses isolated early during the 2005–2006 influenza season in the United States. *JAMA* **2006**, *295*, 891–894.

26. Bright, R. A.; Medina, M. J.; Xu, X.; Perez-Oronoz, G.; Wallis, T. R.; Davis, X. M.; Povinelli, L.; Cox, N. J.; Klimov, A. I. Incidence of adamantane resistance among influenza A (H3N2) viruses isolated worldwide from 1994 to 2005: A cause for concern. *Lancet* **2005**, *366* 1175–1181.

27. Weinstock, D. M.; Zuccotti, G. Adamantane resistance in influenza A. *JAMA* **2006**, *295*, 934–936.

28. Cheung, C.-L.; Rayner, J. M.; Smith, G. J. D.; Wang, P.; Naipospos, T. S. P.; Zhang, J.; Yuen, K.-Y.; Webster, R. G.; Peiris, J. S. M.; Chen, H. Distribution of amantadine-resistant H5N1 avian influenza variants in Asia. *J. Infect. Dis.* **2006**, *193*, 1626–129.

29. Shea, K. M. Shift shown in influenza A adamantane resistance. *JAMA* **2006**, *296*, 1585–1587.

30. De Clercq, E. Antivirals and antiviral strategies. *Nature Rev. Microbiol.* **2004**, *2*, 704–720.

31. Moscona, A. Neuraminidase inhibitors for influenza. *N. Engl. J. Med.* **2005**, *353*, 1363–1373.

32. Matrosovich, M. N.; Matrosovich, T. Y.; Gray, T.; Roberts, N. A.; Klenk, H.-D. Neuraminidase is important for the initiation of influenza virus infection in human airway epithelium. *J. Virol.* **2004**, *78*, 12665–12667.

33. Shinya, K.; Ebina, M.; Yamada, S.; Ono, M.; Kasai, N.; Kawaoka, Y. Avian flu: Influenza virus receptors in the human airway. *Nature* **2006**, *440*, 435–436.

34. van Riel, D.; Munster, V. J.; de Wit, E.; Rimmelzwaan, G. F.; Fouchier, R. A.; Osterhaus, A. D.; Kuiken, T. H5N1 virus attachment to lower respiratory tract. *Science* **2006**, *312*, 399.

35. Abdel-Magid, A. F.; Marvanoff, C. A.; Mehrman, S. J. Synthesis of influenza neuraminidase inhibitors. *Curr. Opin. Drug Discov. Devel.* **2001**, *4*, 776–791.

36. von Itzstein, M.; Wu, W.-Y.; Kok, G. B.; Pegg, M. S.; Dyason, J. C.; Jin, B.; Van Phan, T.; Smythe, M. L.; White, H. F.; Oliver, S. W.; Colman, P. M.;

Varghese, J. N.; Ryan, D. M.; Woods, J. M.; Bethell, R. C.; Hotham, V. J.; Cameron, J. M.; Penn, C. R. Rational design of potent sialidase-based inhibitors of influena virus replication. *Nature* **1993**, *363*, 418–423.

37. Kim, C. U.; Lew, W.; Williams, M. A.; Liu, H.; Zhang, L.; Swaminathan, S.; Bischofberger, N.; Chen, M. S.; Mendel, D. B.; Tai, C. Y.; Laver, W. G.; Stevens, R. C. Influenza neuraminidase inhibitors possessing a novel hydrophobic interaction in the enzyme active site: Design, synthesis, and structural analysis of carbocyclic sialic acid analogues with potent anti-influenza activity. *J. Am. Chem. Soc.* **1997**, *119*, 681–690.

38. Aoki, F. Y.; Macleod, M. D.; Paggiaro, P.; Carewicz, O.; El Sawy, A.; Wat, C.; Griffiths, M.; Waalberg, E.; Ward, P. Early administration of oral oseltamivir increases the benefits of influenza treatment. *J. Antimicrob. Chemother.* **2003**, *51*, 123–129.

39. Kaiser, L.; Wat, C.; Mills, T.; Mahoney, P.; Ward, P.; Hayden, F. Impact of oseltamivir treatment on influenza-related lower respiratory tract complications and hospitalizations. *Arch. Intern. Med.* **2003**, *163*, 1667–1672.

40. Welliver, R.; Monto, A. S.; Carewicz, O.; Schatteman, E.; Hassman, M.; Hedrick, J.; Jackson, H. C.; Huson, L.; Ward, P.; Oxford, J. S. Effectiveness of oseltamivir in preventing influenza in household contacts. *JAMA* **2001**, *285*, 748–754.

41. Hayden, F. G.; Belshe, R.; Villanueva, C.; Lanno, R.; Hughes, C.; Small, I.; Dutkowski, R.; Ward, P.; Carr, J. Management of influenza in households: A prospective, randomized comparison of oseltamivir treatment with or without postexposure prophylaxis. *J. Infect. Dis.* **2004**, *189*, 440–449.

42. Kawai, N.; Ikematsu, H.; Iwaki, N.; Maeda, T.; Satoh, I.; Hirotsu, N.; Kashiwagi, S. A comparison of the effectiveness of oseltamivir for the treatment of influenza A and influenza B: A Japanese multicenter study of the 2003–2004 and 2004–2005 influenza seasons. *Clin. Infect. Dis.* **2006**, *43*, 439–444.

43. De Clercq, E. Strategies in the design of antiviral drugs. *Nature Rev. Drug Discov.* **2002**, *1*, 13–25.

44. Russell, R. J.; Haire, L. F.; Stevens, D. J.; Collins, P. J.; Lin, Y. P.; Blackburn, G. M.; Hay, A. J.; Gamblin, S. J.; Skehel, J. J. The structure of H5N1 avian influenza neuraminidase suggests new opportunities for drug design. *Nature* **2006**, *443*, 45–49.

45. Luo, M. Antiviral drugs fit for a purpose. *Nature* **2006**, *443*, 37–38.

46. McKimm-Breschkin, J. L. Resistance of influenza viruses to neuraminidase inhibitors—A review. *Antiviral Res.* **2000**, *47*, 1–17.

47. McKimm-Breschkin, J.; Trivedi, T.; Hampson, A.; Hay, A.; Klimov, A.; Tashiro, M.; Hayden, F.; Zambon, M. Neuraminidase sequence analysis and susceptibilities of influenza virus clinical isolates to zanamivir and oseltamivir. *Antimicrob. Agents Chemother.* **2003**, *47*, 2264–2272.

48. Monto, A. S.; McKimm-Breschkin, J. L.; Macken, C.; Hampson, A. W.; Hay, A.; Klimov, A.; Tashiro, M.; Webster, R. G.; Aymard, M.; Hayden, F. G.; Zambon, M. Detection of influenza viruses resistant to neuraminidase inhibitors in global surveillance during the first 3 years of their use. *Antimicrob. Agents Chemother.* **2006**, *50*, 2395–2402.

49. Kiso, M.; Mitamura, K.; Sakai-Tagawa, Y.; Shiraishi, K.; Kawakami, C.; Kimura, K.; Hayden, F. G.; Sugaya, N.; Kawaoka, Y. Resistant influenza A viruses in children treated with oseltamivir: Descriptive study. *Lancet* **2004**, *364*, 759–765.

50. Zürcher, T.; Yates, P. J.; Daly, J.; Sahasrabudhe, A.; Walters, M.; Dash, L.; Tisdale, M.; McKimm-Breschkin, J. L. Mutations conferring zanamivir resistance in human influenza virus N2 neuraminidases compromise virus fitness and are not stably maintained *in vitro*. *J. Antimicrob. Chemother.* **2006**, *58*, 723–732.

51. Herlocher, M. L.; Carr, J.; Ives, J.; Elias, S.; Truscon, R.; Roberts, N.; Monto, A. S. Influenza virus carrying an R292K mutation in the neuraminidase gene is not transmitted in ferrets. *Antiviral Res.* **2002**, *54*, 99–111.

52. Herlocher, M. L.; Truscon, R.; Elias, S.; Yen, H.-L.; Roberts, N. A.; Ohmit, S. E.; Monto, A. S. Influenza viruses resistant to the antiviral drug oseltamivir: transmission studies in ferrets. *J. Infect. Dis.* **2004**, *190*, 1627–1630.

53. Yen, H.-L.; Herlocher, L. M.; Hoffmann, E.; Matrosovich, M. N.; Monto, A. S.; Webster, R. G.; Govorkova, E. A. Neuraminidase inhibitor-resistant influenza viruses may differ substantially in fitness and transmissibility. *Antimicrob. Agents Chemother.* **2005**, *49*, 4075–4084.

54. Oxford, J.; Balasingam, S.; Lambkin, R. A new millennium conundrum: How to use a powerful class of influenza anti-neuraminidase drugs (NAIs) in the community. *J. Antimicrob. Chemother.* **2004**, *53*, 133–136.

55. Tumpey, T. M.; Garcia-Sastre, A.; Mikulasova, A.; Taubenberger, J. K.; Swayne, D. E.; Palese, P.; Basler, C. F. Existing antivirals are effective against influenza viruses with genes from the 1918 pandemic virus. *Proc. Natl. Acad. Sci. USA* **2002**, *99*, 13849–13854.

56. Ison, M. G.; Gubareva, L. V.; Atmar, R. L.; Treanor, J.; Hayden, F. G. Recovery of drug-resistant influenza virus from immunocompromised patients: A case series. *J. Infect. Dis.* **2006**, *193*, 760–764.

57. Baz, M.; Abed, Y.; McDonald, J.; Boivin, G. Characterization of multi-drug-resistant influenza A/H3N2 viruses shed during 1 year by an immuno-compromised child. *Clin. Infect. Dis.* **2006**, *43*, 1555–1561.

58. Yen, H.-L.; Hoffmann, E.; Taylor, G.; Scholtissek, C.; Monto, A. S.; Webster, R. G.; Govorkova, E. A. Importance of neuraminidase active-site residues to the neuraminidase inhibitor resistance of influenza viruses. *J. Virol.* **2006**, *80*, 8787–8795.

59. Ferraris, O.; Kessler, N.; Lina, B. Sensitivity of influenza viruses to zana-mivir and oseltamivir: A study performed on viruses circulating in France

prior to the introduction of neuraminidase inhibitors in clinical practice. *Antiviral Res.* **2005**, *68*, 43–48.

60. Le, Q. M.; Kiso, M.; Someya, K.; Sakai, Y. T.; Nguyen, T. H.; Nguyen, K. H.; Pham, N. D.; Ngyen, H. H.; Yamada, S.; Muramoto, Y.; Horimoto, T.; Takada, A.; Goto, H.; Suzuki, T.; Suzuki, Y.; Kawaoka, Y. Avian flu: isolation of drug-resistant H5N1 virus. *Nature* **2005**, *437*, 1108.

61. Gubareva, L. V.; Kaiser, L.; Matrosovich, M. N.; Soo-Hoo, Y.; Hayden, F. G. Selection of influenza virus mutants in experimentally infected volunteers treated with oseltamivir. *J. Infect. Dis.* **2001**, *183*, 523–531.

62. Ives, J. A.; Carr, J. A.; Mendel, D. B.; Tai, C. Y.; Lambkin, R.; Kelly, L.; Oxford, J. S.; Hayden, F. G.; Roberts, N. A. The H274Y mutation in the influenza A/H1N1 neuraminidase active site following oseltamivir phosphate treatment leave virus severely compromised both *in vitro* and *in vivo*. *Antiviral Res.* **2002**, *55*, 307–317.

63. de Jong, M. D.; Trann, T. T.; Truong, H. K.; Vo, M. H.; Smith, G. J.; Nguyen, V. C.; Bach, V. C.; Phan, T. Q.; Do, Q. H.; Guan, Y.; Peiris, J. S.; Tran, T. H.; Farrar, J. Oseltamivir resistance during treatment of influenza A (H5N1) infection. *N. Engl. J. Med.* **2005**, *353*, 2667–2672.

64. Govorkova, E. A.; Ilyushina, N. A.; Smith, J.; Webster, R. G. Oseltamivir protects ferrets against lethal H5N1 influenza virus infection. *Antiviral Res.* **2006**, *70*, A29, Abstract 9.

65. Yen, H.-L.; Monto, A. S.; Webster, R. G.; Govorkova, E. A. Virulence may determine the necessary duration and dosage of oseltamivir treatment for highly pathogenic A/Vietnam/1203/04 influenza virus in mice. *J. Infect. Dis.* **2005**, *192*, 665–672.

66. Rameix-Welti, M. A.; Agou, F.; Buchy, P.; Mardy, S.; Aubin, J. T.; Véron, M.; van der Werf, S.; Naffakh, N. Natural variation can significantly alter the sensitivity of influenza A (H5N1) viruses to oseltamivir. *Antimicrob. Agents Chemother.* **2006**, *50*, 3809–3815.

67. Smee, D. F.; Huffman, J. H.; Morrison, A. C.; Barnard, D. L.; Sidwell, R. W. Cyclopentane neuraminidase inhibitors with potent *in vitro* anti-influenza virus activities. *Antimicrob. Agents Chemother.* **2001**, *45*, 743–748.

68. Sidwell, R. W.; Smee, D. F.; Huffman, J. H.; Barnard, D. L.; Bailey, K. W.; Morrey, J. D.; Babu, Y. S. *In vivo* influenza virus-inhibitory effects of the cyclopentane neuraminidase inhibitor RJW-270201. *Antimicrob. Agents Chemother.* **2001**, *45*, 749–757.

69. Chand, P.; Bantia, S.; Kotian, P. L.; El-Kattan, Y.; Lin, T. H.; Babu, Y. S. Comparison of the anti-influenza virus activity of cyclopentane derivatives with oseltamivir and zanamivir *in vivo*. *Bioorg. Med. Chem.* **2005**, *13*, 4071–4077.

70. Chand, P.; Kotian, P. L.; Dehghani, A.; El-Kattan, Y.; Lin, T. H.; Hutchison, T. L.; Babu, Y. S.; Bantia, S.; Elliott, A. J.; Montgomery, J. A. Systematic structure-based design and stereoselective synthesis of novel multisubsti-

tuted cyclopentane derivatives with potent antiinfluenza activity. *J. Med. Chem.* **2001**, *44*, 4379–4392.

71. Chand, P.; Babu, Y. S.; Bantia, S.; Rowland, S.; Dehghani, A.; Kotian, P. L.; Hutchison, T. L.; Ali, S.; Brouillette, W.; El-Kattan, Y.; Lin, T. H. Syntheses and neuraminidase inhibitory activity of multisubstituted cyclopentane amide derivatives. *J. Med. Chem.* **2004**, *47*, 1919–1929.

72. Wang, G. T.; Chen, Y.; Wang, S.; Gentles, R.; Sowin, T.; Kati, W.; Muchmore, S.; Giranda, V.; Stewart, K.; Sham, H.; Kempf, D.; Laver, W. G. Design, synthesis, and structural analysis of influenza neuraminidase inhibitors containing pyrrolidine cores. *J. Med. Chem.* **2001**, *44*, 1192–1201.

73. DeGoey, D. A.; Chen, H.-J.; Flosi, W. J.; Grampovnik, D. J.; Yeung, C. M.; Klein, L. L.; Kempf, D. J. Enantioselective synthesis of antiinfluenza compound A-315675. *J. Org. Cem.* **2002**, *67*, 5445–5453.

74. Hanessian, S.; Bayrakdarian, M.; Luo, X. Total synthesis of A-315675: A potent inhibitor of influenza neuraminidase. *J. Am. Chem. Soc.* **2002**, *124*, 4716–4721.

75. Kati, W. M.; Montgomery, D.; Carrick, R.; Gubareva, L.; Maring, C.; McDaniel, K.; Steffy, K.; Molla, A.; Hayden, F.; Kempf, D.; Kohlbrenner, W. *In vitro* characterization of A-315675, a highly potent inhibitor of A and B strain influenza virus neuraminidases and influenza virus replication. *Antimicrob. Agents Chemother.* **2002**, *46*, 1014–1021.

76. Maring, C. J.; Stoll, V. S.; Zhao, C.; Sun, M.; Krueger, A. C.; Stewart, K. D.; Madigan, D. L.; Kati, W. M.; Xu, Y.; Carrick, R. J.; Montgomery, D. A.; Kempf-Grote, A.; Marsh, K. C.; Molla, A.; Steffy, K. R.; Sham, H. L.; Laver, W. G.; Gu, Y. G.; Kempf, D. J.; Kohlbrenner, W. E. Structure-based characterization and optimization of novel hydrophobic binding interactions in a series of pyrrolidine influenza neuraminidase inhibitors. *J. Med. Chem.* **2005**, *48*, 3980–3990.

77. Wang, G. T.; Wang, S.; Gentles, R.; Sowin, T.; Maring, C. J.; Kempf, D. J.; Kati, W. M.; Stoll, V.; Stewart, K. D.; Laver, G. Design, synthesis, and structural analysis of inhibitors of influenza neuraminidase containing a 2,3-disubstituted tetrahydrofuran-5-carboxylic acid core. *Bioorg. Med. Chem. Lett.* **2005**, *15*, 125–128.

78. Mishin, V. P.; Hayden, F. G.; Gubareva, L. V. Susceptibilities of antiviral-resistant influenza viruses to novel neuraminidase inhibitors. *Antimicrob. Agents Chemother.* **2005**, *49*, 4515–4520.

79. Molla, A.; Kati, W.; Carrick, R.; Steffy, K.; Shi, Y.; Montgomery, D.; Gusick, N.; Stoll, V. S.; Stewart, K. D.; Ng, T. I.; Maring, C.; Kempf, D. J.; Kohlbrenner, W. *In vitro* selection and characterization of influenza A (A/N9) virus variants resistant to a novel neuraminidase inhibitor, A-315675. *J. Virol.* **2002**, *76*, 5380–5386.

80. Gubareva, L. V. Molecular mechanisms of influenza virus resistance to neuraminidase inhibitors. *Virus Res.* **2004**, *103*, 199–203.

81. Bantia, S.; Arnold, C. S.; Parker, C. D.; Upshaw, R.; Chand, P. Anti-influenza virus activity of peramivir in mice with single intramuscular injection. *Antiviral Res.* **2006**, *69*, 39–45.

82. Mishin, V. P.; Hayden, F. G.; Signorelli, K. L.; Gubareva, L. V. Evaluation of methyl inosine monophosphate (MIMP) and peramivir activities in a murine model of lethal influenza A virus infection. *Antiviral Res.* **2006**, *71*, 64–68.

83. Sidwell, R. W.; et al. Effect of single i. m. or i. v. injection of peramivir on an influenza A (H5N1) virus infection in mice. *Antiviral Res.* **2006**, *70*, A50, Abstract 84.

84. Barroso, L.; Treanor, J.; Gubareva, L.; Hayden, F. G. Efficacy and tolerability of the oral neuraminidase inhibitor peramivir in experimental human influenza: Randomized, controlled trials for prophylaxis and treatment. *Antiviral Ther.* **2005**, *10*, 901–910.

85. Macdonald, S. J.; Cameron, R.; Demaine, D. A.; Fenton, R. J.; Foster, G.; Gower, D.; Hamblin, J. N.; Hamilton, S.; Hart, G. J.; Hill, A. P.; Inglis, G. G.; Jin, B.; Jones, H. T.; McConnell, D. B.; McKimm-Breschkin, J.; Mills, G.; Nguyen, V.; Owens, I. J.; Parry, N.; Shanahan, S. E.; Smith, D.; Watson, K. G.; Wu, W.Y.; Tucker, S. P. Dimeric zanamivir conjugates with various linking groups are potent, long-lasting inhibitors of influenza neuraminidase including H5N1 avian influenza. *J. Med. Chem.* **2005**, *48*, 2964–2971.

86. Macdonald, S.J.F.; Watson, K.G.; Cameron, R.; Chalmers, D.K.; Demaine, D. A.; Fenton, R. J.; Gower, D.; Hamblin, J. N.; Hamilton, S.; Hart, G. J.; Inglis, G. G.; Jin, B.; Jones, H.T.; McConnell, D. B.; Mason, A. M.; Nguyen, V.; Owens, I.J.; Parry, N.; Reece, P. A.; Shanahan, S.E.; Smith, D.; Wu, W. Y.; Tucker, S. P. Potent and long-acting dimeric inhibitors of influenza virus neuraminidase are effective at a once-weekly dosing regimen. *Antimicrob. Agents Chemother.* **2004**, *48*, 4542–4549.

87. Sidwell, R. W.; Huffman, J. H.; Khare, G. P.; Allen, L. B.; Witkowski, J. T.; Robins, R. K. Broad-spectrum antiviral activity of virazole: 1-β-D-ribofuranosyl-1,2,4-triazole-3-carboxamide. *Science* **1972**, *177*, 705–706.

88. Sidwell, R. W.; Bailey, K. W.; Wong, M.-H.; Barnard, D. L.; Smee, D. F. *In vitro* and *in vivo* influenza virus-inhibitory effects of viramidine. *Antiviral Res.* **2005**, *68*, 10–17.

89. Leyssen, P.; De Clercq, E.; Neyts, J. The anti-yellow fever virus activity of ribavirin is independent of error-prone replication. *Mol. Pharmacol.* **2006**, *69*, 1461–1467.

90. Smith, C. B.; Charette, R. P.; Fox, J. P.; Cooney, M. K.; Hall, C. E. Lack of effect of oral ribavirin in naturally occurring influenza A virus (H1N1) infection. *J. Infect. Dis.* **1980**, *141*, 548–554.

91. Knight, V.; Gilbert, B. E. Ribavirin aerosol treatment of influenza. *Infect. Dis. Clin. North Am.* **1987**, *1*, 441–457.

92. Hayden, F. G.; Sable, C. A.; Connor, J. D.; Lane, J. Intravenous ribavirin by constant infusion for serious influenza and parainfluenzavirus infection. *Antiviral Ther.* **1996**, *1*, 51–56.

93. McCormick, J. B.; King, I. J.; Webb, P. A.; Scribner, C. L.; Craven, R. B.; Johnson, K. M.; Elliott, L. H.; Belmont-Williams, R. Lassa fever. Effective therapy with ribavirin. *N. Engl. J. Med.* **1986**, *314*, 20–26.

94. Huggins, J. W.; Hsiang, C. M.; Cosgriff, T. M.; Guang, M. Y.; Smith, J. I.; Wu, Z. Q.; LeDuc, J. W.; Zheng, Z. M.; Meegan, J. M.; Wang, Q. N. Prospective, double-blind, concurrent, placebo-controlled clinical trial of intravenous ribavirin therapy of hemorrhagic fever with renal syndrome. *J. Infect. Dis.* **1991**, *164*, 1119–1127.

95. Ge, Q.; Filip, L.; Bai, A.; Nguyen, T.; Eisen, H. N.; Chen, J. Inhibition of influenza virus production in virus-infected mice by RNA interference. *Proc. Natl. Acad. Sci. USA* **2004**, *101*, 8676–8681.

96. Tompkins, S. M.; Lo, C. Y.; Tumpey, T. M.; Epstein, S. L. Protection against lethal influenza virus challenge by RNA interference *in vivo. Proc. Natl. Acad. Sci. USA* **2004**, *101*, 8682–8686.

97. Li, B. J.; Tang, Q.; Cheng, D.; Qin, C.; Xie, F. Y.; Wei, Q.; Xu, J.; Liu, Y.; Zheng, B. J.; Woodle, M. C.; Zhong, N.; Lu, P. Y. Using siRNA in prophylactic and therapeutic regimens against SARS coronavirus in Rhesus macaque. *Nature Med.* **2005**, *11*, 944–951.

98. Vaillant, A.; et al. Rep 9: a potent broad spectrum aerosol prophylaxis and therapy against influenza infection *in vivo. Antiviral Res.* **2006**, *70*, A52, Abstract 94.

99. Iversen, P.; et al. Inhibition of multiple influenza A subtypes in cell culture with antisense phosphorodiamidate morpholino oligomers. *Antiviral Res.* **2006**, *70*, A49, Abstract 80.

100. Ge, Q.; Pastey, M.; Kobasa, D.; Puthavathana, P.; Lupfer, C.; Bestwick, R. K.; Iversen, P. L.; Chen, J.; Stein, D. A. Inhibition of multiple subtypes of influenza A virus in cell cultures with morpholino oligomers. *Antimicrob. Agents Chemother.* **2006**, *50*, 3724–3733.

101. Deng, T.; Sharps, J.; Fodor, E.; Brownlee, G. G. *In vitro* assembly of PB2 with a PB1-PA dimer supports a new model of assembly of influenza A virus polymerase subunits into a functional trimeric complex. *J. Virol.* **2005**, *79*, 8669–8674.

102. Salomon, R.; Franks, J.; Govorkova, E. A.; Ilyushina, N. A.; Yen, H. L.; Hulse-Post, D. J.; Humberd, J.; Trichet, M.; Rehg, J. E.; Webby R. J.; Webster, R. G.; Hoffmann, E. The polymerase complex genes contribute to the high virulence of the human H5N1 influenza virus isolate A/Vietnam/1203/04. *J. Exp. Med.* **2006**, *203*, 689–697.

103. Tuttle, J. V.; Tisdale, M.; Krenitsky, T. A. Purine 2′-deoxy-2′-fluororibosides as antiinfluenza virus agents. *J. Med. Chem.* **1993**, *36*, 119–125.

104. Tisdale, M.; Ellis, M.; Klumpp, K.; Court, S.; Ford, M. Inhibition of influenza virus transcription by 2'-deoxy-2'-fluoroguanosine. *Antimicrob. Agents Chemother.* **1995**, *39*, 2454–2458.

105. Furuta, Y.; Takahashi, K.; Fukuda, Y.; Kuno, M.; Kamiyama, T.; Kozaki, K.; Nomura, N.; Egawa, H.; Minami, S.; Watanabe, Y.; Narita, H.; Shiraki, K. *In vitro* and *in vivo* activities of anti-influenza virus compound T-705. *Antimicrob. Agents Chemother.* **2002**, *46*, 977–981.

106. Takahashi, K.; Furuta, Y.; Fukuda, Y.; Kuno, M.; Kamiyama, T.; Kozaki, K.; Nomura, N.; Egawa, H.; Minami, S.; Shiraki, K. *In vitro* and *in vivo* activities of T-705 and oseltamivir against influenza virus. *Antiviral Chem. Chemother.* **2003**, *14*, 235–241.

107. Furuta, Y.; Takahashi, K.; Kuno-Maekawa, M.; Sangawa, H.; Uehara, S.; Kozaki, K.; Nomura, N.; Egawa, H.; Shiraki; K. Mechanism of action of T-705 against influenza virus. *Antimicrob. Agents Chemother.* **2005**, *49*, 981–986.

108. Tomassini, J.; Selnick, H.; Davies, M. E.; Armstrong, M. E.; Baldwin, J.; Bourgeois, M.; Hastings, J.; Hazuda, D.; Lewis, J.; McClements, W. Inhibition of cap (m^{7}GpppXm)-dependent endonuclease of influenza virus by 4-substituted 2,4-dioxobutanoic acid compounds. *Antimicrob. Agents Chemother.* **1994**, *38*, 2827–2837.

109. Cianci, C.; Chung, T. D. Y.; Meanwell, N.; Putz, H.; Hagen, M.; Colonno, R. J.; Krystal, M. Identification of *N*-hydroxamic acid and *N*-hydroxyimide compounds that inhibit the influenza virus polymerase. *Antiviral Chem. Chemother.* **1996**, *7*, 353–360.

110. Tomassini, J.; Davies, M. E.; Hastings, J. C.; Lingham, R.; Mojena, M.; Raghoobar, S. L.; Singh, S. B.; Tkacz, J. S.; Goetz, M. A. A novel antiviral agent which inhibits the endonuclease of influenza viruses. *Antimicrob. Agents Chemother.* **1996**, *40*, 1189–1193.

111. Sun, C.; Huang, H.; Feng, M.; Shi, X.; Zhang, X.; Zhou, P. A novel class of potent influenza virus inhibitors: Polysubstituted acylthiourea and its fused heterocycle derivatives. *Bioorg. Med. Chem. Lett.* **2006**, *16*, 162–166.

112. Wang, W.-L.; Yao, D. Y.; Gu, M.; Fan, M. Z.; Li, J. Y.; Xing, Y. C.; Nan, F. J. Synthesis and biological evaluation of novel bisheterocycle-containing compounds as potential anti-influenza virus agents. *Bioorg. Med. Chem. Lett.* **2005**, *15*, 5284–5287.

113. Isaacs, A.; Lindenmann, J. Virus interference. I. The interferon. *Proc. R. Soc. Lond. B. Biol. Sci.* **1957**, *147*, 258–267.

114. Isomura, S.; Ichikawa, T.; Miyazu, M.; Naruse, H.; Shibata, M.; Imanishi, J.; Matsuo, A.; Kishida, T.; Karaki, T. The preventive effect of human interferon-alpha on influenza infection; modification of clinical manifestations of influenza in children in a closed community. *Biken J.* **1982**, *25*, 131–137.

115. Phillpotts, R. J.; Higgins, P. G.; Willman, J. S.; Tyrrell, D. A.; Freestone, D. S.; Shepherd, W. M. Intranasal lymphoblastoid interferon ("Wellferon") prophylaxis against rhinovirus and influenza virus in volunteers. *J. Interferon Res.* **1984**, *4*, 535–541.

116. Fried, M. W.; Shiffman, M. L.; Reddy, K.R.; Smith, C.; Marinos, G.; Goncales, F. L., Jr.; Haussinger, D.; Diago, M.; Carosi, G.; Dhumeaux, D.; Craxi, A.; Lin, A.; Hoffman, J.; Yu, J. Peginterferon alfa-2a plus ribavirin for chronic hepatitis C virus infection. *N. Engl. J. Med.* **2002**, *347*, 975–982.

117. Field, A. K.; Tytell, A. A.; Lampson, G. P.; Hilleman, M. R. Inducers of interferon and host resistance. II. Multistranded synthetic polynucleotide complexes. *Proc. Natl. Acad. Sci. USA* **1967**, *58*, 1004–1010.

118. Saravolac, E. G.; Sabuda, D.; Crist, C.; Blasetti, K.; Schnell, G.; Yang, H.; Kende, M.; Levy, H. B.; Wong, J. P. Immunoprophylactic strategies against respiratory influenza virus infection. *Vaccine* **2001**, *19*, 2227–2232.

119. Ichinohe, T.; Watanabe, I.; Ito, S.; Fujii, H.; Moriyama, M.; Tamura, S.; Takahashi, H.; Sawa, H.; Chiba, J.; Kurata, T.; Sata, T.; Hasegawa, H. Synthetic double-stranded RNA poly(I:C) combined with mucosal vaccine protects against influenza virus infection. *J. Virol.* **2005**, *79*, 2910–2919.

120. Hayden, F. G. Antivirals for influenza: Historical perspectives and lessons learned. *Antiviral Res.* **2006**, *71*, 372–378.

121. Lavrov, S. V.; Eremkina, E. I.; Orlova, T. G.; Galegov, G. A.; Soloviev, V. D.; Zhdanov, V. M. Combined inhibition of influenza virus reproduction in cell culture using interferon and amantadine. *Nature* **1968**, *217*, 856–857.

122. Hayden, F. G. Combinations of antiviral agents for treatment of influenza virus infections. *J. Antimicrob. Chemother.* **1986**, *18*, Suppl. 1, 177–183.

123. Hayden, F. G.; Douglas, R. G., Jr.; Simons, R. Enhancement of activity against influenza viruses by combinations of antiviral agents. *Antimicrob. Agents Chemother.* **1980**, *18*, 536–541.

124. Bizollon, T.; Adham, M.; Pradat, P.; Chevallier, M.; Ducerf, C.; Baulieux, J.; Zoulim, F.; Trépo, C. Triple antiviral therapy with amantadine for IFN-ribavirin nonresponders with recurrent posttransplantation hepatitis C. *Transplantation* **2005**, *79*, 325–329.

125. Hayden, F. G.; Schlepushkin, A. N.; Pushkarskaya, N. L. Combined interferon-α_2, rimantadine hydrochloride, and ribavirin inhibition of influenza virus replication *in vitro*. *Antimicrob. Agents Chemother.* **1984**, *25*, 53–57.

126. Smee, D. F.; Wong, M.-H.; Bailey, K. W.; Sidwell, R. W. Activities of oseltamivir and ribavirin used alone and in combination against infections in mice with recent isolates of influenza A (H1N1) and B viruses. *Antiviral Chem. Chemother.* **2006**, *17*, 185–192.

127. Govorkova, E. A.; Fang, H.-B.; Tan, M.; Webster, R. G. Neuraminidase inhibitor-rimantadine combinations exert additive and synergistic anti-

influenza virus effects in MDCK cells. *Antimicrob. Agents Chemother.* **2004**, *48*, 4855–4863.

128. Ilyushina, N. A.; Bovin, N. V.; Webster, R. G.; Govorkova, E. A. Combination chemotherapy, a potential strategy for reducing the emergence of drug-resistant influenza A variants. *Antiviral Res.* **2006**, *70*, 121–131.

129. Ilyushina, N.; Hoffmann, E.; Salomon, R.; Webster, R.; Govorkova, E. Advantages of combination chemotherapy for highly pathogenic A/Vietnam/1203/04 (H5N1) influenza virus in mice. *Antiviral Res.* **2006**, *70*, A29, Abstract 10.

130. Ison, M. G.; Gnann, J. W., Jr.; Nagy-Agren, S.; Treannor, J.; Paya, C.; Steigbigel, R.; Elliott, M.; Weiss, H. L.; Hayden, F. G. Safety and efficacy of nebulized zanamivir in hospitalized patients with serious influenza. *Antiviral Ther.* **2003**, *8*, 183–190.

131. Quigley, E. Influenza therapies: Vaccines and antiviral drugs. *Drug Discovery Today* **2006**, *11*, 478–480.

132. Oxford, J. Oseltamivir in the management of influenza. *Expert Opin. Pharmacother.* **2005**, *6*, 2493–2500.

133. de Jong, M. D.; Hien, T. T.; Farrar, J. Oseltamivir resistance in influenza A (H5N1) infection. *N. Engl. J. Med.* **2006**, *354*, 1423–1424.

134. Jefferson, T.; Demicheli, V.; Rivetti, D.; Jones, M.; Di Pietrantoni, C.; Rivetti, A. Antivirals for influenza in healthy adults: systematic review. *Lancet* **2006**, *367*, 303–313.

135. Cunha, B. A. Amantadine may be lifesaving in severe influenza A. *Clin. Infect. Dis.* **2006**, *43*, 1372–1373.

136. Vernier, V. G.; Harmon, J. B.; Stump, J. M.; Lynes, T. E.; Marvel, J. P.; Smith, D. H. The toxicologic and pharmacologic properties of amatandine hydrochloride. *Toxicol. Appl. Pharmacol.* **1969**, *15*, 642–665.

137. Whitley, R. J.; Monto, A. S. Prevention and treatment of influenza in high-risk groups: Children, pregnant women, immunocompromised hosts, and nursing home residents. *J. Infect. Dis.* **2006**, *194*, Suppl. 2, S133–S138.

2

DEVELOPMENT OF HIGH-THROUGHPUT SCREENING ASSAYS FOR INFLUENZA

DIANA L. NOAH E. LUCILE WHITE, AND JAMES W. NOAH

Drug Discovery Division, Southern Research Institute, Birmingham, AL 35205

INTRODUCTION

Although a typical influenza season poses only a moderate health risk to the general population, large portions of the community are routinely endangered due to age-related susceptibility or compromised immunity, and influenza remains one of the 10 most common causes of death in the United States.[1] Influenza type A and B virus infection in humans results in an estimated 200,000 hospitalizations and 50,000 deaths in the United States annually.[2,3] These annual epidemics have a large economic impact, costing more than 1 billion dollars directly, and 11 billion dollars indirectly, per year in the United States alone.[4] In the event of a pandemic, the Centers for Disease Control and Prevention (CDC) has predicted a three- to sevenfold increase in hospitalization and mortality rates and at least a 20-fold increase in economic impact in the United States alone. The effect would be many times more devastating in regions of the world where the health-care system is not comparably advanced.[5,6] Finally, the potential decimation of the

Combating the Threat of Pandemic Influenza: Drug Discovery Approaches,
Edited by Paul F. Torrence
Copyright © 2007 by John Wiley & Sons, Inc.

domestic fowl population would have a tremendous economic impact on the worldwide poultry industry.[7,8]

Modern research credits the seasonal reoccurrence of influenza to both its nature as a segmented negative-strand RNA virus and the selective pressure to coexist in a dual host system consisting of the natural avian reservoir and a secondary mammalian host such as humans, horses, dogs, cats, and ferrets, all of which can contract the naturally occurring influenza virus.[9] The success of influenza is attributed partially to mutations in the viral surface proteins (antigenic drift) and partially to the ability of the virus to evade immunogenic recognition by shuffling its genetic constellation annually (antigenic shift), resulting in a genetic reassortment that may combine separate strain idiosyncrasies, some of which may be virulence factors, into a single virus. This is why a new vaccine is required every year, and this also rationalizes the need for continued virological surveillance against the rise of particularly virulent influenza strains. Finally, this is the reason for the statistical certainty of another pandemic, a prospect that is continually emphasized by the emergence of the highly pathogenic avian influenza (HPAI) strains in Asia and their spread over a large portion of the world.[10] The potential social and economic disruption ensuing from a human pandemic combined with the economic disaster resulting from the destruction of domesticated bird populations has prompted the NIAID to classify the influenza virus as a Category C priority pathogen and has led the CDC to classify HPAI as a select agent.[11]

The logistical pressure of monitoring potentially millions of environmental samples for influenza strain migration in the avian reservoir, combined with the need to analyze an equal number of isolates for strain movement within the human population during influenza season, demands assay procedures that use high-throughput screening (HTS) formats.[11] The annual need to develop new vaccines against circulating human influenza strains and emerging avian strains again requires a high-throughput approach to rapidly evaluate vaccine efficacy.[12] Lastly, antiviral drugs are available to protect the human population from influenza infection, but only a few approved antivirals are currently effective against circulating strains. Although great success has come from deriving the structures of influenza viral neuraminidase and rationally designing specific inhibitors for the enzymatic active site,[13] the molecular structures of the majority of targeted influenza components have not yet been solved. An alternative to rational design is a systematic survey of small-molecule compound libraries for antiviral properties and development of lead compounds into pharmaceutical drugs. Although this is a time-consuming and costly process, it has become a model strategy and is employed for viruses such as HIV, West Nile, influenza, herpes, and hepatitis viruses.[14,15] The associated cost and time required for comprehensive surveys of small-molecule libraries (which may contain millions of unique compounds) will be greatly reduced by the development and adaptation of influenza antiviral assays to HTS screening formats by a combination of applicative robotics, miniaturization, and efficient management of the resultant large data sets.

HTS approaches to influenza are divided into three areas: diagnostic identification of viral strains, evaluation of vaccines, and development of antiviral prophylactics and therapeutics. These assay formats include recent methods for genotyping and phenotyping, determination of serum neutralizing antibody levels for vaccine evaluation, and cell-based or biochemical antiviral screens of small-molecule libraries. Because these high-throughput methods often employ a "brute force" strategy for blindly evaluating the largest data set possible, the logistics of effort, economy, and time demand a good deal of finesse in the initial stages of assay design, HTS adaptation, assay validation, and library selection. In addition, strategies such as combinatorial and virtual screening have emerged that are able to systematically narrow large screening sets to a practical size for further evaluation by low-throughput methods. This chapter will briefly describe the potential of each influenza component as an assay target and will detail the current state of influenza assays that are adaptable or have already been adapted to HTS formats for diagnostic strain characterization, vaccine evaluation, and identification of potential antivirals.

THE INFLUENZA REPLICATION CYCLE

The influenza A virus (*orthomyxoviridae*) genome contains eight separate segments[16] of negative-sense RNA which encode 11 viral proteins that are essential for the viral replication cycle and packaging of progeny virus. The crucial functions of these proteins during viral replication direct the processes of cell membrane recognition, endosomal fusion and acidification, delivery of the RNP to the nucleus, polymerase holoenzyme catalysis of transcription and replication, the protein and RNA binding activity of nonstructural proteins, and sialidase activity. Each represents a key point for interruption of the replication cycle. Extensive characterization of the influenza A subtype has occurred because this strain represents the greatest threat to civic welfare. It is the only strain to exhibit antigenic shift[17] and has accounted for all known high-mortality epidemics and pandemics.[18] Therefore this chapter will deal primarily with the components of influenza A, with applications to other influenza viral types.

Influenza particles are spherical (~100-nm diameter) with a lipid bilayer derived from the host plasma membrane.[19] The virion contains a matrix protein (M1) and three transmembrane proteins (hemagglutinin [HA], neuraminidase [NA], and a proton channel [M2]). Beneath the matrix coat is the helical ribonucleocapsid, which includes the vRNA genome, nucleoprotein (NP), nuclear export protein (NEP), and the three viral polymerase subunits (PB1, PB2, PA) that form the polymerase holoenzyme. The viral replication cycle begins with infection of the host cell by HA-mediated binding to cell-surface sialic acids (which are ubiquitously present on membrane-associated glycoproteins and glycolipids), followed by internalization by receptor-mediated endocytosis. Viruses with proteolytically activated HA (HA with a cleaved fusion peptide) fuse with the endosomal membrane through an acidic pH-promoted conformational alteration and is followed by the M2 proton channel-controlled acidification of the viral core. This causes disassociation of the M1 coat protein and release of the viral ribonucleoprotein (vRNP) into the cytoplasm. Nuclear-localization signals on the NP facilitate transport of the vRNP to the nucleus, where viral mRNA transcription (vRNA→vmRNA) and genomic replication (vRNA→cRNA→vRNA) occurs. Once translated, one of the virally encoded nonstructural proteins, NS1, binds double-stranded RNA and host mRNA processing factors to inhibit the cellular interferon-induced antiviral response (reviewed in Ref. 20). Another recently discovered nonstructural protein, PB1-F2, is thought to promote host cell apoptosis by insertion into mitochondrial and cell membranes.[21] The polymerase holoenzyme performs host mRNA cap-recognition and -snatching to provide capped mRNA primers for initiation of viral transcription.[22] Replicated vRNPs are exported from the nucleus, assisted by NEP, and transported to the plasma membrane for assembly and with the envelope proteins (NA, M2, HA, M1). Virus budding and release by NA-facilitated cleavage of terminal sialic acid residues on the cell surface glycoligands completes the cycle.[19]

INFLUENZA COMPONENTS AS HTS ASSAY TARGETS

A molecular targeting approach to influenza requires identification of a viral component as a target for viral detection or function inhibition.[23]

Assays are designed to detect target presence and evaluate target function. Targeted low-throughput assays employing enzyme-linked immunosorbent assay (ELISA), RT-PCR, cell-based, or biochemical methods have been developed using whole virus or purified influenza components to rapidly identify strain lineage, vaccine efficacy, and potential antivirals, yet the overwhelming numbers of diagnostic isolates, vaccines, and potential antiviral compounds available for analysis has driven the adaptation and validation of only a few of these assays to HTS.[24] In some cases, extensive assay design modification is required for HTS adaptation, which demands a rationalization of target selection to choose the best adaptation and endpoint detection methods.

The influenza virus components can be classified into three categories: the envelope-associated proteins (HA, NA, M1, M2), the interior ribonucleoproteins (PB1, PB2, PA, NP), and the nonstructural proteins (NS1, NEP, PB1-F2).[19] The functions of these components have been investigated by genetic and *in vitro* methods, and each has been evaluated as a target for strain identification, vaccine generation, or inhibition by antivirals. Figure 2.1 illustrates the viral life cycle and lists the potential HTS assay targets. A brief review of each influenza component follows, focusing on the functional significance and rational justification of each as a diagnostic, immunogenic, or antiviral target.

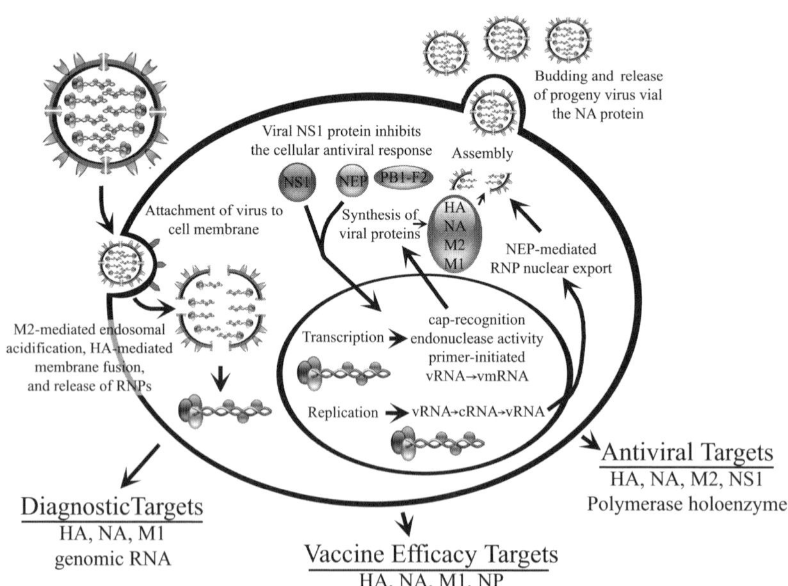

Fig. 2.1. The influenza viral life cycle and targets for HTS assays.

The Envelope-Associated Viral Proteins

During viral infection the envelope proteins work to allow the virus to penetrate mucosal barriers to reach the target cell, bind the cellular membrane to mediate endosomal fusion, and deliver the viral genetic package to the target cell interior. They are also responsible for the promotion of viral uncoating and release of progeny virus. The host-derived viral envelope lipid bilayer encompasses the transmembrane M2 proton channel and the two HA and NA proteins, and it surrounds the M1 coat protein. Three of these components (HA, NA, M1) have been successfully exploited as antigens for strain phenotyping and vaccine development, and two (NA, M2) have been successfully inhibited by small-molecule drugs used as antiviral prophylactics and therapeutics.

Hemagglutinin. Several targets for diagnostic, vaccine evaluation, or inhibition assays exist in HA. These include the sialic acid receptor recognition, the immunogenic potential of the HA1 subunit, the fusiogenic properties of the HA2 fusion peptide, and the proteolytic activation of the HA0 precursor protein. First, 16 influenza A subtypes of HA have been identified, but only three (H1, H2, H3) are adapted to human populations. This specificity is controlled by as few as two critical amino acid residues,[25] making the act of receptor recognition by HA a critical point for antiviral intervention. Second, HA subtyping is based on the affinity of antibodies (derived from hyperimmune anti-HA sera) for varying surface epitopes found predominately in the HA1 domain,[26] which justifies HA1 as a diagnostic assay target. Third, the HA2-mediated endosomal fusion event is a potential target for small-molecule inhibition at the early stages of viral replication. Although the mechanics of fusion are not clearly defined,[27] experiments with fusion peptide mutants have suggested that HA2 employs a "leash-in-groove" mechanism to mediate fusion by packing the N-terminal peptide (the "leash") into the adjacent HA2 coiled-coil structure, thereby bringing conserved hydrophobic leash residues in close proximity with the cell membrane to initiate lipid destabilization.[28] This suggests that these leash residues and their interactions with the coiled coil are viable targets for inhibition of fusion. Lastly, the nature of the protease cleavage site in HA0 is an important virulence determinant for influenza A viruses and a target for antiviral therapies. Activation of HA0 by cleavage into HA1 and HA2 is typically performed by host cell-surface proteases[29] that specifically recognize the multibasic cleavage site, which restricts the spread of most influenza viral strains to lung tissues.[18] It is important to note that the polybasic cleavage site in both the 1918 influenza H1 strain and in recent isolates of highly pathogenic H5 avian influenza viruses is larger than that found in recent human strains and therefore is additionally recognized by furin or furin-like proteases present in the trans-Golgi network of a broad range of cell types.[30] This allows HA activation to occur before assembly and budding, increasing the overall production and spread of infectious virus particles. The high virulence of the H5 virus in domestic birds and the extended tissue tropism in mammals is attributed to the nature of the H5 HA polybasic cleavage site.[18]

Neuraminidase. The NA protein is immunogenic and is therefore a diagnostic target, while the enzymatic activity is an antiviral target. NA is instrumental in both the early and late stages of infection because it cleaves sialic acid residues that are linked to glycoprotein and glyco-lipids on the cell surface[31] and found in mucosal secretions.[32] Inhibition of this process causes an accumulation of attached virus particles at the cell membrane and prevents the spread of the virus to the surrounding cells. NA is also a surface determinant for antibody recognition and viral subtyping. As an antiviral target, NA is one of the most success-fully inhibited influenza proteins, and more than two decades of effort has been spent in NA subtype 1 and 2 crystallization and rational drug design,[13,33] which has yielded two Food and Drug Administration (FDA) approved drugs, zanamivir (Relenza) and oseltamivir (Tamiflu). Based on the assumption that the NA active site is conserved across protein subtypes, these drugs specifically inhibit the viral NA by imitating the substrate transition state, halting release of budding virus.[34] They are currently effective prophylactics[35] and therapeutics, and the present isolation rate of resistant strains is low. However, frequent use of both drugs has the potential to rapidly increase the resistance rate[36,37] (an increasingly disturbing scenario observed in the case of avian influenza[38,39]). Thus NA activity remains a valuable target for antiviral research.

M2 Proton Channel. The M2 proton channel is a well-documented target for inhibition of influenza replication. Influenza A encodes a small (97 amino acids) membrane-bound protein that forms the tetra-meric M2 proton channel. Inhibition of channel function prevents viral uncoating, thereby halting virion release, nuclear localization, and ultimately replication at an early state of infection.[40] Although the M2 protein has not been successfully exploited as a diagnostic or vaccine target, the proton channel is a demonstrated antiviral target. Two M2 channel inhibitors (amantadine and rimantadine) are FDA approved for antiviral therapy, but the high incidence of viral resistance to these drugs restricts their effectiveness[41] and justifies continued antiviral screening. Importantly, some of the H5N1 emergent avian influenza strains are amantadine resistant.[42]

M1 Coat Protein. The M1 viral coat protein is a potential target for diagnostic assays and is a candidate for the development of vaccines.[43] It remains elusive as a therapeutic target due to the insufficient information about the nature and necessity of the interactions between the M1 protein and viral or host factors. The M1 protein is the most abundant component in the virus and plays a well-defined role in RNP coating during viral assembly.[19] As a diagnostic determinant, antibodies to M1 readily recognize the protein, although the lack of antigenic variation does not allow strain determination by M1 protein epitope mapping alone. The same lack of variation instead suggests that the M1 protein might be a good candidate for development of cross-protective vaccines.[43] Finally, antiviral potential might be found in small molecules that inhibit protein–protein interactions,[44] or they might be found in peptides or nucleic acid aptamers, which have been successfully used to inhibit influenza HA receptor recognition.[45]

Ribonucleoproteins

The influenza ribonucleoprotein consists of the genomic vRNA segments in complex with the polymerase protein subunits PB1, PB2, and PA, and the NP. After release into the cytoplasm, the vRNPs are imported into the nucleus for viral transcription and genomic replication. Nuclear transport and import of the vRNPs are directed by multiple and cooperative nuclear localization signals (NLS) located within each of the protein RNP components (see Ref. 46 for review) and controlled by NP-mediated binding of nuclear importins, which actively transport the infectious vRNPs or the newly transcribed polymerase holoenzyme complex and NP into the nucleus for replication or assembly into nascent vRNPs. After assembly, vRNP nuclear export and transport to the cell membrane is necessary for incorporation into new virus particles. The genomic RNA is a major component of the vRNPs and is itself a target for diagnostic screening assays, which are able to determine viral type, subtype, and subfamily (clade) by RNA sequencing and phylogenetic comparisons.[7] However, the genomic RNA is not a candidate for vaccine efficacy or small molecule antiviral screens.

Polymerase Holoenzyme. The polymerase holoenzyme represents three obvious targets for antiviral HTS assay design, and each of them involves the inhibition of substrate recognition or catalysis. Both influenza virus transcription and replication occur in the nucleus through the catalytic action of the three polymerase subunits (PB1, PB2, PA) acting in concert with the RNA organizational ability of the NP. The capping of mRNA with a 5′-m7GpppN-cap structure is essential for efficient export of mRNA from the nucleus and for eukaryotic translation initiation.[47] The cap structure is recognized by eukaryotic initiation factor eIF4E in the eIF4F translation initiation complex,[48] while uncapped mRNAs are restricted to utilizing less efficient, 5′-dependent translation initiation processes.[49] The influenza polymerase holoenzyme possesses no mechanism to cap viral mRNAs (vmRNAs), but instead has evolved an almost unique (shared by *Bunyaviridae*[50]) method for ensuring that vmRNA transcripts all possess host-recognized cap structures. The polymerase holoenzyme employs a specialized cap-snatching mechanism[47] in which it binds a capped host cell mRNA and cleaves the mRNA 9–17 nt downstream from the cap. This short length of host capped mRNA is subsequently used as a primer for viral mRNA transcription.

Based on the evidence indicating that the polymerase subunits are virulence factors,[51] it is clear that cap-recognition and endonuclease functions, as well as transcriptive and replicative polymerization, represent key targets for small-molecule inhibition. Recent experiments have identified (a) compounds that selectively target the influenza polymerase cap-recognition activity and have a lower affinity for cellular cap-recognition proteins that are necessary for cell viability (e.g., eIF4E)[48] and (b) compounds that inhibit endonuclease activity have been investigated for over a decade.[52] Two compounds, ribavirin[53] and T-705,[54] have been shown to affect the holoenzyme polymerase activity. However, neither compound has been approved by the FDA for use as an influenza prophylactic or therapeutic, which highlights the continued need to identify effective antivirals that affect these critical targets.

Nucleoprotein. Nucleoprotein (NP) is a target for diagnostic and vaccine efficacy assays, and evidence suggests that it is also a target for antivirals. NP organizes the vRNA during transcription and replication, functions in packaging and assembly of vRNPs into new virus particles, and associates with the cellular factors required for nuclear cytoplasmic shuttling,[55] including the viral polymerase subunits and the M1 coat protein. NP homo-oligomerizes through the interaction of two independent regions within each monomer and is thought to act as a processivity protein during polymerization, either by regulating the speed of the polymerase holoenzyme complex or by providing additional protein–protein contacts that promote retention of the holoenzyme on the elongating vRNAs.[56,57] It also has been suspected of participating in the primary mechanism that governs the switch from viral mRNA transcription to genomic RNA replication, although the hypothesized manner of this participation ranges from the primary regulatory protein to simply a structural cofactor.[55] Finally, the position of the last NP monomer on the vRNA is associated with the polyadenylation signal.[58]

As an assay target, the early translation and high levels of NP expression make it a candidate for immunodetection of early virus replication in cell-based assays. ELISA-based detection of the early accumulation of NP has been used to determine the amount of neutralizing antibody in the sera of vaccinated individuals.[59] Since the sequence of NP is more than 89% conserved,[60] antibody probes have a large degree of cross-reactivity to conserved NP epitopes and can be used for early multi-strain detection of viral replication. Antiviral targeting potential might be found in disrupting protein–protein interactions that govern the polymerase subunit/NP associations, NP/host protein associations, and the RNA binding potential of NP using peptides, nucleic acid apatmers,[45] or small molecules.[44] Of particular interest is the targeting of the mechanism that governs NP oligomerization, which, if triggered prior to association with vRNPs, could deplete the nuclear store of NP and hamper or prevent the formation of active vRNPs[56,57] and/or their export.

Nonstructural Viral Proteins

Several influenza viral transcription products essential to the replication cycle are not packaged within the virus particles (or are packaged at low levels). These proteins include the NS1 protein, the NEP, and the PB1-F2 fragment. The degree of sequence conservation between the nonstructural viral proteins is greater than that found in the viral envelope proteins, and efforts have been made to develop immunogenic-based diagnostic assays for the NS1 protein from a broad range of avian viral strains, and these proteins might serve as target antigens for diagnostic assays and vaccine efficiency studies.[61] However, the cellular concentrations of the nonstructural proteins are low in comparison with viral immunogenic targets such as the M1 protein or NP,[62] suggesting that ELISA-based diagnostic assays or vaccine development against the former might be less efficient than using the latter. Finally the nonstructural proteins regulate viral and cellular functions not through catalysis but instead through protein–protein or protein–RNA interactions, making them novel targets for antiviral inhibition.

NS1. NS1 has two domains, an RNA-binding domain and a protein-binding domain, both of which are rational targets for antiviral strategies, and NS1 has also been used to generate antibodies for the development of immunogenic diagnostic and neutralization vaccine efficacy assays. It is one of two proteins translated from the NS gene segment during early infection, after which it rapidly localizes to the nucleus, thereafter inhibiting the functions of two host cellular proteins that participate in the 3′-end processing of cellular pre-mRNAs: the poly(A)-binding protein II (PABII) and the 30-kD subunit of the cleavage and polyadenylation specificity factor (CPSF, required for pre-mRNA 3′-end maturation).[63] Also, NS1 binds double-stranded RNA (dsRNA) with low affinity, possibly to antagonize the cellular antiviral dsRNA-induced antiviral response by sequestering and preventing dsRNA-induced activation of 2′-5′oligo (A) synthetase.[64] NS1 has also recently been shown to bind cellular PKR (dsRNA-activated kinase), and this binding likely accounts for the inhibition of PKR during influenza A viral infection.[65] Importantly, NS1 has been identified as a virulence factor in H5N1 strain infections in chickens,[66] increasing its priority as an antiviral target.

The N-terminal 73 amino acids of the NS1A protein comprise the dsRNA-binding domain and possess all the dsRNA binding properties of the full-length protein.[67] Using a reverse genetics system,[68,69] it has been demonstrated that (a) a recombinant influenza A virus encoding an NS1A protein with a mutated RNA-binding domain is highly attenuated and replicates approximately 50-fold less efficiently and (b) dsRNA binding mediated by NS1 is essential for virus replication, making the dsRNA binding potential of the NS1 protein a logical target for antiviral intervention.[70] The NS1A effector domain (aa 74–230) that binds PABII and CPSF is also a target with equal potential for inhibition. Possible inhibitory molecules could be peptide or nucleic acid aptamer-based.[45]

NEP. As a rational diagnostic, vaccine, or antiviral assay target, the influenza NEP has yet to be explored. The NEP is the second gene product of the NS viral segment and is the protein primarily responsible for export of the assembled vRNPs from the nucleus to the cytoplasm for viral packaging.[46,71] It has no documented catalytic function, but instead acts through protein–protein interactions. As a target for diagnostic or vaccine efficacy assays, its cellular expression levels are far lower than that of NP as a marker for cell-based infection assays, although antibodies raised against recombinantly expressed NEP have been shown to alter the nuclear accumulation of NP and vRNPs at late-stage infections,[71] and these same antibodies might prove effective tools in assay development. As a target for antivirals, the protein nuclear export signal (NES) or the interface of NEP/M1 binding might be inhibited by aptamers or peptides specifically designed to bind, sequester, or block these regions.[45]

PB1-F2. PB1-F2 is a recently discovered influenza A virus protein with pro-apoptotic properties that has also only begun to be experimentally explored as a rational assay target.[21] This protein was initially identified in the strain A/PR8/34 (H1N1)[72] and is encoded and conserved in most known human isolates of influenza A subtype viruses, but is not found in influenza B-type viruses.[73] Similar to the polygenic M and NS gene segments, the PB1-F2 sequence is contained within the polymerase subunit PB1 gene segment, and the translation of an alternative (+1) open reading frame within the subunit gene results in an 87-amino-acid protein. The PB1-F2 C-terminal helical region has been shown to promote targeting and insertion of the protein into the cellular mitochondrial membranes.[74] It has been proposed that the apoptotic nature of the protein works to destabilize cells both (a) internally during viral infections by accelerating apoptosis in the cells expressing it[73] and (b) externally once infected cells release the free protein.[21]

INFLUENZA HTS ASSAY DEVELOPMENT AND ADAPTATION TO HTS FORMATS

What does HTS mean? Does it mean screening tens, hundreds, thousands, or hundreds of thousands of points per day? For a small laboratory, an assay format for screening one 96-well microplate/day using a hand-held, multichannel pipette is considered high-throughput, and the corresponding laboratory HTS assays are designed and adapted with human and laboratory limitations in mind. Alternatively, a large industrial laboratory may design and adapt multiple assays that incorporate the use of extreme miniaturization, automated robotics, liquid handlers, and readers for screening 100,000 points/day. Many different assays are capable of screening less than 100 points/day but are labeled as high-throughput, when they are actually moderate- or low-throughput. With the current need to rapidly identify and characterize influenza strains from thousands of avian or human isolates, the urgency to create and evaluate new vaccines for potentially pandemic strains, and the desire to screen uncharacterized small molecule libraries with millions of chemically diverse members for antiviral activity, the development of influenza assays must accommodate these equivalent numbers of available points by adopting HTS. Sophisticated robotics and programming software, along with bioinformatics and statistical computer programs capable of analyzing large data sets, are available. The true bottleneck lies in the difficulty in adapting the many existing benchtop influenza assays to HTS formats.

HTS assays are designed to reproducibly generate a large data set with conservation of time, materials, and manpower. This is accomplished by using assay miniaturization to reduce the ratio of materials consumption to generated data, programmable robotics to decrease the required manpower and increase reproducibility, and bioinformatics programs to efficiently manage and display the resulting large data. Strategies for adapting influenza assays to HTS formats should primarily include reducing the number of assay manipulation steps and developing and validating liquid handling methods and automated detection systems for the reproduction of bench level procedures.[75] Secondary strategies may include assay miniaturization. Following this, a dose–response curve should be established with known assay controls (i.e., oseltamivir carboxylate is an ideal positive control for neuraminidase inhibition assays) to identify the control concentration that balances assay reproducibility with sensitivity. HTS assay design variables can include incubation time and temperature, moderating-edge effects, minimal assay manipulations, and DMSO tolerance (a factor of antiviral compound storage and solubility). Assay quality assessment includes run-to-run and day-to-day reproducibility. Evaluating screening variability takes account of the experimental signal-to-background (S/B) and signal-to-noise (S/N), standard deviation of the mean (σ), coefficient of variation (CV), and Z/Z′ determination (a statistical measure of robustness[76]). Table 2.1 lists the calculations for determination of each of these parameters.

A final step in evaluating the HTS assay performance should include a duplicate pilot screen (on separate days) of a small set of unknown samples ($n = 1000–3000$) to establish the data correlation and historical reproducibility. For antiviral screening, this also establishes optimum compound screening concentration and the cutoff value for compound efficacy (i.e., "hit" qualification). The following section will describe current assay formats for influenza screening and their high-throughput

TABLE 2.1. Parameters for HTS Assay Validation

HTS Validation Parameter	Calculation
S/B[121]	$\mu_p/\mu_n{}^{a}$
S/N[121]	$(\mu_p - \mu_n)/((\sigma_p)^2 + (\sigma_n)^2)^{1/2\,a,b}$
σ	$(1/n\sum(\chi_i - \mu_x)^2)^{1/2\,c}$
CV	σ/μ
Z[76]	$1 - ((3\sigma_p + 3\sigma_n)/|\mu_p - \mu_n|)^{a,d}$
Z'[76]	$1 - ((3\sigma_d + 3\sigma_n)/|\mu_d - \mu_n|)^{b,d}$

[a] μ_p is the mean positive control value, and μ_n is the mean negative control value.
[b] σ_p is the standard deviation of the positive control value, and σ_n is the standard deviation of the negative control value.
[c] n is the number of points, χ_i is the individual point value, and μ_x is the mean of all χ values.
[d] μ_d is the mean drug control value, and σ_d is the standard deviation of the drug control value.

application or adaptation for diagnostic, vaccine, and antiviral screening, with emphasis on target selection, sample throughput, and the adaptation of current low-throughput assays to high-throughput formats.

Influenza Diagnostic HTS assays

In the event of an influenza epidemic or pandemic, early diagnosis is crucial to the success of outbreak management programs and patient therapy. The choice of annual vaccine strains is based on data from surveillance programs that monitor antigenic variation in viral NA and HA viral surface proteins, and the ability and accuracy of these programs in tracking the migration and circulation of influenza viral strains would be greatly increased by the development of diagnostic HTS assays designed to screen thousands of isolates.[12] Of the existing diagnostic influenza assays, only a few of these have been adapted to HTS, and none has yet been rigorously validated or automated. Nonetheless, several of these assays have the potential to greatly increase the power of worldwide influenza surveillance programs once the final steps of automation and validation have been achieved. They include sensitive and strain-specific immunoassays and RT-PCR assays[7], detection of viral protein fragments by mass spectrometry,[1] and microarray technologies.[25]

ELISA Diagnostics. In a pandemic scenario, rapid field detection of influenza virus infection followed by multisample surveys is critical for early subtype identification and outbreak management. Field classifications are done by immunoassays that measure the antibody response to the HA and NA viral surface proteins. The goal of these assays is twofold: to detect the presence of the influenza virus and to determine the type and subtype, but limitations in the assays prevent further viral classification. Strain-specific antibodies for four influenza antigens (HA, NA, NP, and the M1 matrix protein) are commercially available. Several rapid detection kits based on ELISA detection of HA and NA are also commercially available for characterizing virus type and subtype; more recently, assays against the NP[77] have been developed which have proven equally or more sensitive. Subtype specificity for these low-throughput assays frequently reaches 100%,[77] with a sensitivity of 90–99%.[77,78] Adaptation of these methods to completely automated HTS methods has not been accomplished due to the specialized requirements of sample preparation, assay design, and endpoint detection, and the number and type of critical assay steps. Instead, detection kits have been designed for ease of use and rapid readout but are reported to sacrifice sensitivity.[79,80] It is clear that these methods are adequate for field detection but inadequate for adaptation to HTS formats. In light of this, they are rapidly being replaced with more sensitive RT-PCR methods.

RT-PCR Diagnostics. The primary HTS adaptable diagnostic method for influenza virus strain characterization is reverse transcriptase polymerase chain reaction (RT-PCR), which allows for the rapid determination of genomic sequences, surface protein subtyping, and strain classification through phylogenetic comparison of the sample genomic RNA sequences with strains of known sequences. This method requires the identification of a strain-specific viral genomic sequence sandwiched between two conserved regions of the same coding region. Sequence isolation is accomplished by reverse transcription of one or several viral genomic segments with specific DNA primers, followed by PCR amplification of the sequences using DNA primers specific for the conserved regions. The identification of strain-specific sequences flanked by conserved sequences is absolutely critical to the accuracy of the assay; this allows a single set of primers to be used for detection multiple virus subtypes. Using amplification of the HA gene and phylogenetic comparison of the resultant sequences, this method has accurately identified virus strains containing any of the 15 HA subtypes.[7] However, the complex methods currently utilized for the extraction of viral RNA from isolates have proven difficult to automate and remain costly in the time required for sample processing. Adaptation of this assay for higher-throughput could be accomplished by utilizing an HTS real-time RT-PCR method that was previously developed for the Exotic Newcastle Disease (END) virus, a technique that could readily be applied to influenza virus characterization.[81] Briefly, a magnetic bead-based RNA extraction method performed in a 96-well microplate was used to isolate the viral RNA, followed directly by a 96-well real-time RT-PCR assay, which allowed a single technician to process 400 samples per day. The assay demonstrated a sensitivity of ~99% in positive field samples and 100% in negative samples, and it resulted in a 66% reduction in the time required for END virus control and eradication. These methods could be readily adapted to influenza screening and could potentially be coupled to automated DNA sequence analyses for greater efficiency.

Emerging Diagnostic Methods. Significant progress has been made in the last few years on emerging and alternative diagnostic methods for influenza detection and characterization, including the use of nucleic acid and specialized-ligand microarrays as well as mass spectrometry. Stevens et al.[82] have detailed an HTS method using solid-phase glycan ligand microarrays to examine the specificity of the HA protein for different sialic acid ligands using hundreds of different sialic acid linkage combinations.[82] Other microarray assays using immobilized nucleic acids (i.e., a Fluchip) have been designed to provide information for a wide range of viral strains and lineages.[83,84] Assays of this type require the extraction and amplification of the viral RNA, hybridization and fluorescent labeling, and imaging of the chip to determine virus type and subtype. A clinical sensitivity of 95% and clinical specificity of 92% was reported, with errors attributed not to the assay chip performance but rather to the amplification step. Coupled with automated RNA extraction and amplification, these methods can be adapted for HTS to determine both strain specificity and the ability of arrayed small molecules to bind to and possibly inhibit influenza targets.

Lastly, immunoconjugation coupled with a moderate-throughput mass spectrometry assay has been used to identify antigenic influenza HA peptides in a mixture of biological components.[1] This assay requires minimal sample manipulation (consisting of a short tryptic digestion followed by an antibody association step), and the method is able to analyze one sample per minute. It has the potential for HTS adaptation to microplate format using automated liquid handling coupled to matrix-assisted laser desorption/ionization or electrospray mass spectrometry to identify influenza viral type and subtype at femtomolar concentrations of antigenic HA epitopes.

Influenza Vaccine Efficacy HTS Assays

Influenza vaccines are currently the most widely used and most effective means to reduce the severity of yearly influenza infections in the general population. After vaccination, the immunogenic response results in the production of reactive antibodies primarily against the viral HA protein. As part of the pandemic preparedness plan, international scientific communities are developing vaccine candidates to limit spread of a pandemic and reduce morbidity and mortality, or potentially even prevent a pandemic from occurring. Part of the global plan is to analyze patient antibody response titers to vaccines in a uniform, accurate, and reproducible manner at various labs around the world, something that is not currently established.[85] Again, the number of sera samples resulting from multiple vaccine studies involving both human and avian influenza strains requires a validated HTS assay for vaccine efficacy.

An effective, approved vaccine is not yet available for any of the HPAI H5N1 strains, although efforts are currently underway to develop vaccines for both domesticated bird and human populations using LPAI strains [86] or recombinant H5 strains.[87] The spread of HPAI H5N1 strains around the world and the almost 60% current human mortality rate[88] have driven the partial HTS adaptation of two assays, the hemagglutinin inhibition assay and the neutralization assay. Hemagglutinin inhibition has been used for decades as the standard method of vaccine evaluation, but the ELISA-based neutralization assays did not gain wide use until the late 1990s when it provided sensitive results for emerging H5 viruses.[59] Both of these assays are currently performed in 96-well microplates.[87]

Hemagglutinination Inhibition Assay. The primary assay for determining the amount of influenza-specific antibody present in the serum of vaccinated individuals is the hemagglutination inhibition (HAI) assay. It has been known for over 50 years that influenza causes red blood cells (RBCs) to agglutinate in a process called hemagglutination[89] through the binding of the viral hemagglutinin to sialic acid residues present on the RBC surface. When preincubating vaccinated patient sera with the target virus, a sufficient titer of antibodies against the viral HA in the sera results in the binding and sequestering of the virus, thereby preventing agglutination.[90] Because influenza viral strains show a strong species specificity for receptor recognition,[25] the HAI assay has been optimized using RBCs from a variety of avian and mammalian species, depending on the strain of virus assayed. Recently, the sensitivity of the HAI assay for avian viruses has been improved by the use of horse red blood cells,[91] which have species specificity factors similar to avian influenza viruses, including the potentially pandemic H5, H7, and H9 virus strains.

This assay has several critical steps that would hamper a complete adaptation to HTS. First, the HAI assay is labor-intensive because the sera samples require serial dilution for titer determination, although this could be performed by contact liquid handler on an automated robotics platform. Second, antibody standards against potentially pandemic strains of influenza (including pathogenic H5N1 strains) are not available to the international scientific community, making assay standardization difficult. Third, there is a question of the appropriate HTS endpoint detection method. Agglutination is currently determined subjectively by direct visualization, and conversion of this determination to an automated reading system is problematic. Thus the assay, although currently the most widely used method for vaccine efficacy testing, is not amenable to complete HTS adaptation, although some HTS methods (e.g., miniaturization, liquid handling) can be incorporated into sample preparation and assay performance. With a partial HTS adaptation, the assay is highly reproducible (using equivalently trained operators). In a two-month laboratory study, greater than 95% of all assay plates ($n = 450$) had a control titer within one dilution of the historical median.[92]

Neutralization Assay. The neutralization assay is another effective method for determining serum antibody titers against influenza virus as well as against many other viruses, including SARS CoV, cytomegalovirus, and West Nile virus.[93–95] The neutralization assay, like the HAI assay, incubates patient serum with virus to allow for binding and neutralization of the virus. Methods for detection of neutralizing antibody include determining plaque reduction, cytopathic effect (CPE), ELISA-based detection of viral proteins synthesized, and HAI of cell supernatants, each of which is limited in HTS adaptability. The plaque reduction assays are not amenable to a high-throughput format because they require addition and removal of overlay media, and plaques must be either (a) counted manually or (b) stained and read by plate reader. Cell-based CPE assays have been employed in antiviral screening assays[75] using low multiplicity of infection (MOI) ratios and fluorescence or luminescence as the endpoint detection method, and they could be modified for neutralization by shortened incubations to avoid multiple cycles of replication. ELISA-based HTS methods are possible but require specialized equipment such as automated plate washers. Efforts have been made to design an HTS neutralization assay in 96-well microplates that can evaluate up to 400 sera samples/day and can easily meet the requirement of screening thousands of samples from vaccine study participants. This assay follows the same format outlined above, uses manual serial dilution of sera samples into plate wells, and involves automated addition of virus, cells, fixing agents, antibodies, wash solutions, and developing solutions, coupled with an automated reader. In a single 15-month laboratory study, the assay performed consistently and reliably, and greater than 90% of all assay plates ($n = 2500$) had a control titer within one dilution of the historical median.[92]

Influenza Antiviral HTS Assays

The goal of high-throughput antiviral screening is to identify compounds with antiviral potential from pharmacologically uncharacterized, small molecule or natural product libraries. Biochemical investigations have identified several of the viral components as potential targets for inhibition of viral propagation, and multiple HTS assay formats are available for screening against these targets. These can be categorized as cell-based,[75,96] biochemical,[97] or combinatorial assays.[98,99]

A general algorithm for HTS antiviral screening employs a primary assay for determining single-dose efficacy, followed by a secondary assay for efficacy confirmation and dose–response. Finally, a tertiary assay may be used to better define the antiviral activity and mechanism before classification as a lead antiviral.[100] The choice of influenza primary assay depends wholly on the selected assay target. Typically a cell-based primary assay is used when simultaneously screening against several targets during viral replication. Alternatively, a biochemical primary assay is chosen when a single influenza component is targeted. Figure 2.2 outlines an algorithm for screening for influenza antivirals using either cell-based and biochemical primary assays.

Once the primary assay has screened a compound library and identified a smaller subset of effective lead compounds (i.e., "hits"), these are then run through one or several secondary assays to define the compound dose–response and/or toxicity. The accuracy of the primary assay is paramount for identifying hits while simultaneously reducing the number of compounds funneled through the secondary assays and greatly decreasing the amount of time and resources required to evaluate lead antiviral compounds. Following confirmation, structure–activity relationships are defined and parallel chemical synthesis may be done to generate a group of structurally related compounds, which are then evaluated by re-screening using the secondary and tertiary

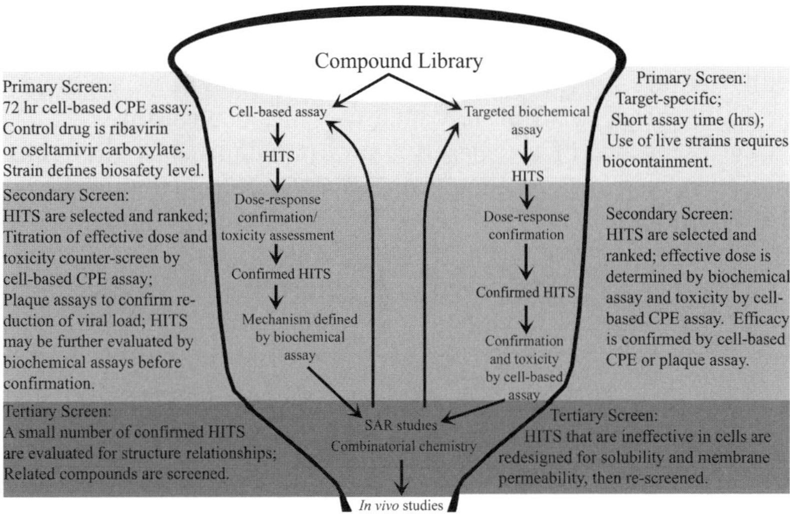

Fig. 2.2. HTS antiviral screening algorithm.

assays. To apply this algorithm, a variety of influenza HTS assays, including both cell-based and biochemical methods, are needed for a complete influenza screening program. This section will discuss cell-based and biochemical influenza assays that have already been adapted to or have the potential for HTS adaptation that can serve as primary, secondary, or tertiary screening assays.

Cell-Based Anti-influenza HTS Assays. Cell-based assays for influenza are commonly used during initial screening efforts to evaluate a diverse compound library against multiple viral targets in a cellular context. One advantage of a cell based assay is that it can identify compounds that are effective against known and unknown targets, as well as identify compounds that are metabolized by the cell into effective antivirals.[101] Compound toxicity can also be established either in the same screen or by secondary counter screens that confirm both dose–response and toxicity. Disadvantages include an inability to recognize effective but toxic compounds, compounds that are excluded from passage through the cellular membrane, or compounds that inhibit through aggregation-based mechanisms.[102] Cell-based screening for influenza has shown that the hit rate is increased by a corresponding increase (10- to 20-fold) in the compound screening concentration,[103] perhaps because the influenza virus replicates in the nucleus and the increased ambient compound screening concentration promotes more efficient penetration of compounds into the nucleus. Alternatively, this may be due to increased compound promoted aggregation and sequestering of viral particles.[102] Finally, in the case of influenza these assays typically require 2–5 days performance time, most of which is incubation time required to accurately measure viral replication.

The growing use of cell-based assays is balanced by the technical challenges in developing robust, large-scale systems—that is, the labor-intensive production of large quantities of cells and the inherent assay variability due to differences in cell passage number and handling.[104] These assays are typically performed in microplates, and the endpoint in most cases is cell death—that is, the CPE induced by viral infection and replication. CPE induced by viral infection is a well-documented and frequently exploited determinant for viral propagation in lytic viruses, but one which requires a reliable method for determining viability.[105] Assays for influenza-induced CPE have previously used the uptake of fluorescent dyes by viable cells as an endpoint.[96,106] This method can determine the efficacy of small numbers of compounds (<400) and is generally conducted in 96-well plate format. Although deemed sufficiently robust for HTS adaptation, this method requires specialized, automated plate washers (for supernatant exchanges and plate well washes), making it unsuitable for screening large numbers (>10,000) of compounds using standard noncontact liquid handlers. As an alternative endpoint detection method, a fully HTS-adapted cell-based primary screening assay that measures the influenza-induced (strain A/Udorn/72) CPE in MDCK cells using luminescence was recently developed and validated.[75] This three-day assay uses 384-well microplates and performs as consistently and reliably as methods using neutral red, with a large signal window (S/B > 30) and low noise level. As a primary screen, it proved effective for blindly identifying control compounds affecting the viral M2 proton channel, NA protein, and polymerase targets while simultaneously evaluating factors such as compound exclusion from the cell and/or toxicity. This HTS assay has also been adapted (at elevated biosafety levels) using HPAI.[107]

A successful cell-based moderate-throughput assay used a *Xenopus laevis* oocyte transient expression system to measure inhibition of the M2 proton channel function.[108] In this assay, cRNA for the influenza M2 protein was microinjected into oocytes followed by a 4- to 6-hr incubation period for protein expression and proton channel insertion into the oocyte lipid bilayer. Compounds were added to the oocyte chamber and were allowed time for potential M2 channel binding, the environmental pH was lowered (to < pH 6.0), and the proton flux was monitored by measuring the electrophysiological potential changes by two-microelectrode voltage clamp technique. Upon activation of the

M2 proton channel, channel blockers (such as amantadine or rimantadine) effectively inhibited channel function. Because this assay is only moderate-throughput (able to screen ~100 compounds/day), it is not amenable for large library screening, but is quite suitable as a secondary confirmation or mechanism evaluation assay. A variation of this assay that could be adapted to screen large libraries has been demonstrated more recently using CV-1 cells that have been infected with a high titer of SV40 virus containing the M2 cDNA sequence.[109] After infection, the cells are plated, allowed time for M2 protein expression, and drugged, and the channel is activated by decreasing the media pH. Constitutive activation of the M2 proton channel causes CPE as the interior of the cell acidifies, which can be accurately measured by methods described above. Compounds that inhibit the M2 channel activity could be identified by a decrease in CPE. This assay format is suitable for miniaturization, as well as for automation of liquid handling and reading, and is fully adaptable to HTS as both a primary or secondary assay.

Biochemical HTS Assays. Biochemical assays for influenza targets have been employed in the past in a low-throughput format as secondary assays to further evaluate compound hits that have shown efficacy in inhibiting viral replication in a primary cell-based assay. For HTS primary antiviral screening, biochemical assays can often be performed in a fraction of the time (hours instead of days) that a cell-based assay can, and they are not bound by compound toxicity issues, making them ideal for targeted primary HTS. For influenza HTS screening, several of the assay formats discussed below are readily adaptable to HTS against targets such as HA2-mediated fusion, NA activity, the polymerase holoenzyme functions, and NS1 RNA binding. The endpoint detection methods use colorimetric, fluorescent, and proximity labels, all of which can be determined by automation.

NA HTS Assays. The influenza NA is bound to the surface of the virus and can be assayed using cell cultured-amplified virus. An effective and sensitive NA assay that directly measures sialidase activity (instead of indirectly by enzyme cascade, as detailed in Ref. 110) has been established for low-throughput use,[111] and it has recently been adapted and validated for HTS in 384-well microplates.[107] Neuraminidase inhibition is measured using 2′-(4-methylumbelliferyl)-a-D-*N*-acetylneuraminic acid, which liberates a quantifiable fluorescent tag (methylumbelliferone) in an enzymatic reaction directly proportional to the amount of sialidase activity. The system uses MDCK cell culture-amplified influenza virus that has been diluted to the appropriate concentration (for linearity of signal) in reaction buffer and added directly to microplates containing the assayed compounds. After a 30-minute incubation to allow for the compounds to potentially bind to the NA on the surface of the virus, the substrate is diluted in reaction buffer and added to the plates, allowed a 30-minute reaction time, and stopped by addition of a high-pH stop buffer. Methylumbelliferone has absorption and fluorescence emission maxima of 365 and 450, respectively, and the signal can be detected with a sensitivity as low as 10^6 H3N2 virus particles/ml within a broad linear range of 10^6–10^8 particles/ml.[107] The assay is robust with S/B > 20 and has been validated in a pilot screen against 10,000 compounds.[107]

Finally, the X-ray crystal structure of the influenza NA protein is known,[112] allowing virtual screening of small-molecule libraries to determine compatibility with the enzyme active site, followed by biochemical screening of candidate inhibitors. This method has recently succeeded in identifying novel NA inhibitors.[113] Virtual screening serves the same purpose as a primary screen by structurally restricting library compounds to a particular pharmacophoric space, although this restriction precludes identification of novel antiviral compounds.

HA HTS Assays. The HA protein is instrumental during the initial stages of infection, and therefore a cell-based primary HTS assay would serve to screen compounds for the target activities that are associated with HA—that is, the surface glycoprotein sialic acid recognition, membrane fusion that is mediated by the HA2 fusion peptide, and activation by protease cleavage of HA0. The lack of HA-associated catalytic activity makes HTS assay development a challenge that depends heavily on the chosen target and method of endpoint. Combinatorial HTS using glycan microarrays has been successfully used to define receptor specificity for both human and avian strains, and it serves as a biochemical method for recognizing inhibitory molecules.[82] The identification of inhibitors of protease cleavage is difficult because the target sequence is variable and is a substrate for a wide variety of proteases that can recognize, cleave, and activate HA0.[114] As of yet, no development has yielded an HTS adaptable HA cleavage assay. Finally, a promising method to determine inhibition of influenza HA-mediated fusion by HTS might be based on a combinatorial assay that has been used to screen for small molecules that inhibit gp41-mediated fusion of the HIV-1 virus with target cells.[99] This work defined a method for selecting short peptides that bind in the hydrophobic surface of the gp41 inner core to guide the binding of an attached small-molecule library that may inhibit viral entry into the cell by blocking gp41-mediated membrane fusion. This method involved attachment of the peptide library to affinity-labeled beads, followed by selection of the members of the peptide library with high affinity for the target site. Once the high-affinity peptides were selected, experiments were done to optimize the formation of a stable gp41-peptide complex and target an attached three position non-peptide small molecule library into the hydrophobic cavity of the gp41 inner core to prevent fusion. The combinatorial approach for influenza may be accomplished by the generation of a biased combinatorial peptide library to identify inhibitors of HA2-mediated viral fusion. This method might be adapted to target small molecules that inhibit membrane fusion of the HA2 peptide, thereby rapidly surveying and identifying effective small molecule combinations from large compound libraries.

Polymerase Holoenzyme HTS Assays. The functions of the individual influenza polymerase subunits (PB1, PB2, PA) and the heterotrimeric holoenzyme have been extensively studied using a series of low-throughput assay systems that have defined the subunits responsible for host mRNA cap-recognition ability, RNA endonuclease activity, and RNA polymerization. These assays have utilized UV-crosslinking to capture RNA-protein binding and electrophoretic detection to examine the reaction products. The largest barriers to adapting these influenza polymerase holoenzyme *in vitro* assay systems for HTS are the availability of purified polymerase and the nature of endpoint detection. Purified polymerase has been efficiently obtained from transiently transfected cells induced to recombinantly express the affinity-tagged polymerase subunits,[115,116] which are then purified as the holoenzyme for assay use. Using purified holoenzyme, low-throughput experiments have shown that polymerase-dependent cap binding and endonuclease activity can be assayed by immobilizing the template RNA, binding the polymerase to the fixed template, and measuring activity upon addition of a short, capped mRNA.[22] In particular, it was found that a 20-nt capped mRNA can be bound to the polymerase complex and cleaved in a magnesium-dependent manner, and quantization of the products is possible. While this assay is extremely useful for measuring a small number of samples, it requires significant adaptation for HTS. This might be accomplished by labeling substrates with fluorescent or affinity proximity labels, which provides a means of rapid endpoint determination. Recently, an HTS fluorescent substrate assay has been used to screen 670,000 compounds against *E. coli* RNA polymerase activity, with a reported hit rate of 0.1%,[117] and might be adapted for influenza polymerase screening. Finally, a promising assay for RNA-dependent RNA polymerization which uses an affinity-labeled primer anchored to a scintillation proximity assay bead has recently been developed for the HCV NS5B polymerase.[118] Initiation of polymerization in the presence of tested compounds and radio-labeled nucleotide substrates allowed determination of the compound effectiveness by measuring the incorporated radio-label in the nascent RNA. This assay has been adapted to a 96-well microplate format, and the addition of automated robotics would allow several thousand com-pounds to be screened by scintillation counting in a single day.

NS1 HTS Assays. The NS1 protein has no defined enzymatic activity but instead regulates the function of host cellular components (CPSF, PABII, PKR, dsRNA) through binding and sequestering of these factors (reviewed in Ref. 20). The protein- and RNA-binding potential of NS1 is an elusive activity to target for inhibition by small molecules, although inhibition by both RNA aptamers and short peptides has been pro-posed.[119] HTS assay designs for inhibition of protein binding have been proposed using proximity-detection systems with fluorescent or affinity labeling of the assayed components (e.g., dsRNA and recombinantly expressed NS1) and measurement of the component association in the presence of potential binding inhibitors. However, these assays have not been developed or validated for HTS at this time. Part of the reason for this is the insoluble nature of the recombinant NS1 protein itself, although truncated versions of the protein containing either the protein-binding potential (C-terminal) or the RNA-binding potential (N-ter-minal) have successfully been affinity-tagged, bacterial-expressed, and purified.[65,119]

SPECIAL CONSIDERATIONS FOR INFLUENZA HTS SCREENING

With the emergence of highly pathogenic avian influenza and the increase in worldwide surveillance of the wild bird and human popula-tions, there is a high probability that a diagnostic HTS screening facility will screen strains with a high lethality and high risk to public security, which requires both administrative and engineering biosafety controls to protect the public, the facility personnel, and the environ-ment. Influenza is not unique in this attribute, but has become extremely high profile as HPAI viruses are identified in avian populations and in isolated human cases. There is also strong demand for HTS vaccine testing and antiviral screening using HPAI H5N1 strains, and the CDC/NIH Biosafety in Microbiological and Biomedical Laboratories requires that this work be performed in at biosafety level 3.[120] HTS screening using HPAI may require additional assay adaptations for performance in a BSL-3 laboratory, and these may include (a) restrictions on the type of equipment used (i.e., equipment that generates aerosol would be a disadvantage when screening respiratory pathogens) and (b) placement of automated robotics and liquid handlers, as well as endpoint readers, inside additional containment facilities, such as a biosafety cabinet. Assay throughput will certainly be reduced at high biosafety in favor of increased safety. The development and adaptation of influenza assays for HTS will continue to force evolution of HTS methodology as the demand for biocontained HTS facilities increases.

CONCLUSION

Influenza is a chronic affliction for the entire world's population, and modern society has enabled the virus to spread and adapt more rapidly than ever before. Adaptation of our diagnostic, vaccine efficacy, and antiviral assays must also occur to meet the demands for heightened surveillance, increased annual vaccine production, and novel antiviral identification. Efforts must be made to continually evaluate new technologies and more fully integrate HTS anticipations into all stages of assay development to (a) speed the rate of influenza diagnosis and vaccine approval and (b) widen the window and options for antiviral therapy. Adaptation of current assays to HTS formats will only partially meet these needs, and future assays must be designed with HTS adaptation in mind to prepare for and combat the statistical certainty of future influenza epidemics and pandemics.

REFERENCES

1. Kiselar, J. G.; Downard, K. M. Antigenic surveillance of the influenza virus by mass spectrometry. *Biochemistry* **1999**, *38*, 14185–14191.
2. Thompson, W. W.; Shay, D. K.; Weintraub, E.; Brammer, L.; Bridges, C. B.; et al. Influenza-associated hospitalizations in the United States. *JAMA* **2004**, *292*, 1333–1340.
3. Thompson, W. W.; Shay, D. K.; Weintraub, E.; Brammer, L.; Cox, N.; et al. Mortality associated with influenza and respiratory syncytial virus in the United States. *JAMA* **2003**, *289*, 179–186.

4. Szucs, T. The socio-economic burden of influenza. *J. Antimicrob. Chemother.* **1999**, *44 Suppl.* B, 11–15.

5. Meltzer, M. I.; Cox, N. J.; Fukuda, K. The economic impact of pandemic influenza in the United States: Priorities for intervention. *Emerg. Infect. Dis.* **1999**, *5*, 659–671.

6. Meltzer, M. I.; Bridges, C. B. Economic analysis of influenza vaccination and treatment. *Ann. Intern. Med.* **2003**, *138*, 608; author reply 608–609.

7. Phipps, L. P.; Essen, S. C.; Brown, I. H. Genetic subtyping of influenza A viruses using RT-PCR with a single set of primers based on conserved sequences within the HA2 coding region. *J. Virol. Methods* **2004**, *122*, 119–122.

8. United States Department of Agriculture. http://www.ars.usda.gov/ Research/docs.htm?docid=11425. **2006**.

9. Vahlenkamp, T. W.; Harder, T. C. Influenza virus infections in mammals. *Berl. Munch. Tierarztl. Wochenschr.* **2006**, *119*, 123–131.

10. Olsen, B.; Munster, V. J.; Wallensten, A.; Waldenstrom, J.; Osterhaus, A. D.; et al. Global patterns of influenza a virus in wild birds. *Science* **2006**, *312*, 384–388.

11. United States Department of Health and Human Services. http://www. pandemicflu.gov/issues/screening.html. **2006**.

12. Layne, S. P. Human influenza surveillance: the demand to expand. *Emerg. Infect. Dis.* **2006**, *12*, 562–568.

13. von Itzstein, M.; Wu, W. Y.; Kok, G. B.; Pegg, M. S.; Dyason, J. C.; Jin, B.; Van Phan, T.; Smythe, M. L.; White, H. F.; Oliver, S. W.; et al. Rational design of potent sialidase-based inhibitors of influenza virus replication. *Nature* **1993**, *363*, 418–423.

14. Hao, W.; Herlihy, K. J.; Zhang, N. J.; Fuhrman, S. A.; Doan, C.; Patick, A. K.; Duggal, R. Development of a novel dicistronic reporter-selectable hepatitis C virus replicon suitable for high-throughput inhibitor screening. *Antimicrob. Agents. Chemother.* **2007**, *51*, 95–102.

15. Kleymann, G.; Werling, H. O. A generally applicable, high-throughput screening-compatible assay to identify, evaluate, and optimize antimicrobial agents for drug therapy. *J. Biomol. Screen.* **2004**, *9*, 578–587.

16. Steinhauer, D. A.; Skehel, J. J. Genetics of influenza viruses. *Annu. Rev. Genet.* **2002**, *36*, 305–332.

17. Hampson, A. W.; Mackenzie, J. S. The influenza viruses. *Med. J. Aust.* **2006**, *185*, S39–S43.

18. Stevens, J.; Blixt, O.; Tumpey, T. M.; Taubenberger, J. K.; Paulson, J. C.; et al. Structure and receptor specificity of the hemagglutinin from an H5N1 influenza virus. *Science* **2006**, *312*, 404–410.

19. Nayak, D. P.; Hui, E. K.; Barman, S. Assembly and budding of influenza virus. *Virus Res.* **2004**, *106*, 147–165.

20. Noah, D. L.; Krug, R. M. Influenza virus virulence and its molecular determinants. *Adv. Virus Res.* **2005**, *65*, 121–145.

21. Bruns, K.; Studtrucker, N.; Sharma, A.; Fossen, T.; Mitzner, D.; et al. Structural characterization and oligomerization of PB1-F2, a pro-apoptotic influenza A virus protein. *J. Biol. Chem.* **2006**.

22. Lee, M. T.; Klumpp, K.; Digard, P.; Tiley, L. Activation of influenza virus RNA polymerase by the 5′ and 3′ terminal duplex of genomic RNA. *Nucleic Acids Res.* **2003**, *31*, 1624–1632.

23. Spector, R.; Vesell, E. S. The heart of drug discovery and development: rational target selection. *Pharmacology* **2006**, *77*, 85–92.

24. Cattoli, G.; Capua, I. Molecular diagnosis of avian influenza during an outbreak. *Dev. Biol. (Basel)* **2006**, *124*, 99–105.

25. Stevens, J.; Blixt, O.; Paulson, J. C.; Wilson, I. A. Glycan microarray technologies: Tools to survey host specificity of influenza viruses. *Nat. Rev. Microbiol.* **2006**, *4*, 857–864.

26. Wiley, D. C.; Skehel, J. J. The structure and function of the hemagglutinin membrane glycoprotein of influenza virus. *Annu. Rev. Biochem.* **1987**, *56*, 365–394.

27. Huang, Q.; Sivaramakrishna, R. P.; Ludwig, K.; Korte, T.; Bottcher, C.; et al. Early steps of the conformational change of influenza virus hemagglutinin to a fusion active state: Stability and energetics of the hemagglutinin. *Biochim. Biophys. Acta* **2003**, *1614*, 3–13.

28. Park, H. E.; Gruenke, J. A.; White, J. M. Leash in the groove mechanism of membrane fusion. *Nat. Struct. Biol.* **2003**, *10*, 1048–1053.

29. Kido, H.; Yokogoshi, Y.; Sakai, K.; Tashiro, M.; Kishino, Y.; et al. Isolation and characterization of a novel trypsin-like protease found in rat bronchiolar epithelial Clara cells. A possible activator of the viral fusion glycoprotein. *J. Biol. Chem.* **1992**, *267*, 13573–13579.

30. Cross, K. J.; Wharton, S. A.; Skehel, J. J.; Wiley, D. C.; Steinhauer, D. A. Studies on influenza haemagglutinin fusion peptide mutants generated by reverse genetics. *EMBO J.* **2001**, *20*, 4432–4442.

31. Nayak, D. P.; Reichl, U. Neuraminidase activity assays for monitoring MDCK cell culture derived influenza virus. *J. Virol. Methods* **2004**, *122*, 9–15.

32. Matrosovich, M. N.; Matrosovich, T. Y.; Gray, T.; Roberts, N. A.; Klenk, H. D. Neuraminidase is important for the initiation of influenza virus infection in human airway epithelium. *J. Virol.* **2004**, *78*, 12665–12667.

33. Fornabaio, M.; Cozzini, P.; Mozzarelli, A.; Abraham, D. J.; Kellogg, G. E. Simple, intuitive calculations of free energy of binding for protein–ligand complexes. 2. Computational titration and pH effects in molecular models of neuraminidase-inhibitor complexes. *J Med. Chem.* **2003**, *46*, 4487–4500.

34. Russell, R. J.; Haire, L. F.; Stevens, D. J.; Collins, P. J.; Lin, Y. P.; et al. The structure of H5N1 avian influenza neuraminidase suggests new opportunities for drug design. *Nature* **2006**, *443*, 45–49.

35. Mungall, B. A.; Xu, X.; Klimov, A. Assaying susceptibility of avian and other influenza A viruses to zanamivir: Comparison of fluorescent and chemiluminescent neuraminidase assays. *Avian Dis.* **2003**, *47*, 1141–1144.

36. Regoes, R. R.; Bonhoeffer, S. Emergence of drug-resistant influenza virus: Population dynamical considerations. *Science* **2006**, *312*, 389–391.

37. Kiso, M.; Mitamura, K.; Sakai-Tagawa, Y.; Shiraishi, K.; Kawakami, C.; et al. Resistant influenza A viruses in children treated with oseltamivir: Descriptive study. *Lancet* **2004**, *364*, 759–765.

38. de Jong, M. D.; Tran, T. T.; Truong, H. K.; Vo, M. H.; Smith, G. J.; et al. Oseltamivir resistance during treatment of influenza A (H5N1) infection. *N. Engl. J. Med.* **2005**, *353*, 2667–2672.

39. Gupta, R. K.; Nguyen-Van-Tam, J. S. Oseltamivir resistance in influenza A (H5N1) infection. *N. Engl. J. Med.* **2006**, *354*, 1423–1424.

40. Pinto, L. H.; Lamb, R. A. Viral ion channels as models for ion transport and targets for antiviral drug action. *FEBS Lett.* **2004**, *560*, 1–2.

41. Bright, R. A.; Shay, D. K.; Shu, B.; Cox, N. J.; Klimov, A. I. Adamantane resistance among influenza A viruses isolated early during the 2005–2006 influenza season in the United States. *JAMA* **2006**, *295*, 891–894.

42. Kandun, I. N.; Wibisono, H.; Sedyaningsih, E. R.; Yusharmen; Hadisoedarsuno, W.; et al. Three Indonesian clusters of H5N1 virus infection in 2005. *N. Engl. J. Med.* **2006**, *355*, 2186–2194.

43. Ozaki, T.; Yauchi, M.; Xin, K. Q.; Hirahara, F.; Okuda, K. Cross-reactive protection against influenza A virus by a topically applied DNA vaccine encoding M gene with adjuvant. *Viral Immunol.* **2005**, *18*, 373–380.

44. Saldanha, S. A.; Kaler, G.; Cottam, H. B.; Abagyan, R.; Taylor, S. S. Assay principle for modulators of protein–protein interactions and its application to non-ATP-competitive ligands targeting protein kinase A. *Anal. Chem.* **2006**, *78*, 8265–8272.

45. Jeon, S. H.; Kayhan, B.; Ben-Yedidia, T.; Arnon, R. A DNA aptamer prevents influenza infection by blocking the receptor binding region of the viral hemagglutinin. *J. Biol. Chem.* **2004**, *279*, 48410–48419.

46. Boulo, S.; Akarsu, H.; Ruigrok, R. W.; Baudin, F. Nuclear traffic of influenza virus proteins and ribonucleoprotein complexes. *Virus Res.* **2007**, *124*, 12–21.

47. Hooker, L.; Sully, R.; Handa, B.; Ono, N.; Koyano, H.; et al. Quantitative analysis of influenza virus RNP interaction with RNA cap structures and comparison to human cap binding protein eIF4E. *Biochemistry* **2003**, *42*, 6234–6240.

48. Fechter, P.; Brownlee, G. G. Recognition of mRNA cap structures by viral and cellular proteins. *J. Gen. Virol.* **2005**, *86*, 1239–1249.

49. De Gregorio, E.; Preiss, T.; Hentze, M. W. Translational activation of uncapped mRNAs by the central part of human eIF4G is 5′ end-dependent. *RNA* **1998**, *4*, 828–836.

50. Hutchinson, K. L.; Peters, C. J.; Nichol, S. T. Sin Nombre virus mRNA synthesis. *Virology* **1996**, *224*, 139–149.

51. Salomon, R.; Franks, J.; Govorkova, E. A.; Ilyushina, N. A.; Yen, H. L.; et al. The polymerase complex genes contribute to the high virulence of the human H5N1 influenza virus isolate A/Vietnam/1203/04. *J. Exp. Med.* **2006**, *203*, 689–697.

52. Tomassini, J.; Selnick, H.; Davies, M. E.; Armstrong, M. E.; Baldwin, J.; et al. Inhibition of cap (m7GpppXm)-dependent endonuclease of influenza virus by 4-substituted 2,4-dioxobutanoic acid compounds. *Antimicrob. Agents Chemother.* **1994**, *38*, 2827–2837.

53. Eriksson, B.; Helgstrand, E.; Johansson, N. G.; Larsson, A.; Misiorny, A.; et al. Inhibition of influenza virus ribonucleic acid polymerase by ribavirin triphosphate. *Antimicrob. Agents Chemother.* **1977**, *11*, 946–951.

54. Furuta, Y.; Takahashi, K.; Kuno-Maekawa, M.; Sangawa, H.; Uehara, S.; et al. Mechanism of action of T-705 against influenza virus. *Antimicrob. Agents Chemother.* **2005**, *49*, 981–986.

55. Portela, A.; Digard, P. The influenza virus nucleoprotein: a multifunctional RNA-binding protein pivotal to virus replication. *J. Gen. Virol.* **2002**, *83*, 723–734.

56. Elton, D.; Medcalf, E.; Bishop, K.; Digard, P. Oligomerization of the influenza virus nucleoprotein: Identification of positive and negative sequence elements. *Virology* **1999**, *260*, 190–200.

57. Elton, D.; Medcalf, L.; Bishop, K.; Harrison, D.; Digard, P. Identification of amino acid residues of influenza virus nucleoprotein essential for RNA binding. *J. Virol.* **1999**, *73*, 7357–7367.

58. Area, E.; Martin-Benito, J.; Gastaminza, P.; Torreira, E.; Valpuesta, J. M.; et al. 3D structure of the influenza virus polymerase complex: Localization of subunit domains. *Proc. Natl. Acad. Sci. USA* **2004**, *101*, 308–313.

59. Rowe, T.; Abernathy, R. A.; Hu-Primmer, J.; Thompson, W. W.; Lu, X.; et al. Detection of antibody to avian influenza A (H5N1) virus in human serum by using a combination of serologic assays. *J. Clin. Microbiol.* **1999**, *37*, 937–943.

60. Shu, L. L.; Bean, W. J.; Webster, R. G. Analysis of the evolution and variation of the human influenza A virus nucleoprotein gene from 1933 to 1990. *J. Virol.* **1993**, *67*, 2723–2729.

61. Tumpey, T. M.; Alvarez, R.; Swayne, D. E.; Suarez, D. L. Diagnostic approach for differentiating infected from vaccinated poultry on the basis

of antibodies to NS1, the nonstructural protein of influenza A virus. *J. Clin. Microbiol.* **2005**, *43*, 676–683.

62. Davey, J.; Colman, A.; Dimmock, N. J. Location of influenza virus M, NP and NS1 proteins in microinjected cells. *J. Gen. Virol.* **1985**, *66(Pt. 11)*, 2319–2334.

63. Noah, D. L.; Twu, K. Y.; Krug, R. M. Cellular antiviral responses against influenza A virus are countered at the posttranscriptional level by the viral NS1A protein via its binding to a cellular protein required for the 3′ end processing of cellular pre-mRNAS. *Virology* **2003**, *307*, 386–395.

64. Min, J. Y.; Krug, R. M. The primary function of RNA binding by the influenza A virus NS1 protein in infected cells: Inhibiting the 2′-5′ oligo (A) synthetase/RNase L pathway. *Proc. Natl. Acad. Sci. USA* **2006**, *103*, 7100–7105.

65. Li, S.; Min, J. Y.; Krug, R. M.; Sen, G. C. Binding of the influenza A virus NS1 protein to PKR mediates the inhibition of its activation by either PACT or double-stranded RNA. *Virology* **2006**, *349*, 13–21.

66. Li, Z.; Jiang, Y.; Jiao, P.; Wang, A.; Zhao, F.; et al. The NS1 gene contributes to the virulence of H5N1 avian influenza viruses. *J. Virol.* **2006**, *80*, 11115–11123.

67. Qian, X. Y.; Chien, C. Y.; Lu, Y.; Montelione, G. T.; Krug, R. M. An amino-terminal polypeptide fragment of the influenza virus NS1 protein possesses specific RNA-binding activity and largely helical backbone structure. *RNA* **1995**, *1*, 948–956.

68. Neumann, G.; Watanabe, T.; Ito, H.; Watanabe, S.; Goto, H.; et al. Generation of influenza A viruses entirely from cloned cDNAs. *Proc. Natl. Acad. Sci. USA* **1999**, *96*, 9345–9350.

69. Donelan, N. R.; Basler, C. F.; Garcia-Sastre, A. A recombinant influenza A virus expressing an RNA-binding-defective NS1 protein induces high levels of beta interferon and is attenuated in mice. *J. Virol.* **2003**, *77*, 13257–13266.

70. Krug, R. M.; Yuan, W.; Noah, D. L.; Latham, A. G. Intracellular warfare between human influenza viruses and human cells: The roles of the viral NS1 protein. *Virology* **2003**, *309*, 181–189.

71. O'Neill, R. E.; Talon, J.; Palese, P. The influenza virus NEP (NS2 protein) mediates the nuclear export of viral ribonucleoproteins. *EMBO J.* **1998**, *17*, 288–296.

72. Henklein, P.; Bruns, K.; Nimtz, M.; Wray, V.; Tessmer, U.; et al. Influenza A virus protein PB1-F2: Synthesis and characterization of the biologically active full length protein and related peptides. *J. Pept. Sci.* **2005**, *11*, 481–490.

73. Chen, W.; Calvo, P. A.; Malide, D.; Gibbs, J.; Schubert, U.; et al. A novel influenza A virus mitochondrial protein that induces cell death. *Nat. Med.* **2001**, *7*, 1306–1312.

74. Yamada, H.; Chounan, R.; Higashi, Y.; Kurihara, N.; Kido, H. Mitochondrial targeting sequence of the influenza A virus PB1-F2 protein and its function in mitochondria. *FEBS Lett.* **2004**, *578*, 331–336.

75. Noah, J. W., Severson, W., Noah, D. L., Rasmussen, L., White, E. L., Jonsson, C. B. A cell-based luminescence assay is effective for high-throughput screening of potential influenza antivirals. *Antiviral Res.* **2006**, doi:10.1016/j.antiviral.2006.07.006.

76. Zhang, J. H.; Chung, T. D.; Oldenburg, K. R. A Simple Statistical Parameter for Use in Evaluation and Validation of High Throughput Screening Assays. *J. Biomol. Screen.* **1999**, *4*, 67–73.

77. Zhang, A.; Jin, M.; Liu, F.; Guo, X.; Hu, Q.; et al. Development and evaluation of a DAS-ELISA for rapid detection of avian influenza viruses. *Avian Dis.* **2006**, *50*, 325–330.

78. Starick, E.; Werner, O.; Schirrmeier, H.; Kollner, B.; Riebe, R.; et al. Establishment of a competitive ELISA (cELISA) system for the detection of influenza A virus nucleoprotein antibodies and its application to field sera from different species. *J. Vet. Med. B. Infect. Dis. Vet. Public Health* **2006**, *53*, 370–375.

79. Bai, G. R.; Sakoda, Y.; Mweene, A. S.; Fujii, N.; Minakawa, H.; et al. Improvement of a rapid diagnosis kit to detect either influenza A or B virus infections. *J. Vet. Med. Sci.* **2006**, *68*, 35–40.

80. Woolcock, P. R.; Cardona, C. J. Commercial immunoassay kits for the detection of influenza virus type A: evaluation of their use with poultry. *Avian Dis.* **2005**, *49*, 477–481.

81. Crossley, B. M.; Hietala, S. K.; Shih, L. M.; Lee, L.; Skowronski, E. W.; et al. High-throughput real-time RT-PCR assay to detect the exotic Newcastle Disease Virus during the California 2002–2003 outbreak. *J. Vet. Diagn. Invest.* **2005**, *17*, 124–132.

82. Stevens, J.; Blixt, O.; Glaser, L.; Taubenberger, J. K.; Palese, P.; et al. Glycan microarray analysis of the hemagglutinins from modern and pandemic influenza viruses reveals different receptor specificities. *J. Mol. Biol.* **2006**, *355*, 1143–1155.

83. Dawson, E. D.; Moore, C. L.; Smagala, J. A.; Dankbar, D. M.; Mehlmann, M.; et al. MChip: A Tool for Influenza Surveillance. *Anal. Chem.* **2006**, *78*, 7610–7615.

84. Townsend, M. B.; Dawson, E. D.; Mehlmann, M.; Smagala, J. A.; Dankbar, D. M.; et al. Experimental evaluation of the FluChip diagnostic microarray for influenza virus surveillance. *J. Clin. Microbiol.* **2006**, *44*, 2863–2871.

85. World Health Organization. WHO activities in avian influenza and pandemic influenza preparedness. In *Epidemic and Pandemic Alert and Response*, January–May 2006.

86. Qiao, C.; Tian, G.; Jiang, Y.; Li, Y.; Shi, J.; et al. Vaccines developed for h5 highly pathogenic avian influenza in china. *Ann. N. Y. Acad. Sci.* **2006**, *1081*, 182–192.

87. Treanor, J. J.; Campbell, J. D.; Zangwill, K. M.; Rowe, T.; Wolff, M. Safety and immunogenicity of an inactivated subvirion influenza A (H5N1) vaccine. *N. Engl. J. Med.* **2006**, *354*, 1343–1351.

88. World Health Organization. (http://www.who.int/csr/disease/avian_influenza/country/cases_table_2006_11_29/en/index.html). **2006**.

89. Bateman, J. B.; Davis, M. S.; McCaffrey, P. A. Rate of reaction of red blood cells with influenza virus hemagglutinin. *Am. J. Hyg.* **1955**, *62*, 342–348.

90. Auewarakul, P.; Kositanont, U.; Sornsathapornkul, P.; Tothong, P.; Kanyok, R.; et al. Antibody responses after dose-sparing intradermal influenza vaccination. *Vaccine* **2006**.

91. Stephenson, I.; Wood, J. M.; Nicholson, K. G.; Charlett, A.; Zambon, M. C. Detection of anti-H5 responses in human sera by HI using horse erythrocytes following MF59-adjuvanted influenza A/Duck/Singapore/97 vaccine. *Virus Res.* **2004**, *103*, 91–95.

92. Noah, D. L. Unpublished data.

93. Reynolds, M. G.; Anh, B. H.; Thu, V. H.; Montgomery, J. M.; Bausch, D. G.; et al. Factors associated with nosocomial SARS-CoV transmission among healthcare workers in Hanoi, Vietnam, 2003. *BMC Public Health* **2006**, *6*, 207.

94. Choi, K. S.; Ko, Y. J.; Nah, J. J.; Kim, Y. J.; Kang, S. Y.; Yoon, K. J.; Joo, Y. S. Monoclonal antibody-based competitive enzyme-linked immunosorbent assay for detecting and quantifying West Nile virus-neutralizing antibodies in horse sera. *Clin. Vaccine Immunol.* **2007**, *14*, 134–138.

95. Gupta, C. K.; Leszczynski, J.; Gupta, R. K.; Siber, G. R. An enzyme immunoassay based micro-neutralization test for titration of antibodies to human cytomegalovirus (CMV) and its correlation with direct ELISA measuring CMV IgG antibodies. *Biologicals* **1996**, *24*, 41–49.

96. Sidwell, R. W.; Smee, D. F. *In vitro* and *in vivo* assay systems for study of influenza virus inhibitors. *Antiviral Res.* **2000**, *48*, 1–16.

97. Gubareva, L. V.; Webster, R. G.; Hayden, F. G. Comparison of the activities of zanamivir, oseltamivir, and RWJ-270201 against clinical isolates of influenza virus and neuraminidase inhibitor-resistant variants. *Antimicrob. Agents Chemother.* **2001**, *45*, 3403–3408.

98. Zhou, G.; Ferrer, M.; Chopra, R.; Kapoor, T. M.; Strassmaier, T.; et al. The structure of an HIV-1 specific cell entry inhibitor in complex with the HIV-1 gp41 trimeric core. *Bioorg. Med. Chem.* **2000**, *8*, 2219–2227.

99. Ferrer, M.; Kapoor, T. M.; Strassmaier, T.; Weissenhorn, W.; Skehel, J. J.; et al. Selection of gp41-mediated HIV-1 cell entry inhibitors from

biased combinatorial libraries of non-natural binding elements. *Nat. Struct. Biol.* **1999**, *6*, 953–960.

100. Fox, S.; Farr-Jones, S.; Sopchak, L.; Boggs, A.; Nicely, H. W.; et al. High-throughput screening: update on practices and success. *J. Biomol. Screen.* **2006**, *11*, 864–869.

101. Westby, M.; Nakayama, G. R.; Butler, S. L.; Blair, W. S. Cell-based and biochemical screening approaches for the discovery of novel HIV-1 inhibitors. *Antiviral Res.* **2005**, *67*, 121–140.

102. Shoichet, B. K. Screening in a spirit haunted world. *Drug Discov. Today* **2006**, *11*, 607–615.

103. Severson, W. E., and Jonsson, C. B. Unpublished data.

104. Digan, M. E.; Pou, C.; Niu, H.; Zhang, J. H. Evaluation of division-arrested cells for cell-based high-throughput screening and profiling. *J. Biomol. Screen.* **2005**, *10*, 615–623.

105. McCoy, M. H.; Wang, E. Use of electric cell-substrate impedance sensing as a tool for quantifying cytopathic effect in influenza A virus infected MDCK cells in real-time. *J. Virol. Methods* **2005**, *130*, 157–161.

106. Smee, D. F.; Morrison, A. C.; Barnard, D. L.; Sidwell, R. W. Comparison of colorimetric, fluorometric, and visual methods for determining anti-influenza (H1N1 and H3N2) virus activities and toxicities of compounds. *J. Virol. Methods* **2002**, *106*, 71–79.

107. Noah, J. W. Unpublished data.

108. Giffin, K.; Rader, R. K.; Marino, M. H.; Forgey, R. W. Novel assay for the influenza virus M2 channel activity. *FEBS Lett.* **1995**, *357*, 269–274.

109. Mould, J. A.; Drury, J. E.; Frings, S. M.; Kaupp, U. B.; Pekosz, A.; et al. Permeation and activation of the M2 ion channel of influenza A virus. *J. Biol. Chem.* **2000**, *275*, 31038–31050.

110. Invitrogen. Amplex Red neuraminidase (Sialidase) Assay. *Molecular Probes* **2004**, *A22178*, 1–3.

111. Blick, T. J.; Tiong, T.; Sahasrabudhe, A.; Varghese, J. N.; Colman, P. M.; et al. Generation and characterization of an influenza virus neuraminidase variant with decreased sensitivity to the neuraminidase-specific inhibitor 4-guanidino-Neu5Ac2en. *Virology* **1995**, *214*, 475–484.

112. Varghese, J. N.; Colman, P. M. Three-dimensional structure of the neuraminidase of influenza virus A/Tokyo/3/67 at 2.2 Å resolution. *J. Mol. Biol.* **1991**, *221*, 473–486.

113. Liu, A.; Cao, H.; Du, G. Drug screening for influenza neuraminidase inhibitors. *Sci. China C. Life Sci.* **2005**, *48*, 1–5.

114. Szecsi, J.; Drury, R.; Josserand, V.; Grange, M. P.; Boson, B.; et al. Targeted retroviral vectors displaying a cleavage site-engineered hemagglutinin (HA) through HA-protease interactions. *Mol. Ther.* **2006**, *14*, 735–744.

115. Deng, T.; Sharps, J.; Fodor, E.; Brownlee, G. G. *In vitro* assembly of PB2 with a PB1-PA dimer supports a new model of assembly of influenza A virus polymerase subunits into a functional trimeric complex. *J. Virol.* **2005**, *79*, 8669–8674.

116. Brownlee, G. G.; Sharps, J. L. The RNA polymerase of influenza a virus is stabilized by interaction with its viral RNA promoter. *J. Virol.* **2002**, *76*, 7103–7113.

117. Bhat, J.; Rane, R.; Solapure, S. M.; Sarkar, D.; Sharma, U.; Harish, M. N.; Lamb, S.; Plant, D.; Alcock, P.; Peters, S.; Barde, S.; Roy, R. K. High-throughput screening of RNA polymerase inhibitors using a fluorescent UTP analog. *J. Biomol. Screen.* **2006**, *11*, 968–976.

118. Wang, Y. K.; Rigat, K. L.; Roberts, S. B.; Gao, M. A homogeneous, solid-phase assay for hepatitis C virus RNA-dependent RNA polymerase. *Anal. Biochem.* **2006**, *359*, 106–111.

119. Chien, C. Y.; Xu, Y.; Xiao, R.; Aramini, J. M.; Sahasrabudhe, P. V.; et al. Biophysical characterization of the complex between double-stranded RNA and the N-terminal domain of the NS1 protein from influenza A virus: Evidence for a novel RNA-binding mode. *Biochemistry* **2004**, *43*, 1950–1962.

120. Prevention, C. f. D. C. a. http://www.cdc.gov/flu/h2n2backgroundqa.htm. **2006**.

121. Ghosh, R. N.; DeBiasio, R.; Hudson, C. C.; Ramer, E. R.; Cowan, C. L.; et al. Quantitative cell-based high-content screening for vasopressin receptor agonists using transfluor technology. *J. Biomol. Screen.* **2005**, *10*, 476–484.

3

MECHANISMS OF IFN RESISTANCE BY INFLUENZA VIRUS

HEATHER J. EZELLE

Marlene and Stewart Greenebaum Cancer Center, University of Maryland, Baltimore School of Medicine, Baltimore, MD 21201

BRET A. HASSEL

Marlene and Stewart Greenebaum Cancer Center and Department of Microbiology and Immunology, University of Maryland, Baltimore School of Medicine, Baltimore, MD 21201

INTRODUCTION

Since the beginning of the twentieth century, influenza has caused three pandemics and multiple epidemics. The 1918 Spanish flu, a product of genetic mutation of avian influenza, killed over 40 million people worldwide.[1] Conversely, the 1957 Asian flu and the 1968 Hong Kong flu viruses were the result of genetic reassortment between human and avian strains.[2,3] In this light, the potential adaptation to permit human-to-human transmission of the current H5N1 avian influenza, either by reassortment or mutation, poses a serious health threat worldwide.

Influenza is a segmented, negative-stranded RNA virus and is a member of the *Orthomyxoviridae* family. It can be divided into three types, A, B, and C, of which A is the primary pathogen for humans. The influenza A genome contains eight RNA segments that encode 10 proteins: the matrix (M1), envelope glycoproteins neuraminidase (NA)

Combating the Threat of Pandemic Influenza: Drug Discovery Approaches,
Edited by Paul F. Torrence

and hemagglutinin (HA), nucleoprotein (NP), a polymerase complex composed of PB1, PB2, and PA, an ion channel protein (M2), and nonstructural proteins (NS1 and NS2).[4] Variances in the envelope proteins HA and NA are used to further subclassify flu into classes H1 to H16 and N1 to N9 (e.g., H3N2 for the 1968 Hong Kong flu). Influenza predominantly infects epithelial cells in the upper respiratory tract, as well as macrophages and other leukocytes; however, because its receptor, sialic acid, is so prevalent, many other cell types can also be infected in culture.[5]

Unlike most other RNA viruses that replicate in the cytoplasm, influenza replicates in the cell nucleus. Upon binding to the cell surface receptor, the virus enters by endocytosis. Once in the endosome, low pH mediates the fusion of the viral and endosome membranes so that the viral nucleocapsids are released into the cytoplasm and then imported into the cell nucleus. Here, the viral polymerase initiates primary mRNA transcription in order to synthesize new polymerase, NP, NS1, and NS2 proteins. After translation in the cytoplasm, the viral proteins are then transported back to the nucleus to initiate replication of the genome and secondary mRNA transcription. Subsequently, viral ribonucleoprotein complexes are assembled in the nucleus and then transported to the plasma membrane where budding of mature virions occurs.[4]

In order to facilitate this productive replication, influenza has devised several mechanisms for inhibiting normal cellular processes, as well as the innate antiviral response to infection. For instance, the viral polymerase complex engages in "cap snatching" of the 5′ caps of host mRNA, leading to their degradation.[6,7] The NS1 protein can also inhibit mRNA splicing of cellular mRNAs as well as prevent their export from the nucleus.[8] In addition, influenza is known to inhibit translation of cellular protein yet selectively translate viral proteins, and ultimately, after hijacking the cell's machinery to replicate, it leads to cell death by cytolysis or apoptosis.[9,10] During the course of infection, numerous chemokines and proinflammatory cytokines are produced not only to recruit and modulate the adaptive immune response, but also to control the immediate infection. One of the key players in this innate immune response is type I interferon (IFNα/β).

TYPE I INTERFERON

One of the key components of innate immunity, particularly against viral infection, are the interferons (IFNs), a family of pleiotropic cytokines that are divided into two major subtypes referred to as type I

(IFNα/β) and type II (IFNγ). Type I interferon is immediately induced upon viral infection and subsequently leads to the induction of hundreds of genes that collectively create an antiviral state in the cell. This inhibitory state can potentially control the infection until a virus-specific adaptive immune response can be generated. IFNα may also serve as a link between innate and adaptive immunity by modulating dendritic cell (DC) maturation, activating T cells, and stimulating the antibody response.[11]

Recent findings have provided greater insight into how influenza and other viruses stimulate IFN production. dsRNA, in the form of dsRNA genomes, replication intermediates, or transcripts with significant secondary structure, has been known to trigger a signaling cascade leading to the activation of the transcription factors interferon regulatory factor 3 (IRF-3), nuclear factor kappa-B (NF-κB), and adaptor-related protein complex-1 (AP-1). These components transcriptionally upregulate IFNβ, leading to its subsequent secretion and autocrine and paracrine signaling cascades.[12] Until recently, it was unknown how viral dsRNA was detected and what signaling events lead to IRF-3 activation. The intracellular viral RNA (vRNA) sensors have now been identified as two putative RNA helicases, retinoic acid inducible gene-I (RIG-I) and melanoma differentiation-associated gene-5 (MDA-5).[13,14] MDA-5 has been shown to recognize dsRNA from viruses such as EMCV, while RIG-I was recently found to be activated by viral RNA possessing 5'-triphosphates generated by the viral polymerases from influenza, VSV, Sendai virus, and Newcastle disease virus.[15–17] Upon binding vRNA, RIG-I and MDA-5 recruit VISA/IPS-1/MAVS/Cardif and activate the IRF-3 kinases, TANK binding kinase-1 (TBK-1) and inhibitor of NF-κB kinase ε (IKKε).[18–23] This leads to the phosphorylation and dimerization of IRF-3 and ultimately to the induction of IFNβ (Fig. 3.1).[24] Influenza has also been shown to be recognized by Toll-like receptor (TLR)-7, and possibly the dsRNA receptor TLR-3, which can lead to IFN induction.[25–27] Presumably, flu's ssRNA genome is detected by cell-surface-bound TLR-7 during endocytosis.

After infection, IFNβ is secreted and binds, in either an autocrine or paracrine fashion, to its cognate receptor, the IFN-α/β receptor (IFNAR). IFNAR signaling can then amplify the production of IFNα, which, like IFNβ, is then secreted and binds to the same IFNAR. Upon binding, the receptor subunits dimerize and signaling proceeds through a well-characterized Jak1/Tyk2 and STAT1/STAT2 signaling cascade. The STAT1/2 heterodimer then complexes with IFN-stimulated gene factor 3 gamma (ISGF-3γ/IRF9), forming the ISGF-3 complex.[12,28,29] This complex then translocates into the nucleus, where it binds IFN

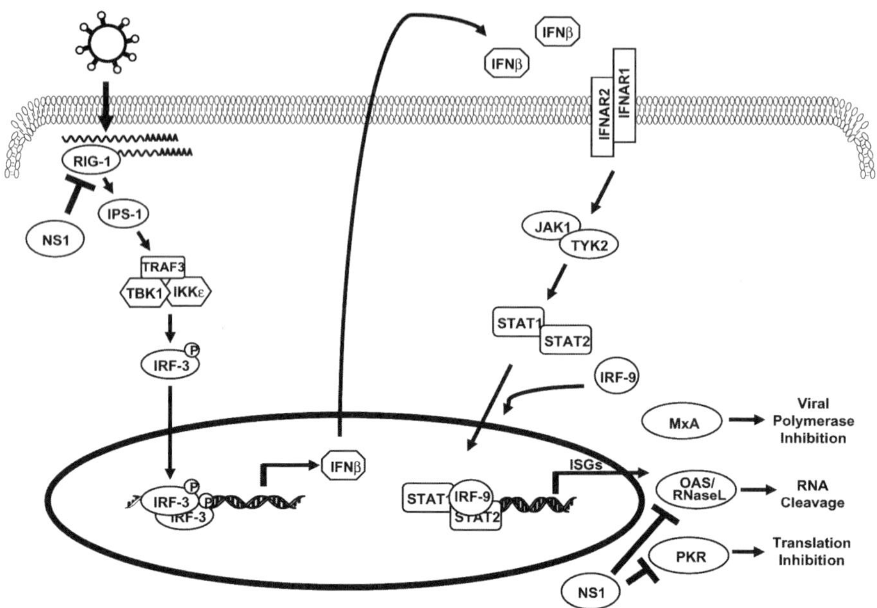

Fig. 3.1. Diagram of type I interferon signaling and targets of inhibition by the influenza NS1 protein.

stimulated response elements (ISREs) found in the promoters of hundreds of IFN stimulated genes (ISGs; Fig. 3.1). Through this pathway, IFN can induce the many genes necessary for producing IFN's antiviral effects. Many of these IFN stimulated genes are cellular components such as MHC class I, LMP-2, and the TAPs, which are required for the processing and presentation of viral antigens to the immune system. In addition, components of the signaling cascade itself, such as STAT-1, are also highly inducible, as are many antiviral effector proteins such as 2′,5′-oligoadenylate sythetase (OAS), Mx proteins, and the dsRNA-activated serine/threonine kinase, PKR.[30]

THE MX FAMILY

The Mx family members are type I IFN-induced GTPases that are part of the superfamily of dynamin-like GTPases. There are two Mx proteins in both mouse and human, and while three of the four display antiviral activity, their mechanisms appear to differ based on subcellular localization and virus specificity. Knockout and transgenic mouse studies demonstrate that both Mx1 and MxA can mediate sufficient antiviral activity to inhibit virus replication, even in the absence of other IFN-mediated effects.[31,32] Mouse Mx1 selectively inhibits members of the *Orthomyxoviridae* family, which includes influenza virus.[32,33] It is localized in the nucleus and blocks influenza's primary transcription by the viral-associated polymerase.[34–36] Mouse Mx2, unlike Mx1, is found in the cytoplasm and can mediate resistance to VSV but not influenza.[37,38] The human Mx proteins have differential antiviral activity. MxA has broad resistance to influenza, VSV, measles virus, Thogoto virus, and Semliki forest virus.[39–41] Likely due to its cytoplasmic localization, rather than through direct inhibition of transcription like Mx1, MxA inhibits replication by binding to the viral nucleocapsid and preventing its entry into the nucleus where viral transcription occurs.[36,42] MxB is the only family member with no known antiviral activity. It resides in the perinuclear region and is believed to inhibit nuclear import and cell-cycle progression.[43] While it is currently unknown whether flu encodes any inhibitors of the Mx proteins, it is well documented that its NS1 protein can inhibit several ISGs and appears to be a key mediator of IFN resistance.

PKR INHIBITION BY NS1

PKR is a well-characterized, key component of the host antiviral response. It exists at low levels in most cell types and is potently induced by IFN. PKR's N-terminus contains two canonical dsRNA binding domains (dsRBD) which, following infection, bind to viral dsRNA, leading to activation of the kinase.[44–46] PKR then autophosphorylates and forms a homodimer that is capable of phosphorylating target substrates, the most well-characterized being the alpha subunit of eukaryotic initiation factor 2 (eIF2α).[47,48] Phosphorylation of eIF2α on Ser-51 causes an inhibition of protein synthesis in the cell by preventing the exchange of eIF2-bound GDP for GTP by eIF2B. This exchange is required for eIF2 to bind methionyl-tRNA to the 40S ribosomal subunit during translation initiation.[49,50] Studies have shown that this translational repression not only leads to a global inhibition of protein synthesis in the cell, but also inhibits viral protein production, thereby inhibiting replication.[51] Other potential PKR targets include the alternatively spliced nuclear proteins NFAR-1 and NFAR-2, histone 2a, and IKKβ.[52,53] These substrates, as well as others, likely facilitate PKR's many roles in the cell including the regulation of translation, the induction of virus associated cell death, and the regulation of growth factor signaling pathways and in the activation of NF-κB through modulation of IκB kinase, IKKβ.[52,54–56]

Due to PKR's antiviral activity, numerous viruses have developed different methods for inhibiting its activity. It has been demonstrated that influenza A's NS1 protein is a potent inhibitor of PKR activity both *in vitro* and *in vivo*. NS1 is a 26.8-kDa protein that contains a dsRBD in its N-terminus, two nuclear localization signals, and one nuclear export signal to allow for shuttling.[57–59] It is expressed early and to very high levels in the nucleus of infected cells and is the most abundant of the nonstructural proteins.[60] Crystallographic structures and mutation analysis indicate that it functions as a homodimer and that dimerization is required for RNA binding.[61] Despite its abundant expression, however, NS1 is not believed to be incorporated into the virion structure. Aside from inhibiting the IFN response, it also has other roles in influenza's pathogenicity. First, NS1 can inhibit the export of cellular poly(A)-containing mRNAs from the nucleus by directly binding the 3′ poly(A) sequence.[8,62,63] Second, it can inhibit pre-mRNA splicing of host mRNAs. NS1 mediates this by binding a purine-containing bulge in a stem structure of the splicesomal U6 small nuclear RNA.[8,64,65] Third, NS1 can enhance viral protein translation by binding and recruiting cellular translation initiation factors, such as eIF-4GI and poly(A) binding protein, to the 5′UTRs of viral mRNAs.[66,67] While NS1's inhibition of cellular protein expression is not a direct IFN inhibitory mechanism, the IFN response requires *de novo* protein expression of ISGs following IFNAR ligation. Therefore, inhibition of total cellular gene expression would also inhibit ISG induction. The overall relevance of these cellular functions is somewhat tempered, however, by studies involving influenza virus lacking NS1 (delNS1). When this virus is grown in cells with a deficient IFN system, viral replication is comparable to wild-type virus, indicating that either (a) NS1's major function is inhibition of the IFN response or (b) compensatory mechanisms exist that mask the other functions of NS1 in this setting.[68,69]

NS1's inhibition of PKR has been continuously well-documented *in vitro* and *in vivo* for over a decade. Though NS1's ability to bind dsRNA was originally documented in 1992, Lu et al. were the first to demonstrate *in vitro* that NS1 could inhibit the dsRNA mediated activation of PKR.[70,71] This was shown at the level of both autophosphorylation and phosphorylation of the PKR substrate eIF2α.[70,72,73] Subsequent experiments utilizing delNS1 or a ts NS1 influenza mutant confirmed these findings by demonstrating that PKR could be activated by infection with these NS1 defective viruses, but not wild-type virus, and this phenotype could be complemented by *trans* expression of intact NS1.[68,74] Studies have also been conducted in mice deficient in either STAT1 or PKR using either wild-type or delNS1 influenza viruses.[68,69,75] In these studies, delNS1 replication in the lungs of infected mice was inhibited in wild-type mice, but not the knockouts, signifying NS1's importance for inhibiting the IFN response and PKR in particular. In fact, replication of delNS1 was similar to wild-type influenza in PKR –/– mice, indicating that NS1's primary function was the inhibition of PKR rather than regulating mRNA processing or translation. In addition, wild-type flu replicated only marginally better in the STAT1 –/– mice, which are defective in all ISG induction, than in the PKR –/– mice.[68] This would suggest that the most significant ISG inhibited in the STAT1 –/– mice is PKR. While these results indicate that other ISGs are involved in inhibiting influenza infections, it should also be mentioned that the STAT1 –/– mice were on a C57BL/6 background, which does not express functional Mx protein. This may suggest that conducting similar experiments in other strains of mice may provide more insight into other potential mediators of host defense. Due to PKR's multiple roles in the IFN response, its inhibition may affect not only eIF2α-mediated translation regulation, but also IFN induction by IRF1, IFNγ signaling through STAT1, and dsRNA-induced cell death.[54,55,76] Further studies would be beneficial to more finely determine which PKR activities are required for inhibiting flu.

The mechanism of NS1's inhibition was originally thought to be dependent on its ability to bind dsRNA. It was hypothesized that NS1 would bind dsRNA and retain it in the nucleus. Although some PKR protein is nuclear, it is predominantly detected in the cytoplasm, and therefore nuclear sequestration of dsRNA could effectively prevent it from activating PKR.[70] In fact, a number of viral inhibitors, such as vaccinia virus E3L, utilize this tactic for preventing PKR activation.[77] Recent evidence, however, has indicated an alternative mechanism of inhibition involving NS1's ability to bind directly to PKR.[72,73] Li et al. have shown that NS1 can inhibit not only dsRNA-induced PKR activation, but also activation by PACT.[72] PACT is a cellular protein that encodes two functional dsRBDs and a third domain that binds directly to PKR in order to activate it, irrespective of the presence or absence of dsRNA.[78,79] When a point mutation was introduced to abrogate NS1's dsRNA binding activity (R38A), NS1 was still able to bind to and inhibit PKR activation by both dsRNA and PACT. It is hypothesized that the binding of NS1 to PKR prevents the conformational change induced by dsRNA binding, which is required for activation. This may be a more plausible mechanism for NS1 since it has also been demonstrated that the NS1 dsRBD has a lower affinity for dsRNA than for PKR's dsRBDs, and therefore may not be capable of outcompeting it.[74,80,81]

Although most research into NS1 inhibition of PKR has been conducted with influenza A NS1 protein, some studies have been performed utilizing influenza B and C viruses. There is little homology between the NS1 proteins of these viruses, but NS1 from influenza B is capable of binding dsRNA and inhibiting PKR.[82,83] It has also been reported to inhibit IRF-3 and subsequent IFNβ transcriptional activation.[84]

ACTIVATION OF THE CELLULAR PKR INHIBITOR, P58[IPK]

P58[IPK] is a cellular inhibitor of PKR that is activated upon influenza infection to suppress PKR's catalytic activity. It contains nine tandemly arranged tetratricopeptide repeats (TPR) as well as a J-domain that shares homology with the DnaJ heat shock family of proteins. There is also limited, localized homology to the PKR substrate eIF2α which may facilitate binding to PKR.[85] Its association with PKR is dependent on TPR6, and direct protein–protein interaction is required for inhibition of PKR dimerization, a required step for activation.[86] P58[IPK] was first discovered in experiments in which influenza infections were conducted in series after mutant adenovirus infections. The adenoviruses were deficient in the PKR inhibitor VAI RNA; therefore, PKR was activated by the viral infection and competent to inhibit translation. In the cultures infected with both mutated adenovirus and influenza however, PKR was inhibited, indicating the induction or activation of a PKR inhibitor by influenza.[87] This novel protein was later purified and identified as the host encoded inhibitor P58[IPK].[88]

P58[IPK] is normally inactive in the cell and is reportedly inhibited by two separate proteins, Hsp40 and P52[rIPK] (repressor of inhibitor of protein kinase). P52[rIPK] has been shown to block P58[IPK]'s suppression of PKR, thereby permitting eIF2α phosphorylation and growth suppression in yeast.[89] The exact mechanism for this regulation has yet to be elucidated; however, the interaction domain has been mapped. Hsp40 inhibition of PKR may involve a third component, Hsp70. Prior to infection, Hsp40, Hsp70, and P58[IPK] reside in a complex that is dissociated following influenza infection. Once Hsp40 is removed from the complex, this allows Hsp70 and P58[IPK] to associate with PKR and inhibit activation.[90,91]

Recently, P58[IPK]-deficient mice have been generated, and their response to influenza and other virus infections are currently being analyzed. Preliminary results have been noted in a review by Kash et al., indicating that knockout mice infected with influenza virus show decreased levels of viral protein synthesis and increased eIF2α phosphorylation, as would be expected by uninhibited PKR.[85] Their data are supported by findings in P58[IPK]-null plants in which infections with Tomato mosaic virus and Tobacco etch virus demonstrate increased cell death and reduced viral titers.[92] The P58[IPK] knockout mouse does have a significant phenotype that has been characterized relating to its roles in stress response. In addition to being an inhibitor of PKR, P58[IPK] is also capable of inhibiting another eIF2α kinase, PERK. PERK is activated by the build-up of misfolded proteins in the endoplasmic reticulum, which is known to induce the unfolded protein response (UPR). One of the general reactions to the UPR is activation of PERK, which phosphorylates eIF2α and induces a global inhibition of protein synthesis, reducing the burden on the ER.[93] A second role for P58[IPK] in the UPR has also been recently elucidated. These studies show that P58[IPK] binds to the ER protein translocation channel, Sec61, and mediates ER protein degradation during the stress response.[94] The absence of P58[IPK] produces a diabetic phenotype in mice, including hyperglycemia and increased apoptosis of pancreatic β-cells, not unlike the PERK−/− phenotype.[95–97]

ISGYLATION INHIBITION BY NS1B

Most of this chapter involves data obtained using the influenza A virus and its NS1 protein (NS1A). Though some of NS1A's functions are shared with its counterpart NS1B, the two proteins are not identical. Unique to influenza B virus is its ability to induce ISG15 expression during infection and to inhibit its conjugation to other proteins.[98]

ISG15 is one of the most highly induced ISGs. Like ubiquitin and other ubiquitin-like proteins such as SUMO-1, Nedd-8, and Rub1, ISG15 is covalently linked by its C-terminal glycine residue to target proteins upon IFN induction.[99] This ISGylation process has three steps that utilize activating (Ube1L), conjugating (UbcH8), and ligating (Efp and Herc5) enzymes to conjugate ISG15 to its substrates.[98,100–103] Though no broad function such as protein degradation or localization have been ascribed to ISGylation, it has been demonstrated to disrupt protein function and prevent thioester bond formation between ubiquitin and its E2 conjugating enzymes, UbcH6 and Ubc13.[104–106] ISG15−/− mice have been generated and show no overt phenotype in development, lymphocyte populations, or resistance to VSV or LCMV infection.[107] However, detailed experiments involving Sindbis virus and HIV have demonstrated a clear role for ISG15 in antiviral immunity.[108,109]

Unlike NS1A, which is able to inhibit ISG15 induction by suppressing IFN production, influenza B virus upregulates ISG15 and ISGylation. In order to combat this IFN induced response by the cell, NS1B has been shown to inhibit the conjugation of ISG15 to its targets by preventing the activation step required for ISGylation. The N-terminus of NS1B binds ISG15 and prevents its thioester bond formation with Ube1L.[98] This interaction with ISG15 is dependent on residues contained in large, N-terminal loops that overlap the dsRNA binding domain of NS1B and that are missing from NS1A. Despite the overlap, ISG15 and dsRNA can bind simultaneously and the binding of one has no appreciable effect on the other.[110] Experiments examining the enhancement of viral fitness due to the presence of NS1B have not been published; however, influenza's susceptibility to the ISG15 targets PKR, MxA, and RIG-I would make it a prime candidate for being vulnerable to ISGylation-mediated antiviral activity.[111]

A NEW TARGET FOR NS1?

Recently, a new potential target for NS1 inhibition of the IFN response has been identified.[112] Although it is a well-characterized antiviral pathway, the 2′-5′ oligoadenylate synthetase (OAS)/RNase L pathway has never been shown to antagonize influenza virus. The OAS and RNase L proteins function in tandem as a sensor and effector mechanism, respectively, that ultimately leads to the cleavage of both cellular and viral RNAs to inhibit virus replication.

The OAS family contains three members in humans (OAS1, OAS2, and OAS3), of which OAS1 and OAS2 are differentially spliced. Though they are all induced by both type I and II IFNs and possess sythetase activity, they vary in their subcellular localization, the size pattern of the 2′-5′ phosphodiester-linked oligoadenylates (2-5A) produced, and their dsRNA requirements. OAS is activated by viral dsRNA, typically produced during viral genome replication or the transcription of viral genes. Upon activation, OAS catalyzes the polymerization of ATP to generate 2-5A oligomers, which are capable of activating RNase L.[113,114]

RNase L (also known as 2-5A-dependent RNase, RNS4, or RNase F) is an endoribonuclease that possesses antiviral, proapoptotic, antiproliferative, tumor-suppressive, and senescence-inducing activity.[115] It contains a 2-5A binding domain and nine ankyrin repeats in its N-terminus, as well as RNase and kinase-like domains in the catalytic C-terminus.[116,117] Binding of 2-5A is believed to release the negative regulatory activity of the N-terminus and enable homodimerization to form an active complex.[118,119] The RNase L homodimer is then capable of cleaving cellular and viral RNAs to inhibit virus replication and presumably mediate its other activities. Although RNase L does not significantly inhibit viruses such as VSV, influenza, or herpesviruses, it is a potent inhibitor of picornavirus replication.[120–123] To emphasize this, RNase L –/– mice were generated and infected with EMCV, a prototypical member of the *Picornaviridae* family. RNase L-deficient mice were found to succumb more rapidly than wild-type mice to EMCV, as well as possess defects in apoptosis.[124]

Recently, Min et al. have identified RNase L as a target of the influenza NS1 protein.[112] In their studies, recombinant influenza virus was generated that possesses a NS1 protein encoding a point mutation (R38A) that renders it unable to bind dsRNA.[71] They demonstrated that this recombinant virus was able to replicate 100- to 200-fold more in RNase L –/– mice than in wild-type mice possessing functional RNase L. Wild-type influenza replicated equally in both RNase L –/– and +/+ mice.[112] These results indicate that fully functional NS1 is capable of inhibiting RNase L activity in a dsRNA-dependent manor. However, if NS1 is unable to bind dsRNA and therefore unable to inhibit RNase L, then RNase L can suppress virus replication. Given that RNase L activity is dependent on OAS activation by dsRNA, it is likely that NS1 sequesters dsRNA away from OAS, preventing its activation. Indeed, possible OAS inhibition by NS1 has been previously suggested.[125]

TACKLING HUNDREDS OF BIRDS WITH ONE STONE

Inhibition of IFN-induced effector proteins has been proven to be a valuable mechanism for virus survival. However, inhibiting even a fraction of the hundreds of ISGs is inefficient, so many viruses have evolved means of inhibiting the IFN response further upstream by impeding IFN production itself. Many studies have documented the diminished IFN production by influenza-virus-infected cells. Though microarray analysis has demonstrated that influenza can stimulate sufficient IFNβ production to cause some ISG induction, significant data also exist showing that influenza can dramatically limit the amount of IFNβ made.[84,126,127] This inhibition is believed to be a result of the multifunctional NS1 protein.

Several studies have explored influenza's role in IFN induction, and recent publications have begun to tease out a possible mechanism for this inhibition. One of the first major achievements was the use of reverse genetics to generate influenza virus lacking the NS1 gene (delNS1).[69] Utilizing this viable, but attenuated, virus, delNS1 has been shown to stimulate severalfold more IFNβ than wild-type virus, and this phenotype can be rescued by transient expression of NS1 or a truncated version composed of the N-terminal 73 amino acids.[127,128] This inhibition of IFNβ is attributed to findings indicating that NS1 can inhibit IRF-3 activation and prevent its translocation to the nucleus where it binds to the IFNβ promoter.[129] Though direct inhibition could have been plausible, evidence also existed that NF-κB activation by virus infection is also inhibited, suggesting that NS1 suppresses a factor upstream of both NF-κB and IRF-3.[127]

Given that only the N-terminus of NS1, which encodes the dsRNA binding domain, was required for inhibition of IFN, it seemed logical that NS1 was inhibiting the viral dsRNA sensor that activates both IRF-3 and NF-κB. Early efforts to prove that NS1 was binding dsRNA and sequestering it were hampered by the fact that at the time, RIG-I and MDA-5 had not yet been identified. Nonetheless, a recombinant virus containing two point mutations (R38A, K41A) that abrogated dsRNA binding was generated.[84] The R38A, K41A virus was shown to be incapable of suppressing IFNβ production and attenuated in mice, indicating a role for dsRNA sequestration in the inhibition of IFN induction. A subsequent study has challenged these findings by generating a single-point mutation in NS1, R38A, which alone is sufficient for preventing dsRNA binding. This analysis showed no inhibition by the mutated virus and concluded that dsRNA binding was not involved in the suppression of IFN.[112] The discrepancy in these findings may be a result of the two mutants being generated in different strains of influenza A, WSN/33 versus Udorn/72, which contain one versus two functional NLSs, respectively. The R38A mutation used in both studies is located in the common NLS and therefore may differentially affect subcellular localization of the two mutant NS1 proteins.[84,112,130]

In 2004, both RIG-I and MDA-5 were identified as intracellular sensors for viral infection that activated a signaling cascade resulting in IRF-3 phosphorylation and IFNβ transcription.[13,14,131] Each helicase was individually stimulated by different viruses, and influenza was found to induce IFN in a RIG-I-dependent fashion.[16] Though originally believed to detect viral dsRNA, recent publications have demonstrated that RIG-I is actually activated by the 5′-triphosphate found on the end of virally transcribed RNA.[15,17] Specifically, flu vRNA is sufficient to stimulate RIG-I, and this activation can be inhibited by NS1.[17,132,133]

Though previously posited to sequester viral dsRNA, NS1 was shown to bind directly to RIG-1 and prevent IRF-3 translocation to the nucleus.[17,133] Although the studies differ in regard to possible inhibition of IPS-1, which is directly downstream of RIG-I, it is clear that NS1 is a potent inhibitor of RIG-I-mediated IFN induction.[132,133]

POTENTIAL THERAPEUTIC TARGETS

Influenza is capable of inhibiting multiple aspects of the IFN-induced innate immune response; however, it is still susceptible to IFN's antiviral activity. In fact, the original discovery of interferon was made using influenza as an inducer and demonstrated that it could inhibit influenza replication.[134,135] In fatal cases of influenza, interferon was not detectable in patients' lungs, perhaps emphasizing its importance in controlling infection.[136] Given flu's susceptibility to IFN's pleiotropic activity, it is reasonable to assert that IFN could be used as an antiviral agent against influenza.

Early attempts to evaluate IFN as an anti-flu therapeutic and prophylactic yielded unsatisfactory results. IFN was able to prevent influenza infection to a limited extent; however, complete protection was not obtained and unwanted side effects were observed.[137–139] Advances in research and technology, and to some degree emphasis on biodefense, have provided a renewed effort toward utilizing IFN as an antiviral drug.

IFN, in combination with the nucleoside analogue ribavirin, is currently the primary therapeutic regimen for hepatitis C virus. Due to the efficacy and side effects of chronic use (flu-like symptoms, fatigue, weight loss, nausea, and depression), pegylated IFN was developed and has become standard therapy for HCV. This modification stabilizes IFN in the body and lessens the side effects in some people.[140] Though usage for flu would be of shorter duration, pegylated IFN could allow for lower doses, better efficacy, and perhaps better tolerance.

A number of new drugs under investigation activate the Toll-like receptors (TLRs), specifically TLRs 3, 4, 7, 8, and 9, which are all capable of inducing IFN production.[141] In mice, these agonists or manufactured mimics can mediate protective effects against flu and many other pathogens.[142] For example, the TLR3 agonist polyI:C is a synthetic dsRNA that would not only activate TLR signaling and MDA-5 to produce IFN, but also could activate two key anti-influenza mechanisms, PKR and the OAS/RNase L pathway. Previous studies have shown that prophylactic polyIC:LC pre-treatment can confer complete protection against lethal influenza infection in mice and partial protection post-exposure.[143]

Along these lines, two drugs have been found to activate IFN effector mechanisms. Geranylgeranylacetone (GGA) is an antiulcer drug that has been shown to upregulate MxA, OAS, and PKR and induce PKR phosphorylation in cultured cells.[144,145] In addition, Hemispherx is developing the drug Oragen, which is a 2-5A analogue that would potentially activate RNase L.[142] Use of these drugs as prophylaxis or therapy could potentially outcompete NS1's inhibition of these key anti-influenza proteins and prevent infection. Likewise, targeting the NS1 protein directly could also be a key strategy. NS1 inhibits RIG-I, PKR, and the OAS/RNase L pathway, and deletion of NS1 renders influenza greatly attenuated in mice (Fig. 3.1).[84] In fact, the current pandemic threat of avian H5N1 is resistant to IFN and TNFα, and this enhanced pathogenesis is mediated by the NS1 protein.[146] Suppression of NS1 would likely allow for full induction of IFN and normal PKR and RNase L antiviral activity to inhibit replication.

Since the discovery of IFN in 1957, influenza and IFN have been investigated as mutual antagonists, each revealing insight into the other's biology.[135] It seems unlikely that flu would have evolved multiple, overlapping mechanisms for inhibiting IFN, if IFN was not effective at suppressing replication. This may implicate the IFN response as a key target for antiviral therapy, specifically PKR, RIG-I, and OAS/RNase L. Enhancement of these antiviral proteins or inhibition of their suppressor may provide adequate protection against influenza without the need for strain identification and vaccine development, key barriers in the event of a pandemic outbreak. Clearly, the threat of pandemic flu and the importance of IFN in influenza's pathogenesis warrant further investigation into the development of IFN and its antiviral proteins as therapeutic targets.

REFERENCES

1. Taubenberger, J. K.; Reid, A. H.; Lourens, R. M.; Wang, R.; Jin, G.; et al. Characterization of the 1918 influenza virus polymerase genes. *Nature* **2005**, *437*, 889–893.

2. Russell, C. J.; Webster, R. G. The genesis of a pandemic influenza virus. *Cell* **2005**, *123*, 368–371.

3. Kilbourne, E. D. Influenza pandemics of the 20th century. *Emerg. Infect. Dis.* **2006**, *12*, 9–14.

4. Lamb, R. A. K., R.M. Orthomyxoviridae: The viruses and their replication. *Fields Virology*, Lippincott, Williams, and Wilkins, Philadelphia, **2001**, pp. 1487–1531.

5. Ronni, T.; Sareneva, T.; Pirhonen, J.; Julkunen, I. Activation of IFN-alpha, IFN-gamma, MxA, and IFN regulatory factor 1 genes in influenza A virus-infected human peripheral blood mononuclear cells. *J. Immunol.* **1995**, *154*, 2764–2774.

6. Plotch, S. J.; Bouloy, M.; Ulmanen, I.; Krug, R. M. A unique cap(m7GpppXm)-dependent influenza virion endonuclease cleaves capped RNAs to generate the primers that initiate viral RNA transcription. *Cell* **1981**, *23*, 847–858.

7. Plotch, S. J.; Bouloy, M.; Krug, R. M. Transfer of 5′-terminal cap of globin mRNA to influenza viral complementary RNA during transcription *in vitro*. *Proc. Natl. Acad. Sci. USA* **1979**, *76*, 1618–1622.

8. Fortes, P.; Beloso, A.; Ortin, J. Influenza virus NS1 protein inhibits pre-mRNA splicing and blocks mRNA nucleocytoplasmic transport. *EMBO J.* **1994**, *13*, 704–712.

9. Park, Y. W.; Katze, M. G. Translational control by influenza virus. Identification of cis-acting sequences and trans-acting factors which may regulate selective viral mRNA translation. *J. Biol. Chem.* **1995**, *270*, 28433–28439.

10. Hinshaw, V. S.; Olsen, C. W.; Dybdahl-Sissoko, N.; Evans, D. Apoptosis: A mechanism of cell killing by influenza A and B viruses. *J. Virol.* **1994**, *68*, 3667–3673.

11. Ikeda, H.; Chamoto, K.; Tsuji, T.; Suzuki, Y.; Wakita, D.; et al. The critical role of type-1 innate and acquired immunity in tumor immunotherapy. *Cancer Sci.* **2004**, *95*, 697–703.

12. Stark, G. R.; Kerr, I. M.; Williams, B. R.; Silverman, R. H.; Schreiber, R. D. How cells respond to interferons. *Annu. Rev. Biochem.* **1998**, *67*, 227–264.

13. Andrejeva, J.; Childs, K. S.; Young, D. F.; Carlos, T. S.; Stock, N.; et al. The V proteins of paramyxoviruses bind the IFN-inducible RNA helicase, mda-5, and inhibit its activation of the IFN-beta promoter. *Proc. Natl. Acad. Sci. USA* **2004**, *101*, 17264–17269.

14. Yoneyama, M.; Kikuchi, M.; Natsukawa, T.; Shinobu, N.; Imaizumi, T.; et al. The RNA helicase RIG-I has an essential function in double-stranded RNA-induced innate antiviral responses. *Nat. Immunol.* **2004**, *5*, 730–737.

15. Hornung, V.; Ellegast, J.; Kim, S.; Brzozka, K.; Jung, A.; et al. 5′-Triphosphate RNA is the ligand for RIG-I. *Science* **2006**, *314*, 994–997.

16. Kato, H.; Takeuchi, O.; Sato, S.; Yoneyama, M.; Yamamoto, M.; et al. Differential roles of MDA5 and RIG-I helicases in the recognition of RNA viruses. *Nature* **2006**, *441*, 101–105.

17. Pichlmair, A.; Schulz, O.; Tan, C. P.; Naslund, T. I.; Liljestrom, P.; et al. RIG-I-mediated antiviral responses to single-stranded RNA bearing 5'-phosphates. *Science* **2006**, *314*, 997–1001.

18. Meylan, E.; Curran, J.; Hofmann, K.; Moradpour, D.; Binder, M.; et al. Cardif is an adaptor protein in the RIG-I antiviral pathway and is targeted by hepatitis C virus. *Nature* **2005**, *437*, 1167–1172.

19. Kawai, T.; Takahashi, K.; Sato, S.; Coban, C.; Kumar, H.; et al. IPS-1, an adaptor triggering RIG-I- and Mda5-mediated type I interferon induction. *Nat. Immunol.* **2005**, *6*, 981–988.

20. Fitzgerald, K. A.; McWhirter, S. M.; Faia, K. L.; Rowe, D. C.; Latz, E.; et al. IKKepsilon and TBK1 are essential components of the IRF3 signaling pathway. *Nat. Immunol.* **2003**, *4*, 491–496.

21. Sharma, S.; tenOever, B. R.; Grandvaux, N.; Zhou, G. P.; Lin, R.; et al. Triggering the interferon antiviral response through an IKK-related pathway. *Science* **2003**, *300*, 1148–1151.

22. Xu, L. G.; Wang, Y. Y.; Han, K. J.; Li, L. Y.; Zhai, Z.; et al. VISA is an adapter protein required for virus-triggered IFN-beta signaling. *Mol. Cell* **2005**, *19*, 727–740.

23. Seth, R. B.; Sun, L.; Ea, C. K.; Chen, Z. J. Identification and characterization of MAVS, a mitochondrial antiviral signaling protein that activates NF-kappaB and IRF 3. *Cell* **2005**, *122*, 669–682.

24. Lin, R.; Heylbroeck, C.; Pitha, P. M.; Hiscott, J. Virus-dependent phosphorylation of the IRF-3 transcription factor regulates nuclear translocation, transactivation potential, and proteasome-mediated degradation. *Mol. Cell. Biol.* **1998**, *18*, 2986–2996.

25. Alexopoulou, L.; Holt, A. C.; Medzhitov, R.; Flavell, R. A. Recognition of double-stranded RNA and activation of NF-kappaB by Toll-like receptor 3. *Nature* **2001**, *413*, 732–738.

26. Guillot, L.; Le Goffic, R.; Bloch, S.; Escriou, N.; Akira, S.; et al. Involvement of toll-like receptor 3 in the immune response of lung epithelial cells to double-stranded RNA and influenza A virus. *J. Biol. Chem.* **2005**, *280*, 5571–5580.

27. Lund, J. M.; Alexopoulou, L.; Sato, A.; Karow, M.; Adams, N. C.; et al. Recognition of single-stranded RNA viruses by Toll-like receptor 7. *Proc. Natl. Acad. Sci. USA* **2004**, *101*, 5598–5603.

28. Perry, A. K.; Chen, G.; Zheng, D.; Tang, H.; Cheng, G. The host type I interferon response to viral and bacterial infections. *Cell Res.* **2005**, *15*, 407–422.

29. O'Shea, J. J.; Gadina, M.; Schreiber, R. D. Cytokine signaling in 2002: New surprises in the Jak/Stat pathway. *Cell* **2002**, *109 Suppl.*, S121–131.

30. Der, S. D.; Zhou, A.; Williams, B. R.; Silverman, R. H. Identification of genes differentially regulated by interferon alpha, beta, or gamma using

oligonucleotide arrays. *Proc. Natl. Acad. Sci. USA* **1998**, *95*, 15623–15628.

31. Hefti, H. P.; Frese, M.; Landis, H.; Di Paolo, C.; Aguzzi, A.; et al. Human MxA protein protects mice lacking a functional alpha/beta interferon system against La crosse virus and other lethal viral infections. *J. Virol.* **1999**, *73*, 6984–6991.

32. Staeheli, P.; Haller, O.; Boll, W.; Lindenmann, J.; Weissmann, C. Mx protein: Constitutive expression in 3T3 cells transformed with cloned Mx cDNA confers selective resistance to influenza virus. *Cell* **1986**, *44*, 147–158.

33. Haller, O.; Arnheiter, H.; Gresser, I.; Lindenmann, J. Virus-specific interferon action. Protection of newborn Mx carriers against lethal infection with influenza virus. *J. Exp. Med.* **1981**, *154*, 199–203.

34. Krug, R. M.; Shaw, M.; Broni, B.; Shapiro, G.; Haller, O. Inhibition of influenza viral mRNA synthesis in cells expressing the interferon-induced Mx gene product. *J. Virol.* **1985**, *56*, 201–206.

35. Aebi, M.; Fah, J.; Hurt, N.; Samuel, C. E.; Thomis, D.; et al. cDNA structures and regulation of two interferon-induced human Mx proteins. *Mol. Cell. Biol.* **1989**, *9*, 5062–5072.

36. Pavlovic, J.; Haller, O.; Staeheli, P. Human and mouse Mx proteins inhibit different steps of the influenza virus multiplication cycle. *J. Virol.* **1992**, *66*, 2564–2569.

37. Jin, H. K.; Takada, A.; Kon, Y.; Haller, O.; Watanabe, T. Identification of the murine Mx2 gene: Interferon-induced expression of the Mx2 protein from the feral mouse gene confers resistance to vesicular stomatitis virus. *J. Virol.* **1999**, *73*, 4925–4930.

38. Zurcher, T.; Pavlovic, J.; Staeheli, P. Mouse Mx2 protein inhibits vesicular stomatitis virus but not influenza virus. *Virology* **1992**, *187*, 796–800.

39. Frese, M.; Kochs, G.; Meier-Dieter, U.; Siebler, J.; Haller, O. Human MxA protein inhibits tick-borne Thogoto virus but not Dhori virus. *J. Virol.* **1995**, *69*, 3904–3909.

40. Schnorr, J. J.; Schneider-Schaulies, S.; Simon-Jodicke, A.; Pavlovic, J.; Horisberger, M. A.; et al. MxA-dependent inhibition of measles virus glycoprotein synthesis in a stably transfected human monocytic cell line. *J. Virol.* **1993**, *67*, 4760–4768.

41. Landis, H.; Simon-Jodicke, A.; Kloti, A.; Di Paolo, C.; Schnorr, J. J.; et al. Human MxA protein confers resistance to Semliki Forest virus and inhibits the amplification of a Semliki Forest virus-based replicon in the absence of viral structural proteins. *J. Virol.* **1998**, *72*, 1516–1522.

42. Kochs, G.; Haller, O. Interferon-induced human MxA GTPase blocks nuclear import of Thogoto virus nucleocapsids. *Proc. Natl. Acad. Sci. USA* **1999**, *96*, 2082–2086.

43. King, M. C.; Raposo, G.; Lemmon, M. A. Inhibition of nuclear import and cell-cycle progression by mutated forms of the dynamin-like GTPase MxB. *Proc. Natl. Acad. Sci. USA* **2004**, *101*, 8957–8962.

44. Patel, R. C.; Sen, G. C. Characterization of the interactions between double-stranded RNA and the double-stranded RNA binding domain of the interferon induced protein kinase. *Cell Mol. Biol. Res.* **1994**, *40*, 671–682.

45. Bevilacqua, P. C.; George, C. X.; Samuel, C. E.; Cech, T. R. Binding of the protein kinase PKR to RNAs with secondary structure defects: Role of the tandem A-G mismatch and noncontiguous helixes. *Biochemistry* **1998**, *37*, 6303–6316.

46. Clemens, M. J.; Elia, A. The double-stranded RNA-dependent protein kinase PKR: structure and function. *J. Interferon Cytokine Res.* **1997**, *17*, 503–524.

47. Levin, D.; London, I. M. Regulation of protein synthesis: Activation by double-stranded RNA of a protein kinase that phosphorylates eukaryotic initiation factor 2. *Proc. Natl. Acad. Sci. USA* **1978**, *75*, 1121–1125.

48. Galabru, J.; Hovanessian, A. Autophosphorylation of the protein kinase dependent on double-stranded RNA. *J. Biol. Chem.* **1987**, *262*, 15538–15544.

49. Kimball, S. R. Regulation of translation initiation by amino acids in eukaryotic cells. *Prog. Mol. Subcell. Biol.* **2001**, *26*, 155–184.

50. Panniers, R.; Henshaw, E. C. A GDP/GTP exchange factor essential for eukaryotic initiation factor 2 cycling in Ehrlich ascites tumor cells and its regulation by eukaryotic initiation factor 2 phosphorylation. *J. Biol. Chem.* **1983**, *258*, 7928–7934.

51. Perkins, D. J.; Barber, G. N. Defects in translational regulation mediated by the alpha subunit of eukaryotic initiation factor 2 inhibit antiviral activity and facilitate the malignant transformation of human fibroblasts. *Mol. Cell. Biol.* **2004**, *24*, 2025–2040.

52. Chu, W. M.; Ostertag, D.; Li, Z. W.; Chang, L.; Chen, Y.; et al. JNK2 and IKKbeta are required for activating the innate response to viral infection. *Immunity* **1999**, *11*, 721–731.

53. Saunders, L. R.; Perkins, D. J.; Balachandran, S.; Michaels, R.; Ford, R.; et al. Characterization of two evolutionarily conserved, alternatively spliced nuclear phosphoproteins, NFAR-1 and -2, that function in mRNA processing and interact with the double-stranded RNA-dependent protein kinase, PKR. *J. Biol. Chem.* **2001**, *276*, 32300–32312.

54. Balachandran, S.; Kim, C. N.; Yeh, W. C.; Mak, T. W.; Bhalla, K.; et al. Activation of the dsRNA-dependent protein kinase, PKR, induces apoptosis through FADD-mediated death signaling. *EMBO J.* **1998**, *17*, 6888–6902.

55. Kumar, A.; Yang, Y. L.; Flati, V.; Der, S.; Kadereit, S.; et al. Deficient cytokine signaling in mouse embryo fibroblasts with a targeted deletion in the PKR gene: role of IRF-1 and NF-kappaB. *EMBO J.* **1997**, *16*, 406–416.

56. Yang, Y. L.; Reis, L. F.; Pavlovic, J.; Aguzzi, A.; Schafer, R.; et al. Deficient signaling in mice devoid of double-stranded RNA-dependent protein kinase. *EMBO J.* **1995**, *14*, 6095–6106.

57. Krug, R. M. Unique functions of the NS1 protein. In *Textbook of Influenza*, Blackwell Science, Oxford, **1998**, pp. 82–92.

58. Yoshida, T.; Shaw, M. W.; Young, J. F.; Compans, R. W. Characterization of the RNA associated with influenza A cytoplasmic inclusions and the interaction of NS1 protein with RNA. *Virology* **1981**, *110*, 87–97.

59. Chien, C. Y.; Tejero, R.; Huang, Y.; Zimmerman, D. E.; Rios, C. B.; et al. A novel RNA-binding motif in influenza A virus non-structural protein 1. *Nat. Struct. Biol.* **1997**, *4*, 891–895.

60. Shapiro, G. I.; Gurney, T., Jr.; Krug, R. M. Influenza virus gene expression: control mechanisms at early and late times of infection and nuclear-cytoplasmic transport of virus-specific RNAs. *J. Virol.* **1987**, *61*, 764–773.

61. Bornholdt, Z. A.; Prasad, B. V. X-ray structure of influenza virus NS1 effector domain. *Nat. Struct. Mol. Biol.* **2006**, *13*, 559–560.

62. Qiu, Y.; Krug, R. M. The influenza virus NS1 protein is a poly(A)-binding protein that inhibits nuclear export of mRNAs containing poly(A). *J. Virol.* **1994**, *68*, 2425–2432.

63. Qian, X. Y.; Alonso-Caplen, F.; Krug, R. M. Two functional domains of the influenza virus NS1 protein are required for regulation of nuclear export of mRNA. *J. Virol.* **1994**, *68*, 2433–2441.

64. Qiu, Y.; Nemeroff, M.; Krug, R. M. The influenza virus NS1 protein binds to a specific region in human U6 snRNA and inhibits U6-U2 and U6-U4 snRNA interactions during splicing. *RNA* **1995**, *1*, 304–316.

65. Lu, Y.; Qian, X. Y.; Krug, R. M. The influenza virus NS1 protein: A novel inhibitor of pre-mRNA splicing. *Genes. Dev.* **1994**, *8*, 1817–1828.

66. Enami, K.; Sato, T. A.; Nakada, S.; Enami, M. Influenza virus NS1 protein stimulates translation of the M1 protein. *J. Virol.* **1994**, *68*, 1432–1437.

67. Burgui, I.; Aragon, T.; Ortin, J.; Nieto, A. PABP1 and eIF4GI associate with influenza virus NS1 protein in viral mRNA translation initiation complexes. *J. Gen. Virol.* **2003**, *84*, 3263–3274.

68. Bergmann, M.; Garcia-Sastre, A.; Carnero, E.; Pehamberger, H.; Wolff, K.; et al. Influenza virus NS1 protein counteracts PKR-mediated inhibition of replication. *J. Virol.* **2000**, *74*, 6203–6206.

69. Garcia-Sastre, A.; Egorov, A.; Matassov, D.; Brandt, S.; Levy, D. E.; et al. Influenza A virus lacking the NS1 gene replicates in interferon-deficient systems. *Virology* **1998**, *252*, 324–330.

70. Lu, Y.; Wambach, M.; Katze, M. G.; Krug, R. M. Binding of the influenza virus NS1 protein to double-stranded RNA inhibits the activation of the protein kinase that phosphorylates the elF-2 translation initiation factor. *Virology* **1995**, *214*, 222–228.

71. Wang, W.; Riedel, K.; Lynch, P.; Chien, C. Y.; Montelione, G. T.; et al. RNA binding by the novel helical domain of the influenza virus NS1 protein requires its dimer structure and a small number of specific basic amino acids. *RNA* **1999**, *5*, 195–205.

72. Li, S.; Min, J. Y.; Krug, R. M.; Sen, G. C. Binding of the influenza A virus NS1 protein to PKR mediates the inhibition of its activation by either PACT or double-stranded RNA. *Virology* **2006**, *349*, 13–21.

73. Tan, S. L.; Katze, M. G. Biochemical and genetic evidence for complex formation between the influenza A virus NS1 protein and the interferon-induced PKR protein kinase. *J. Interferon Cytokine Res.* **1998**, *18*, 757–766.

74. Hatada, E.; Saito, S.; Fukuda, R. Mutant influenza viruses with a defective NS1 protein cannot block the activation of PKR in infected cells. *J. Virol.* **1999**, *73*, 2425–2433.

75. Garcia-Sastre, A. Inhibition of interferon-mediated antiviral responses by influenza A viruses and other negative-strand RNA viruses. *Virology* **2001**, *279*, 375–384.

76. Ramana, C. V.; Grammatikakis, N.; Chernov, M.; Nguyen, H.; Goh, K. C.; et al. Regulation of c-myc expression by IFN-gamma through Stat1-dependent and -independent pathways. *EMBO J.* **2000**, *19*, 263–272.

77. Jagus, R.; Joshi, B.; Barber, G. N. PKR, apoptosis and cancer. *Int. J. Biochem. Cell. Biol.* **1999**, *31*, 123–138.

78. Patel, R. C.; Sen, G. C. PACT, a protein activator of the interferon-induced protein kinase, PKR. *EMBO J.* **1998**, *17*, 4379–4390.

79. Ito, T.; Yang, M.; May, W. S. RAX, a cellular activator for double-stranded RNA-dependent protein kinase during stress signaling. *J. Biol. Chem.* **1999**, *274*, 15427–15432.

80. Chien, C. Y.; Xu, Y.; Xiao, R.; Aramini, J. M.; Sahasrabudhe, P. V.; et al. Biophysical characterization of the complex between double-stranded RNA and the N-terminal domain of the NS1 protein from influenza A virus: Evidence for a novel RNA-binding mode. *Biochemistry* **2004**, *43*, 1950–1962.

81. Liu, J.; Lynch, P. A.; Chien, C. Y.; Montelione, G. T.; Krug, R. M.; et al. Crystal structure of the unique RNA-binding domain of the influenza virus NS1 protein. *Nat. Struct. Biol.* **1997**, *4*, 896–899.

82. Wang, W.; Krug, R. M. The RNA-binding and effector domains of the viral NS1 protein are conserved to different extents among influenza A and B viruses. *Virology* **1996**, *223*, 41–50.

83. Dauber, B. S. J.; Wolff, T. Double-stranded RNA binding of influenza B virus nonstructural NS1 protein inhibits protein kinase R but is not essential to antagonize production of alpha/beta interferon. *J. Virol.* **2006**, *80*, 11667–11677.

84. Donelan, N. R.; Basler, C. F.; Garcia-Sastre, A. A recombinant influenza A virus expressing an RNA-binding-defective NS1 protein induces high levels of beta interferon and is attenuated in mice. *J. Virol.* **2003**, *77*, 13257–13266.

85. Kash, J. C.; Goodman, A. G.; Korth, M. J.; Katze, M. G. Hijacking of the host-cell response and translational control during influenza virus infection. *Virus Res.* **2006**, *119*, 111–120.

86. Tang, N. M.; Ho, C. Y.; Katze, M. G. The 58-kDa cellular inhibitor of the double stranded RNA-dependent protein kinase requires the tetratricopeptide repeat 6 and DnaJ motifs to stimulate protein synthesis *in vivo*. *J. Biol. Chem.* **1996**, *271*, 28660–28666.

87. Katze, M. G.; Detjen, B. M.; Safer, B.; Krug, R. M. Translational control by influenza virus: Suppression of the kinase that phosphorylates the alpha subunit of initiation factor eIF-2 and selective translation of influenza viral mRNAs. *Mol. Cell. Biol.* **1986**, *6*, 1741–1750.

88. Lee, T. G.; Tang, N.; Thompson, S.; Miller, J.; Katze, M. G. The 58,000-dalton cellular inhibitor of the interferon-induced double-stranded RNA-activated protein kinase (PKR) is a member of the tetratricopeptide repeat family of proteins. *Mol. Cell. Biol.* **1994**, *14*, 2331–2342.

89. Gale, M., Jr.; Blakely, C. M.; Darveau, A.; Romano, P. R.; Korth, M. J.; et al. P52rIPK regulates the molecular cochaperone P58IPK to mediate control of the RNA-dependent protein kinase in response to cytoplasmic stress. *Biochemistry* **2002**, *41*, 11878–11887.

90. Melville, M. W.; Hansen, W. J.; Freeman, B. C.; Welch, W. J.; Katze, M. G. The molecular chaperone hsp40 regulates the activity of P58IPK, the cellular inhibitor of PKR. *Proc. Natl. Acad. Sci. USA* **1997**, *94*, 97–102.

91. Melville, M. W.; Tan, S. L.; Wambach, M.; Song, J.; Morimoto, R. I.; et al. The cellular inhibitor of the PKR protein kinase, P58(IPK), is an influenza virus-activated co-chaperone that modulates heat shock protein 70 activity. *J. Biol. Chem.* **1999**, *274*, 3797–3803.

92. Bilgin, D. D.; Liu, Y.; Schiff, M.; Dinesh-Kumar, S. P. P58(IPK), a plant ortholog of double-stranded RNA-dependent protein kinase PKR inhibitor, functions in viral pathogenesis. *Dev. Cell* **2003**, *4*, 651–661.

93. Fels, D. R.; Koumenis, C. The PERK/eIF2alpha/ATF4 module of the UPR in hypoxia resistance and tumor growth. *Cancer Biol. Ther.* **2006**, *5*, 723–728.

94. Oyadomari, S.; Yun, C.; Fisher, E. A.; Kreglinger, N.; Kreibich, G.; et al. Cotranslocational degradation protects the stressed endoplasmic reticulum from protein overload. *Cell* **2006**, *126*, 727–739.

95. Harding, H. P.; Zeng, H.; Zhang, Y.; Jungries, R.; Chung, P.; et al. Diabetes mellitus and exocrine pancreatic dysfunction in perk–/– mice reveals a role for translational control in secretory cell survival. *Mol. Cell* **2001**, *7*, 1153–1163.

96. Harding, H. P.; Ron, D. Endoplasmic reticulum stress and the development of diabetes: A review. *Diabetes* **2002**, *51* Suppl. 3, S455–S461.

97. Ladiges, W. C.; Knoblaugh, S. E.; Morton, J. F.; Korth, M. J.; Sopher, B. L.; et al. Pancreatic beta-cell failure and diabetes in mice with a deletion mutation of the endoplasmic reticulum molecular chaperone gene P58IPK. *Diabetes* **2005**, *54*, 1074–1081.

98. Yuan, W.; Krug, R. M. Influenza B virus NS1 protein inhibits conjugation of the interferon (IFN)-induced ubiquitin-like ISG15 protein. *EMBO J.* **2001**, *20*, 362–371.

99. Loeb, K. R.; Haas, A. L. The interferon-inducible 15-kDa ubiquitin homolog conjugates to intracellular proteins. *J. Biol. Chem.* **1992**, *267*, 7806–7813.

100. Zou, W.; Zhang, D. E. The interferon-inducible ubiquitin-protein isopeptide ligase (E3) EFP also functions as an ISG15 E3 ligase. *J. Biol. Chem.* **2006**, *281*, 3989–3994.

101. Wong, J. J.; Pung, Y. F.; Sze, N. S.; Chin, K. C. HERC5 is an IFN-induced HECT-type E3 protein ligase that mediates type I IFN-induced ISGylation of protein targets. *Proc. Natl. Acad. Sci. USA* **2006**, *103*, 10735–10740.

102. Zhao, C.; Beaudenon, S. L.; Kelley, M. L.; Waddell, M. B.; Yuan, W.; et al. The UbcH8 ubiquitin E2 enzyme is also the E2 enzyme for ISG15, an IFN-alpha/beta-induced ubiquitin-like protein. *Proc. Natl. Acad. Sci. USA* **2004**, *101*, 7578–7582.

103. Dastur, A.; Beaudenon, S.; Kelley, M.; Krug, R. M.; Huibregtse, J. M. Herc5, an interferon-induced HECT E3 enzyme, is required for conjugation of ISG15 in human cells. *J. Biol. Chem.* **2006**, *281*, 4334–4338.

104. Takeuchi, T.; Iwahara, S.; Saeki, Y.; Sasajima, H.; Yokosawa, H. Link between the ubiquitin conjugation system and the ISG15 conjugation system: ISG15 conjugation to the UbcH6 ubiquitin E2 enzyme. *J. Biochem. (Tokyo)* **2005**, *138*, 711–719.

105. Takeuchi, T.; Yokosawa, H. ISG15 modification of Ubc13 suppresses its ubiquitin-conjugating activity. *Biochem. Biophys. Res. Commun.* **2005**, *336*, 9–13.

106. Zou, W.; Papov, V.; Malakhova, O.; Kim, K. I.; Dao, C.; et al. ISG15 modification of ubiquitin E2 Ubc13 disrupts its ability to form thioester bond with ubiquitin. *Biochem. Biophys. Res. Commun.* **2005**, *336*, 61–68.

107. Knobeloch, K. P.; Utermohlen, O.; Kisser, A.; Prinz, M.; Horak, I. Reexamination of the role of ubiquitin-like modifier ISG15 in the phenotype of UBP43-deficient mice. *Mol. Cell. Biol.* **2005**, *25*, 11030–11034.

108. Lenschow, D. J.; Giannakopoulos, N. V.; Gunn, L. J.; Johnston, C.; O'Guin, A. K.; et al. Identification of interferon-stimulated gene 15 as an antiviral molecule during Sindbis virus infection in vivo. *J. Virol.* **2005**, *79*, 13974–13983.

109. Okumura, A.; Lu, G.; Pitha-Rowe, I.; Pitha, P. M. Innate antiviral response targets HIV-1 release by the induction of ubiquitin-like protein ISG15. *Proc. Natl. Acad. Sci. USA* **2006**, *103*, 1440–1445.

110. Yuan, W.; Aramini, J. M.; Montelione, G. T.; Krug, R. M. Structural basis for ubiquitin-like ISG 15 protein binding to the NS1 protein of influenza B virus: A protein–protein interaction function that is not shared by the corresponding N-terminal domain of the NS1 protein of influenza A virus. *Virology* **2002**, *304*, 291–301.

111. Zhao, C.; Denison, C.; Huibregtse, J. M.; Gygi, S.; Krug, R. M. Human ISG15 conjugation targets both IFN-induced and constitutively expressed proteins functioning in diverse cellular pathways. *Proc. Natl. Acad. Sci. USA* **2005**, *102*, 10200–10205.

112. Min, J. Y.; Krug, R. M. The primary function of RNA binding by the influenza A virus NS1 protein in infected cells: Inhibiting the 2′-5′ oligo (A) synthetase/RNase L pathway. *Proc. Natl. Acad. Sci. USA* **2006**, *103*, 7100–7105.

113. Player, M. R.; Torrence, P. F. The 2–5A system: Modulation of viral and cellular processes through acceleration of RNA degradation. *Pharmacol. Ther.* **1998**, *78*, 55–113.

114. Samuel, C. E. Antiviral actions of interferons. *Clin. Microbiol. Rev.* **2001**, *14*, 778–809, table of contents.

115. Silverman, R. H. Implications for RNase L in prostate cancer biology. *Biochemistry* **2003**, *42*, 1805–1812.

116. Tanaka, N.; Nakanishi, M.; Kusakabe, Y.; Goto, Y.; Kitade, Y.; et al. Structural basis for recognition of 2′,5′-linked oligoadenylates by human ribonuclease L. *EMBO J.* **2004**, *23*, 3929–3938.

117. Zhou, A.; Hassel, B. A.; Silverman, R. H. Expression cloning of 2-5A-dependent RNAase: A uniquely regulated mediator of interferon action. *Cell* **1993**, *72*, 753–765.

118. Dong, B.; Xu, L.; Zhou, A.; Hassel, B. A.; Lee, X.; et al. Intrinsic molecular activities of the interferon-induced 2-5A-dependent RNase. *J. Biol. Chem.* **1994**, *269*, 14153–14158.

119. Dong, B.; Silverman, R. H. 2-5A-dependent RNase molecules dimerize during activation by 2-5A. *J. Biol. Chem.* **1995**, *270*, 4133–4137.

120. De Benedetti, A.; Pytel, B. A.; Baglioni, C. Loss of (2′-5′)oligoadenylate synthetase activity by production of antisense RNA results in lack of protection by interferon from viral infections. *Proc. Natl. Acad. Sci. USA* **1987**, *84*, 658–662.

121. Hassel, B. A.; Zhou, A.; Sotomayor, C.; Maran, A.; Silverman, R. H. A dominant negative mutant of 2-5A-dependent RNase suppresses antiproliferative and antiviral effects of interferon. *EMBO J.* **1993**, *12*, 3297–3304.

122. Meurs, E.; Hovanessian, A. G.; Montagnier, L. Interferon-mediated antiviral state in human MRC5 cells in the absence of detectable levels of 2-5A synthetase and protein kinase. *J. Interferon Res.* **1981**, *1*, 219–232.

123. Taylor, J. L.; Witt, P. L.; Irizarry, A.; Tom, P.; O'Brien, W. J. 2′,5′-Oligoadenylate synthetase in interferon-alpha- and acyclovir-treated herpes simplex virus-infected cells. *J. Interferon Cytokine Res.* **1995**, *15*, 27–30.

124. Zhou, A.; Paranjape, J.; Brown, T. L.; Nie, H.; Naik, S.; et al. Interferon action and apoptosis are defective in mice devoid of 2′,5′-oligoadenylate-dependent RNase L. *EMBO J.* **1997**, *16*, 6355–6363.

125. Donelan, N. a. G.-S., A. Inhibition of the 2-5A synthetase activity by the NS1 protein of influenza A virus. *19th Annual Meeting of the American Society for Virology*, Fort Collins, CO, **2000**.

126. Baskin, C. R.; Garcia-Sastre, A.; Tumpey, T. M.; Bielefeldt-Ohmann, H.; Carter, V. S.; et al. Integration of clinical data, pathology, and cDNA microarrays in influenza virus-infected pigtailed macaques (*Macaca nemestrina*). *J. Virol.* **2004**, *78*, 10420–10432.

127. Wang, X.; Li, M.; Zheng, H.; Muster, T.; Palese, P.; et al. Influenza A virus NS1 protein prevents activation of NF-kappaB and induction of alpha/beta interferon. *J. Virol.* **2000**, *74*, 11566–11573.

128. Fernandez-Sesma, A.; Marukian, S.; Ebersole, B. J.; Kaminski, D.; Park, M. S.; et al. Influenza virus evades innate and adaptive immunity via the NS1 protein. *J. Virol.* **2006**, *80*, 6295–6304.

129. Talon, J.; Horvath, C. M.; Polley, R.; Basler, C. F.; Muster, T.; et al. Activation of interferon regulatory factor 3 is inhibited by the influenza A virus NS1 protein. *J. Virol.* **2000**, *74*, 7989–7996.

130. Greenspan, D.; Palese, P.; Krystal, M. Two nuclear location signals in the influenza virus NS1 nonstructural protein. *J. Virol.* **1988**, *62*, 3020–3026.

131. Kang, D. C.; Gopalkrishnan, R. V.; Wu, Q.; Jankowsky, E.; Pyle, A. M.; et al. mda-5: An interferon-inducible putative RNA helicase with double-stranded RNA-dependent ATPase activity and melanoma growth-suppressive properties. *Proc. Natl. Acad. Sci. USA* **2002**, *99*, 637–642.

132. Guo, Z.; Chen, L. M.; Zeng, H.; Gomez, J. A.; Plowden, J.; et al. NS1 Protein of influenza A virus inhibits the function of intracytoplasmic pathogen sensor, RIG-I. *Am. J. Respir. Cell. Mol. Biol.* **2006**, *36*, 263–269.

133. Mibayashi, M.; Martinez-Sobrido, L.; Loo, Y. M.; Cardenas, W. B.; Gale, M., Jr.; et al. Inhibition of Retinoic Acid-Inducible Gene-I-Mediated

Induction of Interferon-{beta} by the NS1 protein of influenza A virus. *J. Virol.* **2006**, *81*, 514–524.

134. Isaacs, A.; Lindenmann, J. Virus interference. I. The interferon. *Proc. R. Soc. Lond. B Biol. Sci.* **1957**, *147*, 258–267.

135. Isaacs, A.; Lindenmann, J.; Valentine, R. C. Virus interference. II. Some properties of interferon. *Proc. R. Soc. Lond. B Biol. Sci.* **1957**, *147*, 268–273.

136. Baron, S.; Isaacs, A. Absence of interferon in lungs from fatal cases of influenza. *Br. Med. J.* **1962**, *1*, 18–20.

137. Isomura, S.; Ichikawa, T.; Miyazu, M.; Naruse, H.; Shibata, M.; et al. The preventive effect of human interferon-alpha on influenza infection; modification of clinical manifestations of influenza in children in a closed community. *Biken J.* **1982**, *25*, 131–137.

138. Phillpotts, R. J.; Higgins, P. G.; Willman, J. S.; Tyrrell, D. A.; Freestone, D. S.; et al. Intranasal lymphoblastoid interferon ("Wellferon") prophylaxis against rhinovirus and influenza virus in volunteers. *J. Interferon Res.* **1984**, *4*, 535–541.

139. Sperber, S. J.; Levine, P. A.; Innes, D. J.; Mills, S. E.; Hayden, F. G. Tolerance and efficacy of intranasal administration of recombinant beta serine interferon in healthy adults. *J. Infect. Dis.* **1988**, *158*, 166–175.

140. Matthews, S. J.; McCoy, C. Peginterferon alfa-2a: A review of approved and investigational uses. *Clin. Ther.* **2004**, *26*, 991–1025.

141. Akira, S. TLR signaling. *Curr. Top. Microbiol. Immunol.* **2006**, *311*, 1–16.

142. Amlie-Lefond, C.; Paz, D. A.; Connelly, M. P.; Huffnagle, G. B.; Whelan, N. T.; et al. Innate immunity for biodefense: A strategy whose time has come. *J. Allergy Clin. Immunol.* **2005**, *116*, 1334–1342.

143. Wong, J. P.; Saravolac, E. G.; Sabuda, D.; Levy, H. B.; Kende, M. Prophylactic and therapeutic efficacies of poly(IC.LC) against respiratory influenza A virus infection in mice. *Antimicrob. Agents Chemother.* **1995**, *39*, 2574–2576.

144. Ichikawa, T.; Nakao, K.; Nakata, K.; Hamasaki, K.; Takeda, Y.; et al. Geranylgeranylacetone induces antiviral gene expression in human hepatoma cells. *Biochem. Biophys. Res. Commun.* **2001**, *280*, 933–939.

145. Unoshima, M.; Iwasaka, H.; Eto, J.; Takita-Sonoda, Y.; Noguchi, T.; et al. Antiviral effects of geranylgeranylacetone: Enhancement of MxA expression and phosphorylation of PKR during influenza virus infection. *Antimicrob. Agents Chemother.* **2003**, *47*, 2914–2921.

146. Seo, S. H.; Hoffmann, E.; Webster, R. G. Lethal H5N1 influenza viruses escape host anti-viral cytokine responses. *Nat. Med.* **2002**, *8*, 950–954.

4

BROADLY EFFECTIVE ANTI-RESPIRATORY VIRUS AGENTS

SHIRO SHIGETA

Fukushima Medical University and Bureau of Prefectural Hospitals of Fukushima, Fukushima 960-8043, Japan

INTRODUCTION

Multiple viral agents are known to cause acute respiratory infections. Most of those agents belong to the families orthomyxoviridae, paramyxoviridae, picornaviridae, coronaviridae, adenoviridae, and so on. Among them, the orthomyxoviruses and paramyxoviruses share a common nature, that is, they have negative-strand RNA and have viral envelopes with a plasma membrane structure, and they are similar in several steps of viral replication. In Table 4.1, the causative agents of human respiratory infections which belong to ortho- and paramyxoviruses are listed. Influenza virus (FLUV) A, B, and C are orthomyxoviruses; and parainfluenza virus (PFLUV) 1, 2, 3, 4, mumps virus (MPSV), measles virus (MLSV), respiratory syncytial virus (RSV) A and B, and metapneumovirus are paramyxoviruses. Most human viral respiratory infections are highly contagious and sometimes epidemic. Clinical symptoms of the acute respiratory infections vary and are diagnosed as the common cold, rhinitis, pharyngitis, croup, bronchitis, bronchiolitis, pneumonia, influenza and so on. However, etiological diagnosis of respiratory infection from clinical manifestations alone is

Combating the Threat of Pandemic Influenza: Drug Discovery Approaches,
Edited by Paul F. Torrence
Copyright © 2007 by John Wiley & Sons, Inc.

TABLE 4.1. Human Orthomyxovirus and Paramyxovirus

Family *Orthomyxoviridae*	
Influenza virus type A	(H1N1)
	(H2N2)
	(H3N2)
	(H5N1) May change from avian virus to human virus
Influenza virus type B	
Influenza virus type C	
Family *Paramyxoviridae*	
Subfamily Paramyxovirinae	
Genus *Respirovirus*	Human parainfluenza virus type 1
	Human parainfluenza virus type 3
Genus *Rubulavirus*	Human parainfluenza virus type 2
	Human parainfluenza virus type 4
	Mumps virus
Genus *Morbillivirus*	Measles virus
Subfamily Pneumovirinae	
Genus *Pneumovirus*	Human respiratory syncytial virus
Genus *Metapneumovirus*	Human metapneumovirus

very difficult for general practioner physicians. At times, metapneumovirus and even rhinovirus have caused influenza-like disease.[1,2] Although there are several laboratory diagnostic procedures for FLUV and RSV, the reagents are expensive, it takes time to perform the diagnosis, and the patients have to be treated as soon as possible, usually at home. Most of the antiviral drugs developed recently for FLUV and RSV are virus-specific, but I will introduce some broad-spectrum anti-respiratory virus agents found from a random screening for ortho- and paramyxoviruses conducted in our laboratory.[3]

A RAPID *IN VITRO* SCREENING METHOD FOR MYXOVIRUSES

The cytopathic effects (CPE) on tissue culture cells caused by myxovirus infections are not strikingly apparent—if they exist at all—and do not have a sufficient effect to differentiate viable and dead cells on MTT assay. It is also difficult to induce the formation of visible plaques of PFLUV-1, -2, -3 or FLUV C in tissue culture cells. The MTT assay utilizes 3,4,5-diphenyltetrazolium bromide (MTT), which is converted to a water-soluble blue crystal (formazan) in viable cells through mitochondrial dehydrogenese activity. Dead cells are unable to reduce MTT to formazan. Another colorimetric method, the LDH assay which quantifies the infected cells by detection of lactate dehydrogenase activity (LDH) elution from cells, was devised to detect the infection with weakly cytopathogenic myxoviruses such as FLUV C, PFLUV 1, 2, and 3.[4,5] Colorimetric methods are objective and vary less than the plaque reduction assay for evaluation of the antiviral effect of compounds. In addition, colorimetric assays facilitate the mass screening of compounds and computerization of the obtained data. At first we selected a human melanoma cell line (HMV-II) for the LDH and MTT assays to examine the antimyxovirus activity of compounds. We found that the critical points for the sensitive colorimetric method are as follows: First, the cells have to be used in a suspended state; second, cells, virus, and diluted compounds have to be introduced simultaneously to the culture plate; and third, the plate has to be centrifuged at 700 g for 10 min before incubation. We examined the sensitivity of viral titration by comparatively using $LDHID_{50}$ and $MTTID_{50}$ and plaque forming units (PFU) for ortho- and paramyxoviruses. The $LDHID_{50}$ expressed the minimal virus amount that eluted the LDH at 50% of the completely degenerated cells, and the $MTTID_{50}$ expressed the minimal virus amount that reduced MTT in cells at 50% of the mock-infected cells. As shown in Table 4.2, $LDHID_{50}$ was less sensitive than $MTTID_{50}$ for FLUV A, B, PFLUV 2, MPSV, and RSV. On the other hand, $LDHID_{50}$ was more sensitive than $MTTID_{50}$ for FLUV C, PFLUV 1, and MLSV.

TABLE 4.2. Comparative Titration of Virus Infectivity with $LDHID_{50}$, $MTTID_{50}$, and PFU[a]

Virus and Strain	$LDHID_{50}/0.1$ ml $(\log_{10})$	$MTTID_{50}/0.1$ ml $(\log_{10})$	PFU/0.1 ml $(\log_{10})$
FLUV A (Ishikawa H_3N_2)	3.73	4.63	3.58
FLUV B (Singapore)	3.61	4.24	3.11
FLUV C (Ann Arbor)	3.09	1.69	NA
PFLUV 1 (Y91N820)	3.31	1.70	NA
PFLUV 2 (Greer)	5.89	6.24	3.47
PFLUV 3 (C243)	2.45	NA[b]	6.39
MPSV (F1213)	4.49	5.19	5.47
MLSV (Sugiyama)	2.05	NA	2.92
RSV A (Long)	3.45	3.59	4.30
RSV B (SM61-48)	3.02	2.89	4.02

[a]For plaque titration, MDCK cells for FLUV A, B, and C, Vero cells for PFLUV 2, PFLUV 3, MPSV, and MLSV, and HeLa cells for RSV A and B were used.
[b]NA: The corresponding method was not applicable.

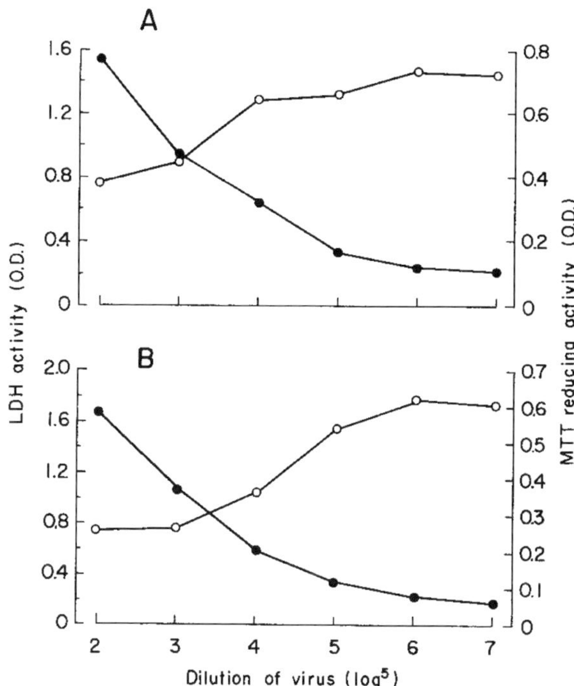

Fig. 4.1. Changes in leaked LDH activity and MTT reducing activity of infected cells with respect to the viral dilution. The correlations between the leaked LDH activity and the mitochondrial reducing activity in (A) PFLUV 1- and (B) FLUV C-infected HMV-II cell cultures were determined. The LDH activity (●) and MTT reducing activity (○) are expressed as the optical density (O.D.) of formazan.

For plaque titration we used MDCK cells for FLUV A and B, Vero cells for PFLUV 2 and 3, and MPSV, MLSV, and HeLa cells for RSV. PFLUV 1 and FLUV C did not form visible plaques in MDCK, Vero, HeLa, or HMV-II cells. Figure 4.1 shows the decrease of LDH elution and increase of MTT reducing activity in HMV-II cells following the dilution of inoculated virus (PFLUV 1 and FLUV C). These viruses were weakest in cytopathogenicity for cells and difficult to determine viral titer by PFU. As shown in the figure, LDH activity and MTT reducing activity by the viral infection varied together with viral dilution while they were reciprocal with each other. Thus, both the LDH and MTT methods were proven to be applicable for the titration and evaluation of the antiviral activity of compounds for these viruses.[5]

From the result of repeated experiments we chose the most susceptible tissue culture cells for each virus, that is, MDCK cells for FLUV A and FLUV B, HEp-2 cells for RSV, HMV-II cells for FLUV C,

PFLUV 1, and PFLUV 2, Vero cells for PFLUV 3 and MPSV, and B95a (a human lymphoid cell line) cells for MLSV. The LDH method was used for FLUV C and PFLUV 1, and the MTT method was used for the other viruses. The use of suspended cells and centrifugation at low speed were requisites for the colorimetric antiviral assay of myxoviruses.

RESULTS OF RANDOM SCREENING OF ANTIVIRAL AGENTS FOR MYXOVIRUSES

Using this efficient colorimetric assay, we examined thousands of compounds for inhibitory activities against ortho- and paramyxoviruses.

Nucleoside Analogues

At first, we examined 20 nucleoside analogues including 3 uridine analogues, 1 cytidine analogue, 7 adenosine analogues, and 6 guanosine analogues for inhibitory activities against RSV *in vitro*. Among these, pyrazofurin, 3-deazaguanine, and ribavirin emerged as selective anti-RSV agents (Fig. 4.2). Their 50% effective dose (EC_{50}) and selectivity

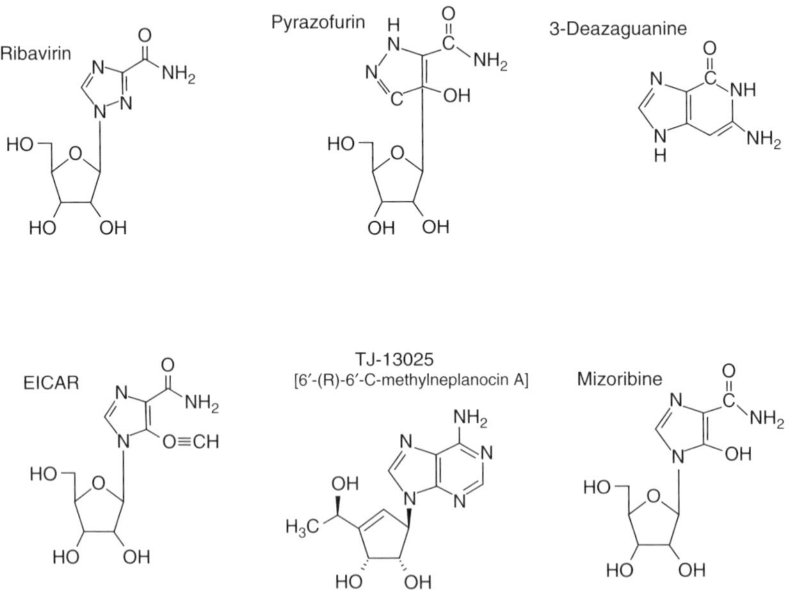

Fig. 4.2. Chemical structures of the nucleoside analogues that have anti-myxovirus activity.

index (SI) were 0.07, 1.65, and 5.82 µg/ml and 1071, >200, 34, respectively. Pyrazofurin and 3-deazaguanine inhibited virus growth in HEp-2 cells at 0.2 and 5 µg/ml, respectively. Ribavirin has been approved for the clinical treatment of RSV infection as aerosol inhalation. Thus pyrazofurin and 3-deazaguanine appeared to be candidate anti-RSV agents in addition to ribavirin.[6] In another experiment, 20 nucleoside analogues (15 were the same as the anti-RSV study) were examined for anti-FLUV (including A/H1N1, A/H3N2, B, and C) activities *in vitro*. After the examination, five compounds—pyrzofurin, 3-deazaguanine, ribavirin, and the two cytidine analogues carbodine and cyclopentenyl cytosine—were found to be potent and selective anti-FLUV agents *in vitro* (Table 4.3). When we calculated SIs as the ratio of the 50% cytotoxic dose (CC_{50}) to the 50% effective dose (EC_{50}), they were more than 96 for all five compounds. The SIs as the ratio of the 50% inhibitory dose for cellular RNA synthesis to the EC_{50} were more than 96 for pyrazofurin, 3-deazagunine, and ribavirin but less than 3 for carbodine and cycolpentenyl cytosine.[7] Hosoya et al. reported an inhibitory effect of ribavirin and pyrazofurin against replication of FLUV A in 8-day-old chick embryos. For ribavirin the SI (TD_{50}/ED_{50}, here ED_{50} = dose for 50% survival of FLUV-infected chick embryos and TD_{50} = dose for 50% survival of mock-infected chick embryos) was calculated as 55, whereas that for pyrazofurin was less than 1. This report indicates that pyrazofurin was more toxic for chick embryos than ribavirin.[8] On the other hand, pyrazofurin displayed a suppressive effect against RSV in the lungs of cotton rats that were infected with 10^3 $TCID_{50}$ of RSV by an intranasal route. As shown in Table 4.4, RSV titers in the lungs of rats that were treated by aerosol exposure with

TABLE 4.3. EC_{50} of Five Nucleoside Analogues for FLUV A, B, and C

| Compound | EC_{50} (µg/ml) | | | SI^a | |
	FLUV A(H3N2, H1N1) (Average of Five Strains)	FLUV B	FLUV C (Single Strain)	a	b
Pyrazofurin	0.17	0.16	0.16	100	365
3-Deazaguanine	3.0	3.3	2.1	>167	>167
Ribavirin	5.2	4.8	2.8	>96	>96
Carbodine	3.0	4.8	2.0	>167	2.3
Cyclopentenyl cytosine	5.2	4.3	2.8	>96	0.6

[a]To determine the SI, cytotoxicity was evaluated by (a) cell viability determined by a trypan blue exclusion test and (b) [5-^{3}H]Urd incorporation into host cell RNA. EC_{50} for SI was determined by an average of that for FLUV A, B, and C.

TABLE 4.4. Aerosol Treatment of RSV-Infected Cotton Rats with Pyrazofurin

Rat No.	RSV Titer ($TCID_{50}$/g) in Lung	
	Untreated	Treated with Pyrazofurin[a,b]
1	$10^{2.6}$	$<10^{1.5}$
2	$10^{2.6}$	$<10^{1.5}$
3	$10^{2.5}$	$<10^{1.5}$
4	$10^{2.5}$	$<10^{1.5}$
5	$10^{2.7}$	$10^{3.6}$
Average	$10^{2.58\pm0.18}$[c]	$<10^{1.93\pm0.9}$

[a] Exposed to 0.5 mg/ml of solution for 48 hr.
[b] There was no obvious toxicity for rats.
[c] Significance between two average titers is $p < 0.01$.

0.5 mg/ml pyrazofurin were significantly less than those in untreated rats, and no obvious toxicity was observed in the treated rats.[9] Thus, the toxic effect of pyrazofurin *in vivo* is still obscure.

5-Ethynyl-1-β-D-ribofuranosylimidazol-4-carboxamide (EICAR) is a potent IMP (inosine monophosphate) dehydrogenase inhibitor, and 6′-(*R*)-6′-C-methyl neplanocine A (TJ-13025) is an inhibitor of S-adenosylhomocystein (SAH) hydrolase. EICAR inhibited multiple strains of RSV, PFLUV, MPSV, MLSV, and FLUV at 2 μg/ml or less concentrations *in vitro*. The EC_{50} values of EICAR against ortho- and paramyxoviruses were far less than those of ribavirin. TJ-13025 was also inhibitory against several strains of PFLUV, MPSV, and MLSV at a lower EC_{50} (less than 1 μg/ml) than ribavirin. However, TJ-13025 was not inhibitory against FLUV A and B and less inhibitory against RSV (Table 4.5). It is well known that FLUV does not utilize the SAH cycle to obtain methyl bases for the cap formation of its own mRNA. FLUV obtains methyl residues from a cap of host cell mRNA using its own endonuclease activity. Thus, the inhibition of SAH hydrolase does not affect the methylation of FLUV mRNA. On the other hand, the low susceptibility of RSV to TJ-13025 cannot be explained completely. Probably the efficiency of the SAH hydrolase system in host cells for mRNA cap formation is different among the host cells. As host cells for RSV replication we chose HeLa cells, which form apparent plaques of RSV in this antiviral assay and the difference of the host cells may have influenced the efficacy of TJ-13025 on RSV replication. TJ-13025 was modified at the 6′ position of neplanocin A. This modification made the compound resistant to adenosine deaminase activity and blocked the phosphorylation of the 6′-end of the compound. TJ-13025 exhibited enhanced anti-RNA virus activity and reduced cytotoxicity compared

TABLE 4.5. Inhibitory Effects of Ribavirin, EICAR, and TJ13025 on Replication of Ortho- and Paramyxoviruses *in Vitro*

	EC_{50} (µg/ml)[a]		
Virus Type and Strain	Ribavirin	EICAR	TJ13025
RSV			
A. Long	1.9	0.13	25
A. FM-58-8	3.5	0.09	25
A. NS-100	1.6	0.06	13.4
B. SM-6148	1.6	0.06	14.0
PFLUV			
1. Sendai Fushimi	30.0	0.97	15.0
2. CA Greer	25.8	0.63	0.47
3. HA-1 C243	27.2	0.56	0.16
MPSV			
ECXH-3-II	23.7	1.26	0.62
WV-3	13.9	0.46	0.43
F-1213	28.7	0.49	0.2
BMV-0320	32.8	0.57	0.44
MLSV			
Sugiyama	21.9	0.69	0.15
Toyoshima	9.1	0.9	0.25
Edmonston	66.7	1.51	0.2
SSPE Yamagata 1	8.6	0.32	0.12
FLUV			
A. Bangkok H1N1	1.5	0.4	>100
A. Ishikawa H3N2	5.3	2.3	>100
B. Singapore	1.4	0.44	>100

[a] Average values for three to four independent experiments.

with the original substance, neplanocin A. As shown in Table 4.5, when the EC_{50} values for the paramyxoviruses except RSV (PFLUV, MPSV, and MLSV) were compared, the result was 10- to 330-fold lower in EICAR and TJ-13025 than in ribavirin.[10,11]

In Table 4.6, anti-myxovirus activities of the selected nucleoside analogues are summarized and comparatively listed as EC_{50} (µg/ml) values *in vitro*. As shown in the table, pyrazofurin and 3-deazaguanine exhibited potent anti-RSV, MLSV, SSPE, and FLUV activities. EICAR and TJ-13025 are also broadly effective agents for paramyxoviruses. Their EC_{50}s for paramyxovirus (except for RSV) *in vitro* were 16- to 160-fold less than that of ribavirin. Since antiviral efficacy against PFLUV, MPSV, and MLSV are potent *in vitro*, EICAR and TJ-13025 might be anti-paramyxovirus drugs. However, pyrazorfurin exhibited some toxicity to chicken embryos,[9] and TJ-13025 is toxic for rapidly growing cells[11]; therefore they still have to be examined in animal studies before

TABLE 4.6. Inhibitory Effects of Selected Nucleoside Analogues on Replication of Ortho- and Paramyxoviruses

Virus[a]	EC$_{50}$ (µg/ml)					
	Ribavirin	EICAR	Mizoribin	Pyrazofurin	3-Deazaguanin	TJ13025
RSV	3.0	0.1	2.9	0.09	5.5	19.4
PFLUV	39.5	2.4	16.5	NT[c]	NT	0.33
MPSV	22.3	0.78	30[b]	NT	NT	0.4
MLSV	32.7	1.0	1.8	0.13	0.8	0.2
SSPE[b]	9	0.3	NT	0.12	0.7	0.1
FLUV A	4.25	0.43	8.7	0.3	3.5	>100
FLUV B	6.2	3.0	3.45	0.16	3.9	>100
FLUV C[b]	2.8	NT	NT	0.16	3.3	>100

[a] Data are averages of EC$_{50}$ which are obtained from two to four different strains. RSV contains four strains of type A and B, and PFLUV contains type 1, 2, and 3. MPSV and MLSV each contain three strains. FLUV A includes subtypes H1N1 and H3N2.
[b] Data from only one strain.
[c] Not tested.

the development of these compounds as antiviral drugs. Finally, mizoribin is a compound that has been applied clinically as an immunosuppressive drug. Mizoribine is a strong IMP dehydrogenase inhibitor and inhibitory against RSV, FLUV, and MLSV replication *in vitro*.[12] If short time usage of mizoribin are possible for the respiratory infections and it does not excessively suppress the immune system, this compound may be applicable for the therapy of MLSV and PFLUV infections instead of ribavirin.

Sulfated Polysaccharides

Sulfated polysaccharides such as dextran sulfate have been reported to be potent and selective inhibitors of several envelope viruses.[13,14] Dextran sulfate, polyvinyl alcohol sulfate (PVAS), and polymers of acyclic acid and vinyl alcohol sulfate (PAVAS) have been shown to be potent inhibitors of RSV, FLUV A, and HIV-1 but not of other myxoviruses (FLUV B, PFLUV 3, MLSV) or simian immunodeficiency virus (SIV). Hosoya et al.[15] analyzed an amino acid sequence of HA2 glycoprotein of FLUV, F1 glycoprotein of paramyxoviruses, and the transmembrane glycoproteins of HIV and SIV and found a common amino acid sequence in sulfated polysaccharide-sensitive viruses. A triple sequence of Phe-Leu-Gly is shared in the envelope glycoproteins of RSV, FLUV A, and HIV 1, which were sensitive to dextran sulfate, PVAS, and PAVAS, but not in those of FLUV B, PFLUV 3,

TABLE 4.7. Inhibitory Effect of OKU-40, OKU-41, and DS on the Replication of Enveloped Viruses

Virus (strain)	EC_{50} (μg/ml)		
	OKU-40 (8×10^6)[a]	OKU-41 (5×10^5)	DS (7×10^4)
HSV 1 (KOS)	4.5	0.97	0.1
FLUV A (H3N2 Ishikawa)	1.1	0.25	1.4
FLUV B (Singapore)	8.3	4.0	>100
RSV (Long)	2.0	19.0	0.2
RSV (FM-58-8)	3.0	NT	0.2
MLSV (Edmonston)	40	NT	>100
PFLUV 2 (Greer)	0.8	25.3	NT
PFLUV 3	>100	>100	>100
HIV-1	1.7	1.7	1.1

[a]Values in parentheses molecular weights of polysaccharides.

MLSV, or SIV, which are resistant to the sulfated polysaccharides (polymers).[15]

Sulfated and non-sulfated polysaccharides exist in several natural substances because they comprise a critical substance in the cell wall of microorganisms. A naturally sulfated mucopolysaccharide extracted from a marine plant *Dinoflagellata* (OKU-40) and an artificially sulfated polysaccharide prepared from a marine *Pseudomonas* (OKU-41) displayed antiviral activities against several myxoviruses and HIV-1. OKU-40 and OKU-41 were highly inhibitory against FLUV A, FLUV, B, RSV, and PFLUV 2. Although dextran sulfate (DS) could not inhibit replication of FLUV B, and MLSV, naturally obtained sulfated polysaccharides (OKU-40) were able to inhibit their replication. OKU-40, OKU-41, and DS were not active against PFLUV 3 replication (Table 4.7). Although we were not able to analyze the sugar sequence of the polysaccharide, the composition of the sugar moiety was analyzed. The molar ratio of sugars in OKU-40 is glucose 1.4, galactose 1.0, urinate 1.4, and sulfate 3.7, and that in OKU-41 is galacturonic acid 2, *N*-acetylgalactosamine 2, galactose 1, *N*-acetylglucosamine 1, and alanine 1. OKU-40 and OKU-41 are noncytotoxic substances whereas we were concerned about their anti-coagulating effect on normal plasma. We examined the influence of OKU-40, OKU-41, and DS on prothrombin time (PT) and activated partial thromboplastine time (APTT). As shown in Table 4.8, PT was not affected by 10 μg/ml of OKU-40 or -41, or 100 μg/ml of OKU-40. APTT was almost within the normal range by addition of OKU-40 and -41 at a concentration of 10 μg/ml. On the other hand, DS prolonged APTT at 10 μg/ml and extremely prolonged PT and APTT at 100 μg/ml.[16,17]

TABLE 4.8. Influence of OKU-40, OKU-41, and DS on Anticoagulant Activity of Normal Human Plasma

Compound (Molecular Weight)	Concentration (µg/ml)	PT[a] (seconds)	APTT[b] (seconds)
OKU-40 (8×10^6)	10	10.9	48.8
	100	14.4	>300
OKU-41 (5×10^5)	10	10.5	45.3
DS (5×10^6)	10	13.4	234
	100	>300	>300
Water		10.0	32.5
Normal human plasma		9.9	35.0

[a] PT, prothorombin time.
[b] APTT, activated partial thromboplastin time.

OKU-40 and -41 are nontoxic and broad-spectrum anti-myxovirus substances. They are inhibitory against FLUV B, PFLUV, and MLSV, which were not sensitive to DS or other synthetic sulfated polymers. Since these substances exist abundantly in nature and are easy to extract from microorganisms, it is worth of investigating them further to develop anti-myxovirus drugs from these substances.

Polyoxometalates

Polyoxometalates (POM) are soluble inorganic cluster-like compounds formed principally of an oxide anion and early transition metal cations such as tungsten (W), molybdenium (Mo), niobium(Nb), antimony (Sb), vanadium (V), and so on. Several POMs have been reported to inhibit the replication of HIV, herpes simplex virus (HSV), FLUV, and RSV.[18-21] We examined 25 POMs for anti-ortho-, anti-paramyxo-, and anti-HIV-1 activities *in vitro*. Of the 25 compounds evaluated, 24 showed anti-FLUV A activity, 11 showed anti-RSV, 6 showed anti-MLSV, and 23 showed anti-HIV-1 activities at lower concentrations than those producing cytotoxicity. Among the effective compounds, HS-054 [$Na_{16}Fe_4(H_2O)_2(P_2W_{15}O_{56})_2nH_2O$] and HS-058 [$K_{10}Fe_4(H_2O)_2(PW_9O_{32})_2nH_2O$] exhibited potent and broad-spectrum anti-myxovirus activities. Both compounds were effective for additional myxoviruses including FLUV B, RSV B, and PFLUV 2. HS-054 was inhibitory against MPSV and PFLUV 3 at a relatively high concentration (20–28 µM), whereas HS-058 was not inhibitory at 50 µM. HS-058 inhibited both adsorption and the fusion process of RSV infection, whereas it only inhibited the fusion process of FLUV to the cellular membrane.[22]

We examined further 60 POMs for anti-FLUV A activity and 16 compounds exhibited antiviral activity with SIs within a range of 4–20. Six compounds showed SIs of more than 20. PM-504 [$K_9H_5(Ge_2Ti_6W_{18}O_{77})16H_2O$] and PM-523 [$iPrNH_3]_6H(PTi_2W_{10}O_{38}(O_2)_2)H_2O$] showed SIs of more than 308 and 167, respectively. Their EC_{50}s for FLUV A were 1.3 and 2.4 μM, respectively. PM-523 showed anti-RSV activity (EC_{50} = 3.0 μM), anti-PFLUV 2 activity (EC_{50} = 2.7 μM), and anti-MLSV activity (EC_{50} = 11.0 μM). The anti-FLUV B activity of PM-523 was rather weak but exhibited an EC_{50} of 39 μM.[23] When we investigated the mechanism of anti-FLUV A activity of the compounds by FACScan analysis of FLUV-bound cells for adsorption and by fluorescent dequenching assay for membrane fusion, PM-504 inhibited both viral adsorption and membrane fusion whereas PM-523 inhibited only fusion between the viral envelope and cellular membrane (Figs. 4.3 and 4.4).[23]

During the search for the broad-spectirum antimyxovirus activity of POM, we found that titanium (Ti)- or vanadium (V)-substituted Keggin (or Keggin sandwich)-type polyoxotungstates possess broad-spectrum anti-RNA virus activities. From POMs that were examined for anti-myxovirus activity previously, 7 POMs which have the above-mentioned chemical futures were selected and examined precisely for anti-orthomyxovirus, paramyxovirus, and flavivirus (Dengue fever virus, DFV) and HIV activities. As shown in Table 4.9, all compounds were broadly inhibitory against FLUV A, RSV, PFLUV 2, canine distemper virus (CDV, belonging to the morbilli paramyxovirus in Table 4.1), DFV, and HIV-1. Among these compounds, PM-43, -47, -1001, and -1002 were V-containing polyoxotungstates and PM-518, 520, 523 were Ti-containing polyoxotungstates. Except for PM-1001 and -1002, which had the Keggin sandwich structure, all the other POMs had the Keggin structure.[24] Next, we expanded the research to investigate anti-coronavirus activities of certain Ti- and V-containing POMs. Coronavirus is a positive-strand RNA virus and is covered with an envelope that is obtained at the release of the virus from the cell membrane. Coronaviruses are infectious in a number of animals, namely, pigs, cattle, cats, birds, and so on. A coronavirus that infects humans causes a severe, sometimes mortal respiratory disease called SARS. We examined 13 POMs with the Ti- and V-substituted form for antiviral activities against TGEV (pig gastroenteritis virus), FIPV (feline peritonitis virus), and SARS coronavirus *in vitro*. Table 4.10 shows the EC_{50} values of the selected POMs for coronaviruses. As shown in the table, V-substituted Keggin sandwich-type POMs displayed a high SI for SARS coronavirus. PM-1001, PM-1002, PM-1207, and PM-1208 were all V-containing

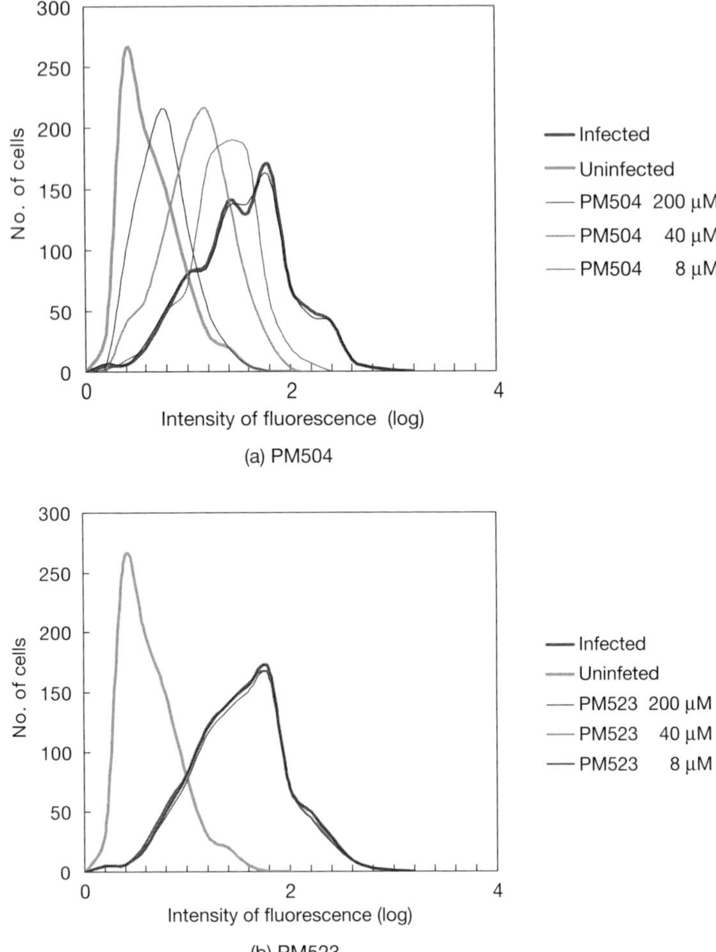

Fig. 4.3. FACS analysis of FLUV A bound cells. MDCK cells were mixed with FLUV A at a MOI of 1 and incubated at 37°C for 1.5 hr. During the incubation, 8–200 µM of compounds were combined with the virus cell mixture. After incubation, binding of FLUV to cells was examined by FACS using indirect immunofluorescence with anti-FLUV A mouse serum and FITC conjugated goat anti-mouse IgG antibody. The abscissa indicates intensity of populations of infected cells and the ordinate indicates the number of cells. The rightmost line is a population of infected cells without compounds, and the leftmost line is that of uninfected cells. See color insert.

Keggin sandwich structured compounds and have the same core structure of $(VO)_3(XW_9O_{33})$(Here X = Sb, As, or Bi). However, the V_3 of 1001, 1207, and 1208 consist of two V^{IV} and one V^V while that of PM1002 consists of three V^V. PM-1001 and PM-1002 have the same core ion of Sb (X = Sb) and exhibited broad-spectrum anti-RNA virus

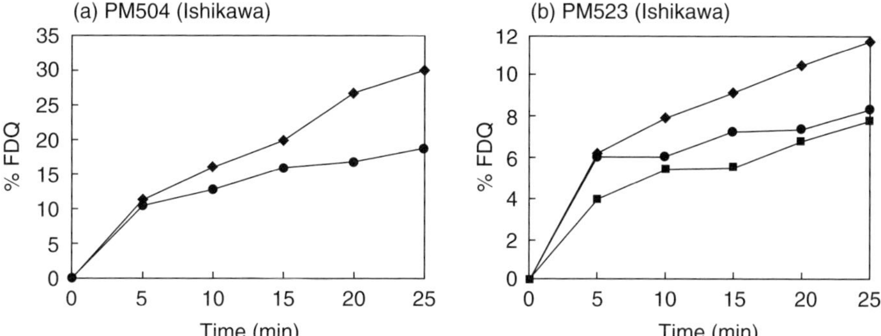

Fig. 4.4. Effect of polyoxometalates on the dequenching of R-18 on FLUV A envelope by fusion with the cellular membrane. The increase in fluorescence was expressed in % FDQ. Control ($\blacklozenge$), 5 μM ($\bullet$), 25 μM ($\blacksquare$) of compounds were added.

TABLE 4.9. Antiviral Activities of Polyoxometalates Against Several RNA Viruses *in Vitro*

	Core Metal	EC_{50} (μM)[a] for					
Compound	Ion	DFV	FLUV A	RSV	PFLUV 2	CDV[b]	HIV-1
PM-43[c]	V, W	10.7	8.4	1.6	>100	7.5	0.3
PM-47	V, W	10.5	11.5	29.0	67.1	6.0	0.03
PM-518	Ti, W	36.8	62.3	26.5	53.2	>50	2.0
PM-520	Ti, W	11.7	45.2	0.74	23.2	7.4	2.0
PM-523	Ti, W	>61.5	5.6	1.3	2.5	7.3	0.3
PM-1001	V, Sb, W	0.45	1.8	<0.16	1.1	5.7	0.14
PM-1002	V, Sb, W	2.0	4.6	0.75	0.75	2.8	0.03
Ribavirin		>100	5.0	3.9	14.0	73.6	NT[d]

[a] Average values for three to seven independent experiments.
[b] EC_{50} was determined by the plaque reduction method. For other viruses it was determined by the MTT method.
[c] PM-43, -47, -518, -520, and -523 had Keggin structures. PM-1001 and PM-1002 had Keggin sandwich structures.
[d] NT, not tested.

activity *in vitro* (Table 4.9) and had low EC_{50} values to FLUV A, RSV, PFLUV 2, as well as SARS coronavirus (Table 4.10).[25] If it were possible to develop gauzes that adhered PM-1001 or -1002 as medical masks during epidemic seasons of respiratory infectious diseases, these compounds may strongly inhibit respiratory infections by a broad spectrum of RNA viruses.

TABLE 4.10. Antiviral Activities of Polyoxometalates Against Coronaviruses

Compound	Core Metal Ions[c]	EC$_{50}$ (µM)[a]			SI[b]		
		TGFV[d]	FIPV[d]	SARS-V[d]	TGEV	FIPV	SARS-V
PM-504	Ge, Ti, W	1.4	0.4	3.5	>12.8	**>46.7**	>14.3
PM-518	Ti, W	2.1	>32.9	>50	>15.6	<1.0	<1.0
PM-520	Ti, W	1.4	0.76	4.9	>20.4	**>38.5**	>10.3
PM-523	Ti, W	2.5	>32.0	>50	**>32**	<1.0	<1.0
PM-802	Eu, Al, Nb	0.5	0.03	>50	4.9	**97.2**	<1.0
PM-1001	V, Sb, W	0.14	0.2	0.7	**83.6**	**84.4**	**>70**
PM-1002	V, Sb, W	0.6	NT	0.25	18.6	—	**>400**
PM-1207	V, As, W	1.9	0.09	0.9	>9.3	**35.2**	**>54**
PM-1208	V, Bi, W	2.0	>3.6	2.7	>8.1	<1.0	>18.4
PM-1210	Bi, W, V	1.6	0.74	0.76	>6.6	>14.3	**>66**
PM-1213	V, W	1.7	>10.5	0.47	>18.2	<1.0	**106**

[a] EC$_{50}$ and CC$_{50}$ (50% cytotoxic concentration) were determined by the average of three independent experiments.

[b] The host cells used for the CC$_{50}$ determination were CPK (derived from porcine kidney) cells for TGFV, fcwf-4 (derived from feline embryo fibroblast) cells for FIPV, and Vero cells for SARS-V, respectively. The SIs greater than 30 are indicated in boldface.

[c] PM-518, -520, and -523 have Keggin structures; PM-1001, -1002, -1207, -1208, and -1213 have Keggin sandwich structures. PM-504, -802, and -1210 have particular structures—that is, Keggin dimmer, Lindqvist triangle, and Keggin triangle, respectively.

[d] TGFV, transmissible gastroenteritis virus of swine; FIPV, feline infectious peritonitis virus; SARS-V, SARS coronavirus.

RESULT OF SCREENING OF INHIBITORS FOR SPECIFIC VIRUS

Influenza A Virus

Recently, the specific anti-FLUV drugs oseltamivir and zanamivir were developed and have been used clinically for the treatment of influenza. These drugs are specific inhibitors of FLUV neuraminidase and inhibit the release of FLUV A and B from infected cells. On the other hand, in spite of the efforts by several workers, detection of specific inhibitors of the RNA polymerase of FLUV is thus far unsuccessful and still in the process of laboratory studies. Antisense oligonucleotides can be utilized as specific inhibitors of targeted viral gene expression—that is, inhibition of RNA (DNA) replication and transcription.

Takaku and his working group synthesized several antisense oligodeoxynucleotide (ODN) targeted to the FLUV RNA polymerase gene—that is PA, PB1, and PB2. Among the several antisense ODN synthesized, they found a 20-mer antisense ODN targeted to the

20 mar nucleotide sequence of PB2 initiation codon

3′ aag aaa   ggu aua   acu uau au 5′

CDRDON-Al-PB2-as

CC TTC TTT CCA TAT TGA ATA TA CC

R   R

CC aag   aaa ggu   aua   acu uau au CC

Fig. 4.5. The structure of circular dumbbell RNA/DNA chimera with antisense ODN targeted to the FLUV A PB2 AUG initiation codon. Capital letters express DNA nucleotide sequence, and lowercase letters express RNA nucleotide sequence. Antisense sequences are underlined. R represents an alkyl loop (hexa-ethylene glycol) structure.

initiation codon of PB2 mRNA which showed specific inhibition for mRNA transcription.[26] There are three problems with antisense ODN therapy. First, antisense ODN must be sufficiently resistant to both 3′ and 5′ exonucleases as well as the endonuclease present in tissue or plasma. Second, antisense ODN must have sufficient affinity for the targeted viral mRNA to bind with a high degree of specificity, and third, the antisense ODN must be delivered to infected cells efficiently and be taken up by the cells in adequate quantities. For the delivery of antisense ODN, they used liposome encapsulation of the materials.[27] For the stability of the nucleotides, they used at first phosphorothioate antisense ODN. However, phosphorothioate antisense ODN hybridized more weakly with the complementary nucleotide than the unmodified antisense ODN. Therefore, they subsequently devised circular dumbbell RNA/DNA chimeras for antisense ODN. The circular dumbbell RNA/DNA chimeras with antisense ODN sequence targeted to FLUV PB2 mRNA (Fig. 4.5) were shown to be resistant to digestion by exonuclease, sustained a sufficient affinity to PB2 mRNA, and efficiently suppressed mRNA expression in FLUV A-infected MDCK cells when delivered to cells by a cationic liposome system.[28] In the figure, R = 18-*o*-dimethoxyltriethylene glycol. When they introduced the antisense ODN into FLUV A-infected mice inravenously with cationic liposomes, the mean survival time of the mice was significantly prolonged.[29] The antisense ODN for PB2 mRNA with the structure of a circular dumbbell RNA/DNA chimera could prove to be an effective and specific therapeutic agent for FLUV infection.

Respiratory Syncytial Virus

For the treatment of RSV infections, aerosol ribavirin has been approved in the United States. As specific anti-RSV agents, antisense RNA conjugated with 2′,5′-oligoadenylate (2-5A) and humanized monoclonal antibody for the RSV F-glycoprotein have been reported. The former is designated RBI-034 and the latter is commercialized as palivizumab.[30–33]

From a random screening of anti-RSV compounds, we found a sulfated sialyl lipid (NMSO3) and a benzodithiin derivative (RD3-0028) to be potent and selective anti-RSV agents *in vitro* and *in vivo* (Fig. 4.6). When we examined the EC_{50} value of these compounds and ribavirin for several laboratory and clinical strains of RSV, the EC_{50}s of NMSO3 were almost 50- to 165-fold less and those of RD3-0028 were 2.3- to 8-fold less than the EC_{50}s of ribavirn (Table 4.11). Both compounds interacted with the early (adsorption) and late stages (probably fusion and penetration) of virus replication. We also examined the anti-RSV activity of both compounds *in vivo*, using intranasal infection of RSV to cotton rats or immunosuppressed mice (by cyclophosphamide injection). NMSO3 was injected intraperitoneally at a dose of 100 mg/ kg once a day 1–3 days after viral infection. RD3-0028 was administrated as an aerosol for 2 hours twice daily (1.25–7 mg/ml). After 3 days of treatments, the animals were sacrificed and the viral titer in the lungs

NMSO3

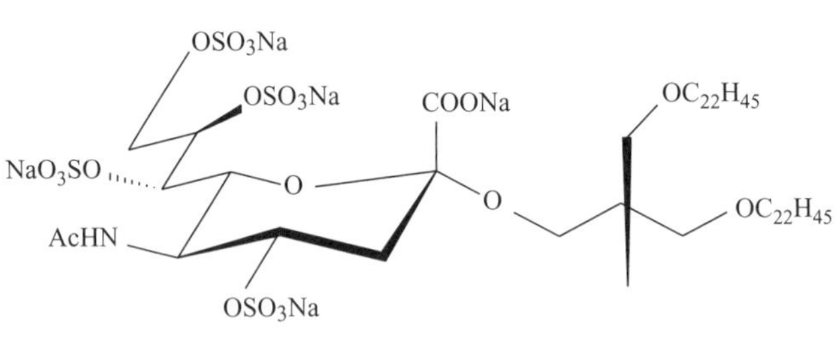

RD-3-0028

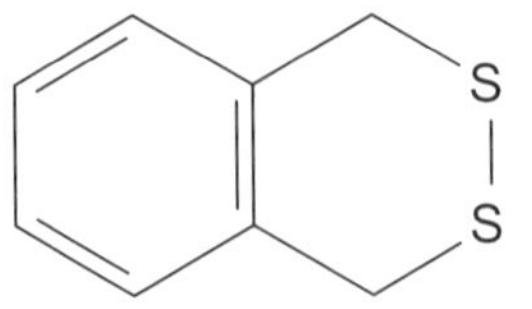

Fig. 4.6. Anti-RSV compounds. Top: NMSO3. Bottom: RD-3-0028.

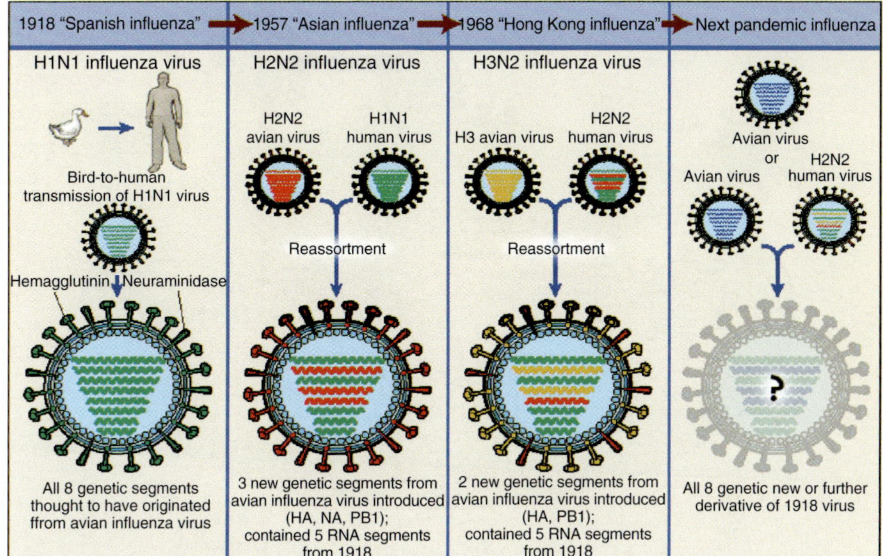

Fig. 1.1. The two mechanisms whereby pandemic influenza originates. In 1918, the "Spanish influenza" H1N1 virus closely related to an avian virus adapted to replicate efficiently in humans. In 1957 and 1968, reassortment events led to, respectively, the "Asian influenza" H2N2 virus and the "Hong Kong influenza" H3N2 virus. The "Asian influenza" H2N2 virus acquired three genetic segments from an avian species [a hemagglutinin, a neuraminidase, and a polymerase (PB1) gene]. The "Hong Kong influenza" H3N2 virus acquired two genetic segments from an avian species (hemagglutinin and PB1). Future pandemic strains could arise through either mechanism.[10] (Taken from Belshe.[10])

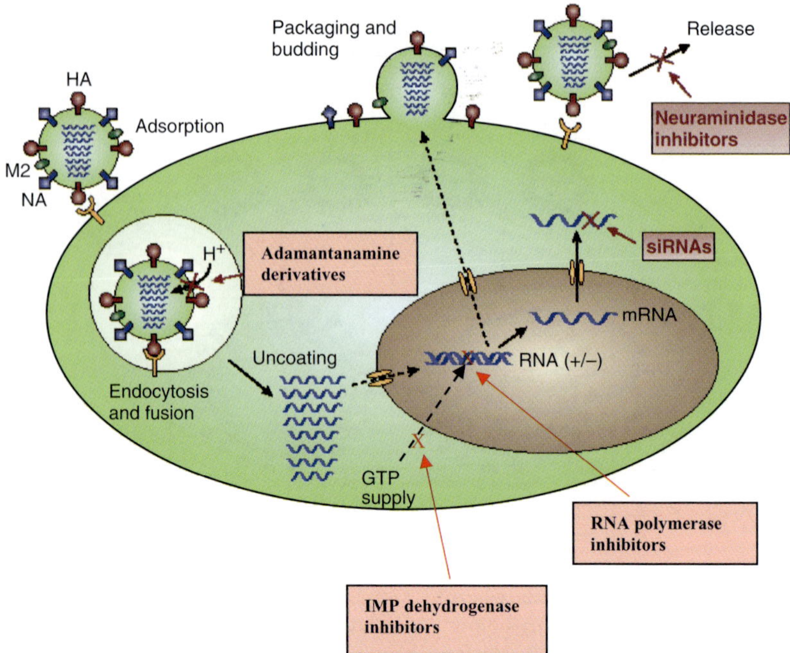

Fig. 1.2. Inhibition of influenza virus replication cycle by antivirals. After binding to sialic acid receptors, influenza virions are internalized by receptor-mediated endocytosis. The low pH in the endosome triggers the fusion of viral and endosomal membranes, and the influx of H^+ ions through the M2 channel releases the viral RNA genes in the cytoplasm. Adamantanamine derivatives block this uncoating step. RNA replication/ transcription occurs in the nucleus. This process can be blocked by inhibitors of IMP dehydrogenase (a cellular enzyme) or viral RNA polymerase. The stability of the viral mRNA and its translation to viral protein may be prevented by siRNAs. Packaging and budding of virions occur at the cytoplasmic membrane. Neuraminidase inhibitors block the release of the newly formed virions from the infected cells. (Taken from Palese,[11] with modifications.[1])

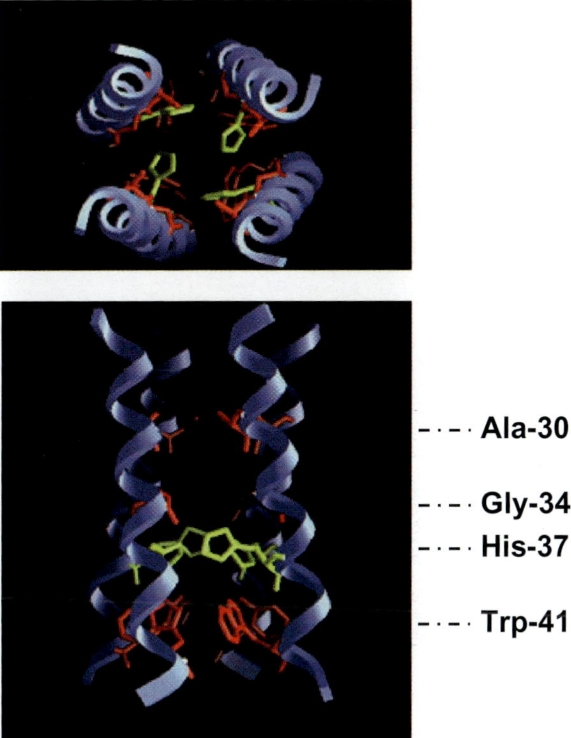

Fig. 1.3. Model of the proposed transmembrane domain of the M2 protein, showing top view as seen from the extracellular side and a cross section in the plane of the lipid layer. Residues that were identified as facing the ion-conducting aqueous pore are indicated. (Taken from Shuck et al.[14])

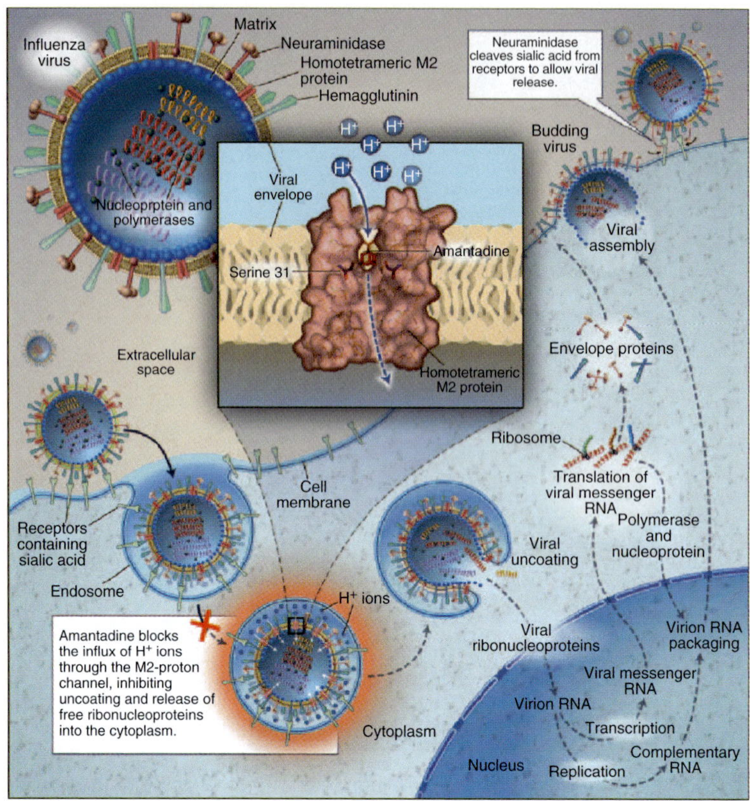

Fig. 1.5. Mechanism of action of and development of resistance to M2 inhibitors. In the absence of amantadine, the proton channel mediates an influex of H[+] ions into the infecting virion early in the viral replication cycle, which facilitates the dissociation of the ribonucleoproteins from the virion interior and allows them to be released into the cytoplasm and transported into the cell nucleus. In highly pathogenic avian viruses (H5 and H7), the M2-proton channel protects the hemagglutinin from acid-induced inactivation in the trans-Golgi network during transport to the cell surface. In the presence of amantadine, the channel is blocked and replication is inhibited. The serine at position 31 lies partially in the protein–protein interface and partially in the channel (see inset). Replacement of serine by a larger asparagine leads to the loss of amantadine binding and the restoration of channel function. Depending on the particular amino acid, other mutations at position 26, 27, 30, or 34 may inhibit amantadine binding or allow binding without the loss of ion-channel function. [Taken from Hayden.[24] Inset courtesy of Rupert Russell, Phillip Spearpoint, and Alan Hay (National Institute for Medical Research, London).]

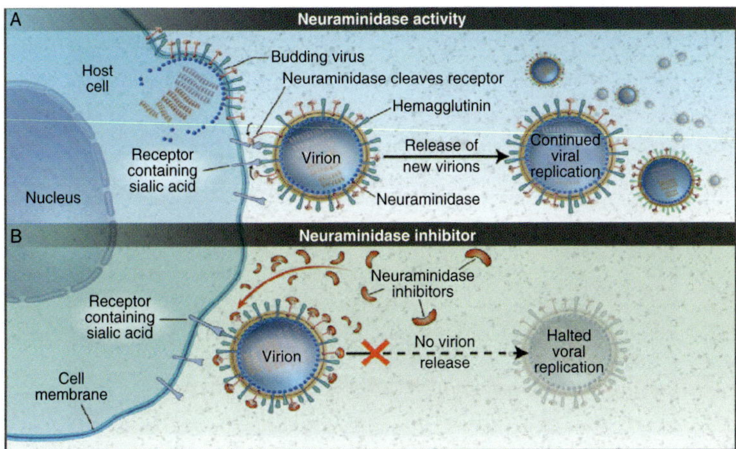

Fig. 1.6. Mechanism of action of neuraminidase inhibitors. Neuraminidase inhibitors, such as zanamivir and oseltamivir (see Fig. 1.8), interfere with the release of progeny influenza virions from the surface of infected host cells. In doing so, the neuraminidase inhibitors prevent virus infection of new host cells and thereby halt the spread of infection in the respiratory tract. The neuraminidase cleaves off sialic acid (*N*-acetylneuraminic acid) from the cell receptor for influenza virus (see Fig. 1.7), so that the newly formed virus particles can be released from the cells. Neuraminidase inhibitors prevent this process. (Taken from Moscona.[31])

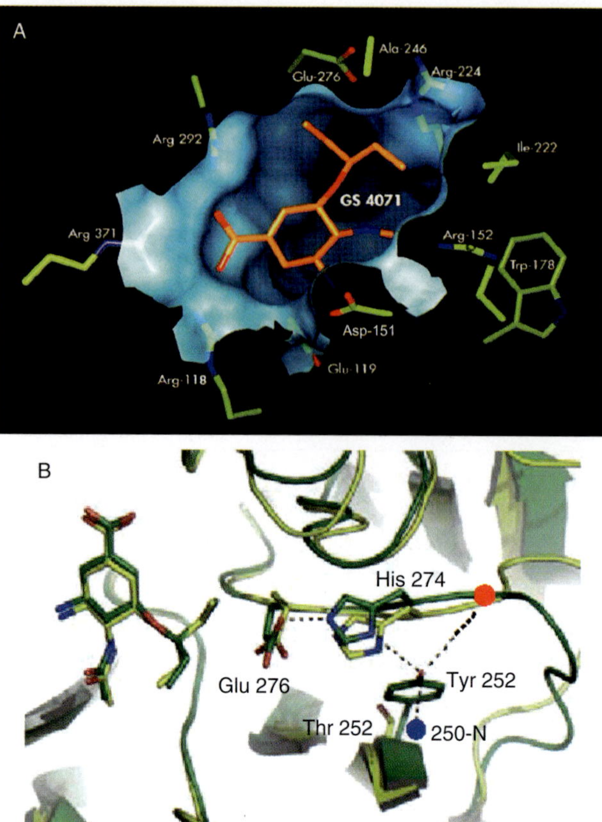

Fig. 1.9. GS4071 within the active site of the influenza A viral neuraminidase. Locations of oseltamivir-resistance mutations (i.e., H274Y) showing that the tyrosine at position 252 is involved in a network of hydrogen bonds in group-1 (H5N1 and H1N1) neuraminidases.[44] (Figure 1.9A was taken from Kim et al.[37] and De Clercq,[43] and Fig. 1.9B was taken from Russell et al.[44])

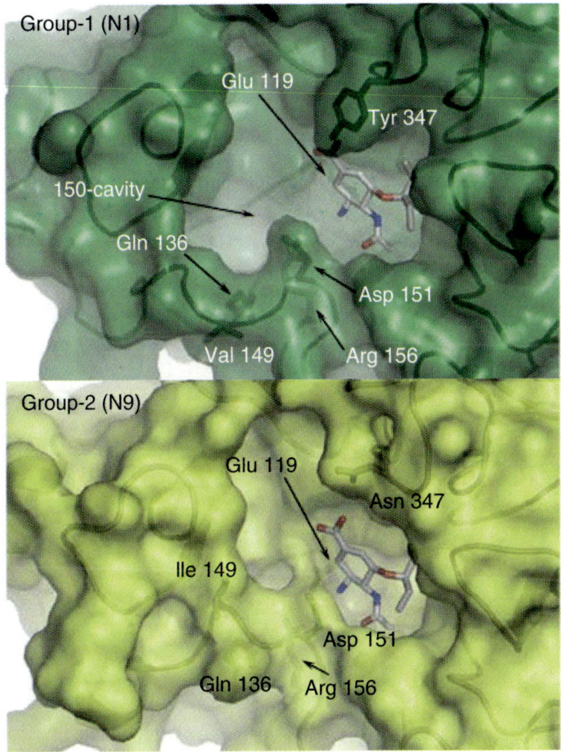

Fig. 1.10. Molecular surfaces of group-1 (N1) and group-2 (N9) neuraminidases with bound oseltamivir showing the 150-cavity in the group-1 (N1) structure that arises because of the distinct conformation of the 150-loop. (Taken from Russell et al.[44])

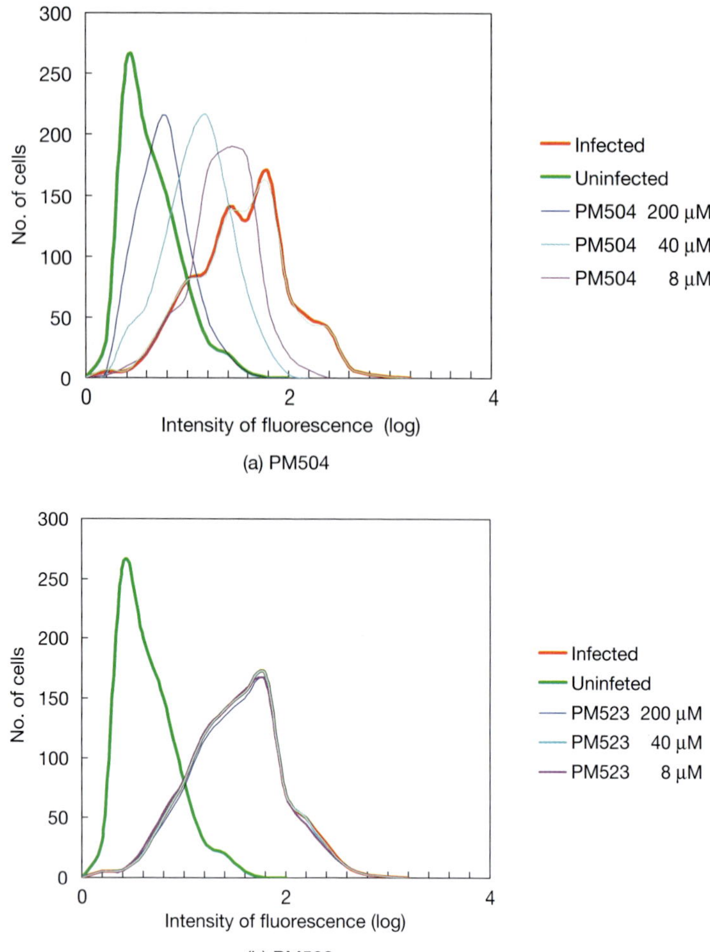

Fig. 4.3. FACS analysis of FLUV A bound cells. MDCK cells were mixed with FLUV A at a MOI of 1 and incubated at 37°C for 1.5 hr. During the incubation, 8–200 µM of compounds were combined with the virus cell mixture. After incubation, binding of FLUV to cells was examined by FACS using indirect immunofluorescence with anti-FLUV A mouse serum and FITC conjugated goat anti-mouse IgG antibody. The abscissa indicates intensity of populations of infected cells and the ordinate indicates the number of cells. The rightmost line is a population of infected cells without compounds, and the leftmost line is that of uninfected cells.

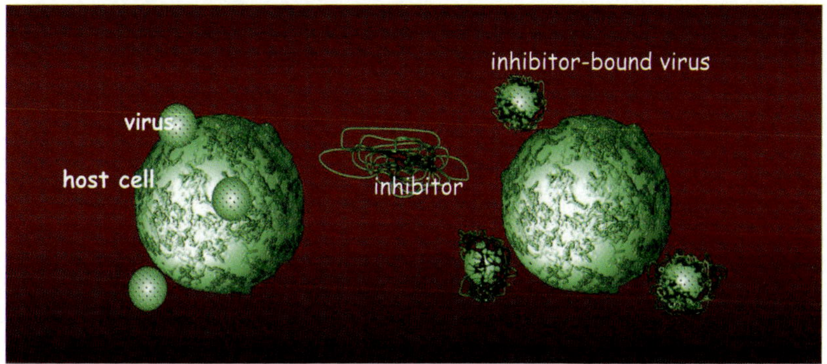

Fig. 8.1. Anti-adhesion principle. Oligosaccharide (OS) of host cell serves as receptor for virus. Natural mucin or synthetic bulky conjugate of this OS able to attain high-affinity binding to virus particle and to inhibit virus-to-cell binding, thus blocking infectivity.

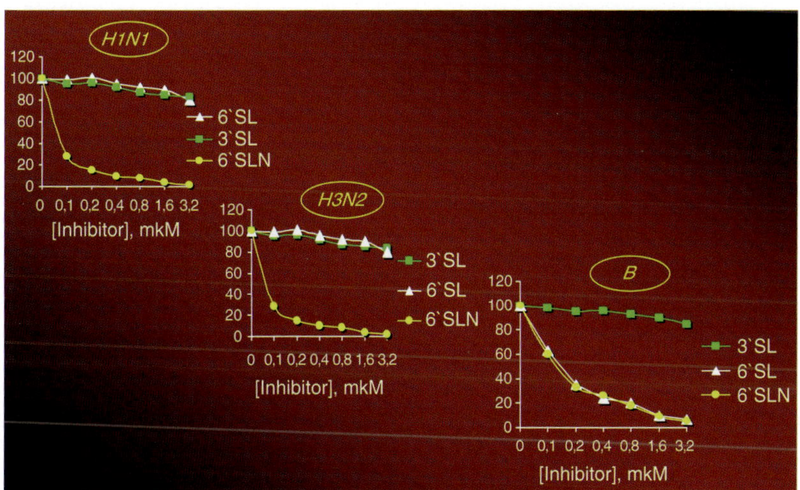

Fig. 8.2. High specificity of modern human H1, H3, and B influenza viruses toward trisaccharide 6′SLN. Solid-phase assay (FBI) in inhibitory mode, polyacrylamide (30 kDa) conjugates of 6′SLN, 6′SL, and 3′SLN as inhibitors. Similar results were observed with all other modern isolates propagated in MDCK or Vero cell culture.

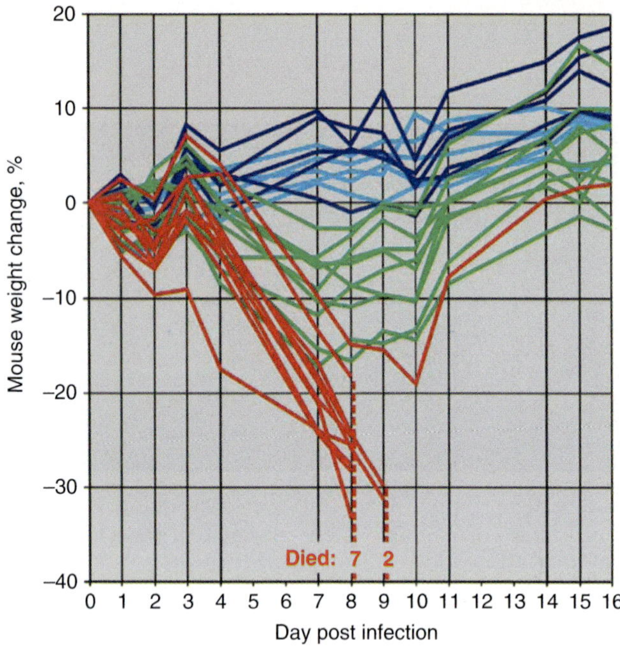

Fig. 8.3. Weight dynamics and survival of A/Sn mice from noninfected control group treated with placebo (blue); noninfected control group treated with 6′-SLN-PAA (cyan); and virus-infected mice treated either with placebo (red, 10 mice) or 6′-SLN-PAA (green). On days 2–5 after infection (10^3 IU of virus), mice were treated by 10-min exposures with 6′-SLN-PAA in aerosol form every 2 hr with 10-hr night break. The preparation dose (for each administration) was ~1 nmol by sialic acid per mouse. *P*-value for WL difference between the two control groups and between the two infected groups was 0.528 and <0.001, respectively. (Adapted from Ref. 14.)

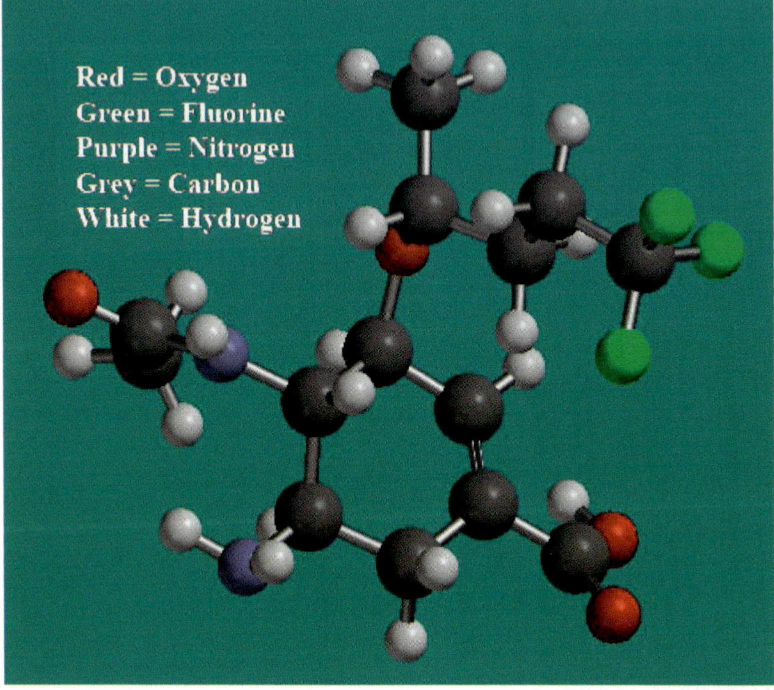

Fig. 9.2. The minimized energy geometry of compound (**II**) obtained from Spartan '06.

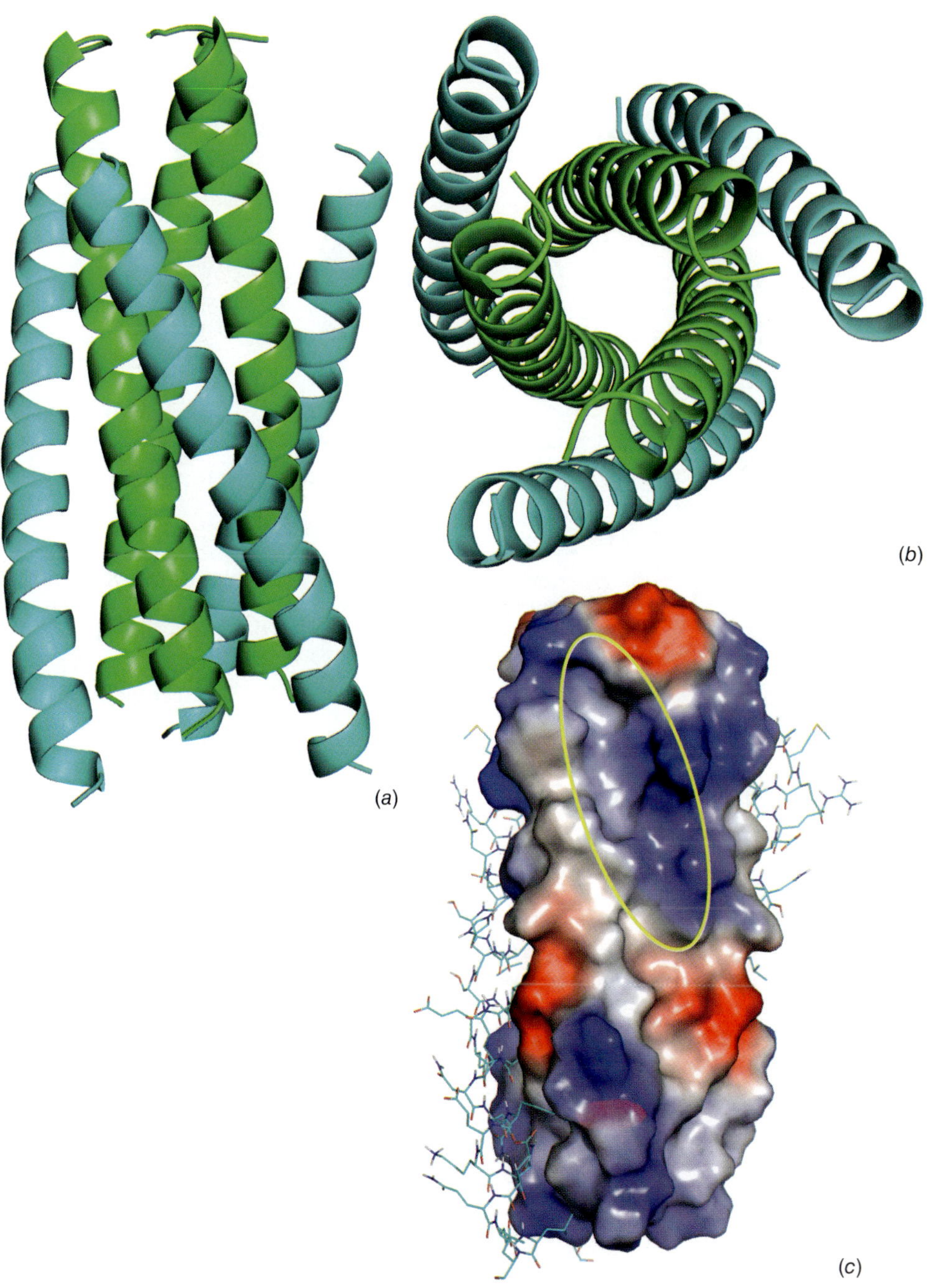

Fig. 10.2. Crystal structure of the fusion core of the HIV HR1/HR2 6-helix bundle. (a) Side view of the α-helix structure. HR1 (green) forms a tightly bound trimer surrounded by three HR2 (cyan). (Source of the structure: PDB code 1AIK.) (b) Top view of the fusion core. (c) Fusion structure (HR1 in space-filling form to show the surface potential and HR2 in stick form) with one HR2 removed to show the cavities (circled), which are targets for small-molecule design.

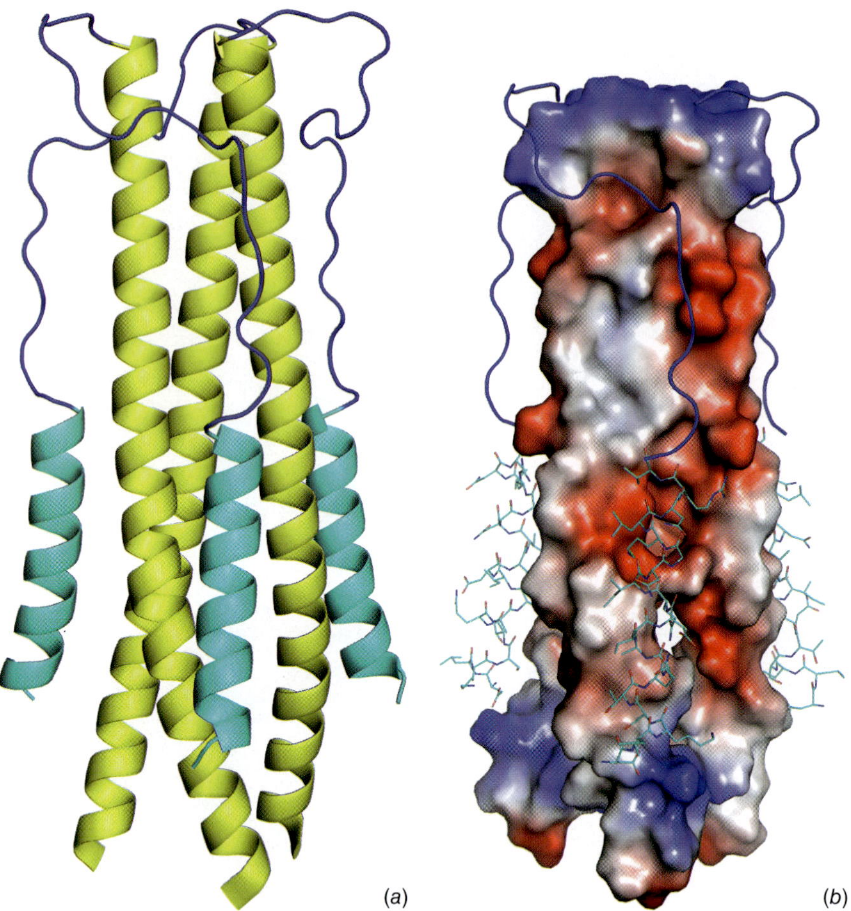

Fig. 10.3. Crystal structure of the HR1/HR2 complex of influenza virus HA. (a) Typical α-helix structure of the three long HR1 (yellow) surrounded by three shorter HR2 (cyan) with some flexible loops shown in blue. (Source of the structure: PDB code 2viu.) (b) Space-filling presentation of the structure in part a to show the HR1 surface potential and the bound HR2 in stick.

TABLE 4.11. Anti-RSV Activities of NMSO3 and RD3-0028 for Several Laboratory and Clinical Strains

Virus Strain (Type)	EC$_{50}$ (µM)			
	NMSO3	Ribavirin	RD3-0028	Ribavirin
Long (A)[a]	0.2	10.5	4.5	36.0
A2 (A)[a]	NT[c]	NT	11.1	35.1
FM-58-8 (A)[b]	0.15	24.1	7.1	47.5
K-656 (A)[b]	0.3	14.7	NT	NT
N-869 (A)[b]	0.12	11.9	NT	NT
NS-100 (A)[b]	NT	NT	8.9	41.4
SM-6148 (B)[b]	0.13	7.7	5.6	13.2
Average	0.18	13.8	7.44	34.6

[a] Laboratory strain.
[b] Fresh clinical strain.
[c] NT, not tested.

of the animals determined. The viral titer in the lungs of the treated animals significantly decreased compared with the untreated animals. When the section of infected lung was observed histologically, the evidence of interstitial pneumonia observed in untreated animals (i.e., mononucleal cell infiltration in peribronchial and perivascular spaces, as well as thickness of the alveolar wall) was markedly suppressed in the treated animals.[34,35]

Small-Molecule Virus-Specific Inhibitors from References

As antiviral agents, small-molecule compounds have advantages over large-molecule compounds because they are easy to synthesize in the laboratory, soluble in water in many cases, and applicable to systemic administration *in vivo*. Against RSV and MLSV virus-specific small-molecule compounds have been reported to be potent inhibitors. The one for RSV was found from a random screening and bound the hydrophobic cavity of the RSV fusion protein, while the one for MLSV was designed to dock in the pocket of the fusion protein of MLSV. The antiviral effects of these compounds designated as VP14637 and AS-48 were highly specific and selective for RSV and MLSV, respectively.[36–39]

Specific inhibitors of myxoviruses may be promising for antiviral treatment in the future. However, I am still adhering to the broad-spectrum anti-respiratory virus agents for the reasons cited above.

COMBINATION AND SYNERGISTIC EFFECTS OF ANTI-RESPIRATORY VIRUS AGENTS

The combination effects of selected antiviral agents were examined for several of the demonstrably effective compounds. Since ribavirn is a broad-spectrum anti-myxovirus compound, synergistic effects were mainly examined between ribavirin and the other compounds. As a result, a Keggin-type POM, PM-523, and ribavirin displayed a synergistic anti-FLUV A activity *in vitro* and *in vivo*. *In vitro* assay was conducted with infection of MDCK cells and evaluated based on the MTT method. The effect of the combination of PM-523 and ribavirin on FLUV replication was evaluated by median-effect principle and isobologram, and it was analyzed by using a microcomputer with dose–effect analysis software. The degree of interaction of the two compounds was determined by calculating the combination index (CI, CI = d1/D1 + d2/D2 + α(d1 × d2/D1 × D2). In this equation, d1 and d2 indicate the fractional dose of compound 1 and 2 in combination, respectively, which are required to produce a median effect or 70% inhibitory effect (e.g., the affected fraction is 50% or 70% that of the control). D1 and D2 are the doses of compounds 1 and 2, respectively, which are required to produce the same median effect or 70% inhibitory effect when these compounds are used singly. α is set at 0 for mutually exclusive drugs, and α is set at 1 for mutually nonexclusive drugs.

When we examined the *in vitro* combination effects and calculated the CI in several ratios of combination of PM-523 and ribavirin, the CI was consistently lower than 1.0 at several endopoints of inhibition (Fa) (Fig. 4.7). This result indicates that PM-523 and ribavirin displayed synergism for inhibition against FLUV A replication. Similar synergistic inhibitory effects were observed by a combination of ribavirin and interferon (IFN) α-2b (Schering Plough) against MLSV (Edmonston strain) and ribavirin and pegilated IFN (PEG-IFN) against MPSV (EXCH-3 strain) (Fig. 4.8a, b).[40,41] Ribavirin and IFN-α (Sumitomo) also showed a combination effect *in vitro* against SSPE virus. As shown in Fig. 4.9, the fractional inhibitory concentration of both drugs was plotted in the synergistic area of the isobologram. Thus the combination effect of ribavirin and IFN α against SSPE virus was evaluated as a synergism.[42] It was reported that paramyxovirus accessory proteins antagonize the interferon promoter signal, and the viruses thus circumvent IFN response.[43,44] However, this activity is directed at innate IFN signaling and exogenous IFN-α might be active as antiviral substance. Ribavirin may act to suppress the production of the accessory proteins of paramyxoviruses and weaken the antagonistic activity to IFN

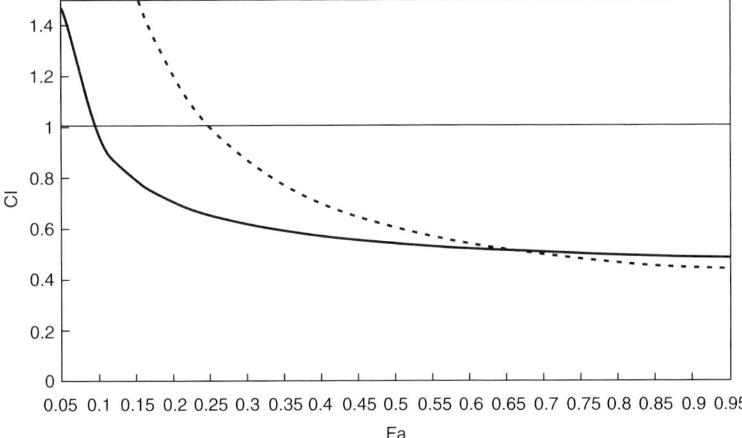

Fig. 4.7. Computer-generated presentation of combination index (CI) with respect to the fraction affected (Fa) for the inhibition of influenza virus A (H1N1) multiplication in MDCK cells. Combination of PM-523 and ribavirin at a ratio of 1:16 (——) and 1:4 (------) were analyzed under mutually nonexclusive assumptions.

production. Thus the combined use of rivabirin and IFN-α may have worked synergistically. The combination effects were also examined in the *in vivo* infection of FLUV and SSPE virus using small animals. For the combination of ribavirin and PM-523, mice were infected with FLUV A (H1N1/PR8 strain) intranasally and treated with the single and combined use of each compound. In another experiment with ribavirn and IFN-α, hamsters were infected intracranially with SSPE virus and treated with the single or combined use of ribavirin and IFN-α. Figures 4.10 and 4.11 show the survival rate of animals after infection and effects of treatments.[40,42] As shown in these figures, the combination use of the antiviral agents enhanced the survival days of the infected animals significantly compared with the single use of each compound.

CONCLUSION

From our own mass-screening trial of anti-myxovirus agents from a large number of synthetic and natural substances, several broad-spectrum anti-myxovirus agents were found. These compounds exceeded ribavirin in the potency and selectivity of their anti-myxovirus effects *in vitro*. Some compounds displayed therapeutic effects on FLUV A- and RSV-infected animals. A naturally obtained sulfated polysaccharide (OKU-40) and synthetic Ti- or V-containing polyoxotungstates

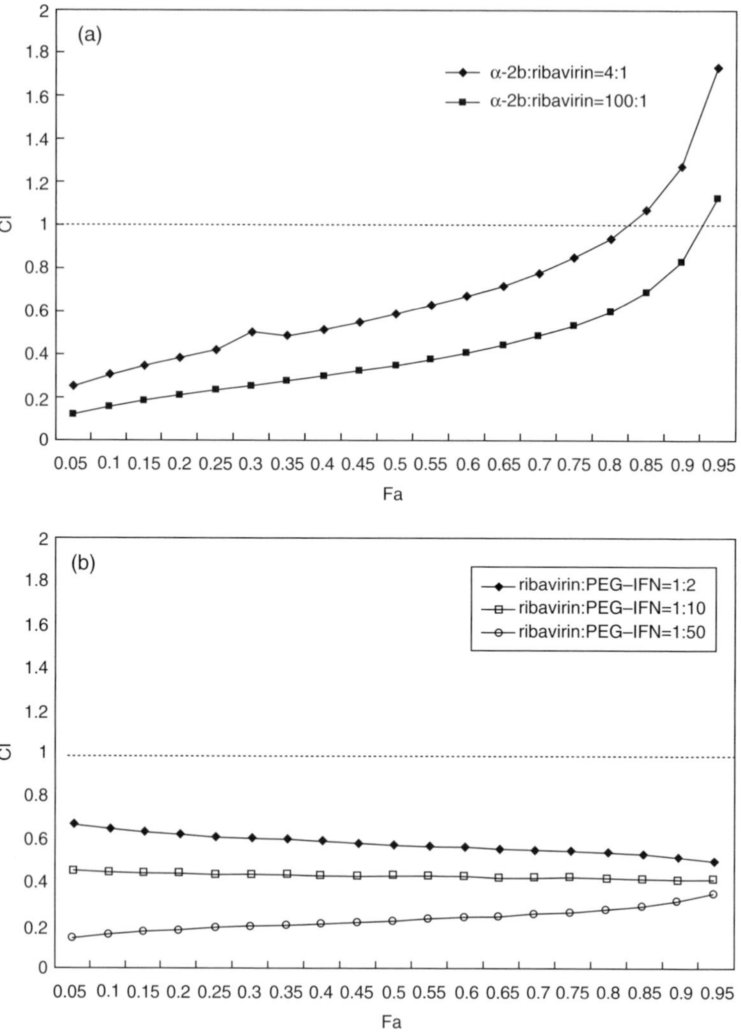

Fig. 4.8. Combination index with respect to the fraction affected by the inhibition of (a) measles virus multiplication in Vero cells and (b) mumps virus in Vero cells. A combination of ribavirin and IFN-α-2b was used for MLSV, and a combination of ribavirin and PEG-IFN was used for MPSV.

(PM-523, PM-1001) showed broad-spectrum antiviral activities for orthomyxo- and paramyxoviruses and HIV-1. Among them, PM-1001 exhibited expanded efficacy to Dengue fever virus and SARS coronavirus. Since these negatively charged compounds interact with different targets of viral replication from nucleoside analogues and neuraminidase inhibitors, a combination use of these compounds with virus-

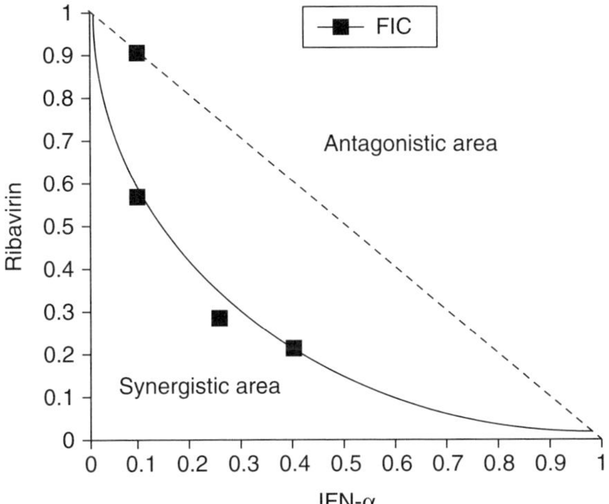

Fig. 4.9. Isobologram of combination effect of ribavirin and IFN-α against SSPE virus infection *in vitro*.

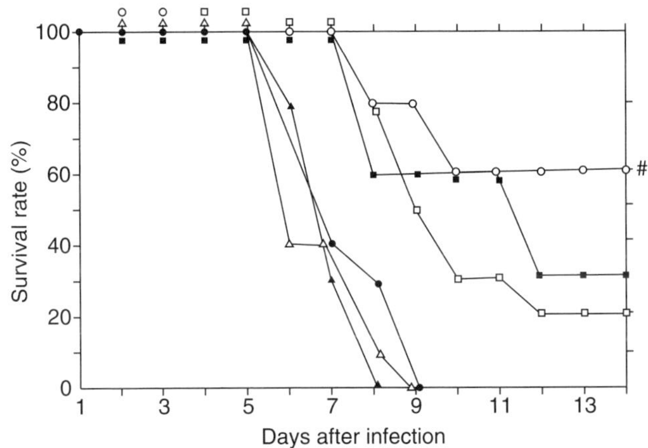

Fig. 4.10. Therapeutic effect of aerosol treatment of FLUV A-infected mice with PM-523 and ribavirin. Mice were infected with virus (1.6×10^4 $TCIC_{50}$) intranasally and were exposed to an aerosol of the compound solutions at the indicated condition for 2 hr. The compounds were given to the infected mice every 12 hr for 4 days starting at 8 hr after viral inoculation. (•) Untreated control; (▲) ribavirin at 40 mM: (■) ribavirin at 80 mM; (△) PM-523 at 2.4 mM; (□) PM-523 ar 4.8 mM; (○) PM-523 at 2.4 mM plus ribavirn at 40 mM; (#) a level of significance of $P < 0.001$ was found against 40 mM ribavirin alone and 2.4 mM PM-523 alone. $P < 0.01$ against 4.8 mM PM-523, $P < 0.05$ against 80 mM ribavirin.

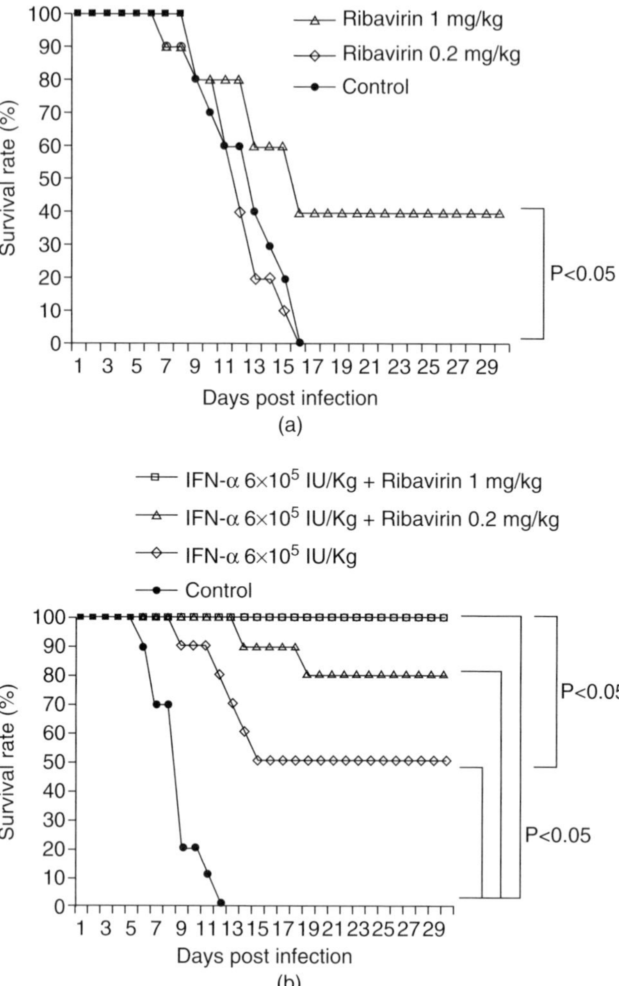

Fig. 4.11. Therapeutic effect of IFN-α and ribavirin for SSPE-virus-infected mice. Mice were inoculated with 50 µl of the virus-infected Vero cell suspension containing approximately 500 PFU of SSPE virus. The materials were injected 2 mm deep with a 27-gauge needle at two 10-hr intervals into the subarachnoid space of hamsters under ether anesthesia. Intracranial administration of IFN-α and ribavirin was started at 12 hr after the initial virus inoculation and then repeated every 48 hr for IFN and every 24 hr for ribavirin for 10 days. (a) Hamsters were treated with ribavirin alone with doses of ($\triangle$) 1 mg/kg and ($\diamond$) 0.2 mg/kg. (b) Hamsters were treated with IFN-α alone and with combinations of IFN-α and ribavirin. ($\diamond$) IFN α 6 × 10⁵ IU/kg; ($\triangle$) IFN-α 6 × 10⁵ IU/kg plus ribavirin 0.2 mg/kg: ($\square$) IFN-α 6 × 10⁵ IU/kg plus ribavirn 1 mg/kg. ($\bullet$) Untreated control.

specific inhibitors may enhance the activity for the specific virus and extend the spectrum to the other myxoviruses. Our findings on the specific inhibitors of FLUV A (antisense ODN for PB2 mRNA) and RSV (NMSO3 and RD-0028) were the result of (a) the cooperative works with other laboratories and (b) the licenses of these compounds to be utilized by commercial companies for the purpose of developing them into therapeutic drugs.

ACKNOWLEDGMENTS

This chapter is dedicated to the memory of our late Dr. T. Yokota.

The author thanks for the technical assistance of Dr. S. Mori for the preparation of figures.

REFERENCES

1. Klein, M. I.; Coviello, S.; Bauer, G.; Benitez, A.; Serra, M. E.; Schatti, M. P.; Delgado, M. F.; Melendi, G. A.; Novalli, L.; Pena, H. G.; Karron, R. A.; Kleeberger, S. R.; Polack, F. P. The impact of infection with human metapneumovirus and other respiratory viruses in young infants and children at high risk for severe pulmonary disease. *J. Infect. Dis.* **2006**, *193*, 1544–1551.

2. Lamson, D.; Renwick, N.; Kapoor, V.; Liu Z.; Palacios, G.; Ju, J.; Dean, A.; St. George, K.; Briese, T.; Lipkin, W. I. MassTag polymerase-chain reaction detection of respiratory pathogens, including a new rhinovirus genotype, that caused influenza-like illness in New York state during 2004–2005. *J. Infect. Dis.* **2006**, *194*, 1398–1402.

3. Yokota, T.; Shigeta, S. The rational drug design laboratories in Fukushima, Japan. *Int. Antiviral News* **1996**, *4*, 60–62.

4. Watanabe, W.; Konno, K.; Ijichi, K.; Inoue, H.; Yokota, T.; Shigeta, S. MTT colorimetric assay system for the screening of anti-orthomyxo- and paramyxoviral agents. *J. Virol. Methods* **1994**, *51*, 185–192.

5. Mori, S.; Watanabe, W.; Shigeta, S. A colorimetric LDH assay for the titration of infectivity and the evaluation of anti-viral activity against ortho- and paramyxoviruses. *Tohoku J. Exp. Med.* **1995**, *177*, 315–325.

6. Kawana, F.; Shigeta, S.; Hosoya, M.; Suzuki, H.; De Clercq, E. Inhibitory effects of antiviral compounds on respiratory syncytial virus replication *in vitro. Antimicrob. Agents Chemother.* **1987**, *31*, 1225–1230.

7. Shigeta, S.; Konno, K.; Yokota, T.; Nakamura, K.; De Clercq, E. Comparative activities of several nucleoside analogs against influenza A, B, and C viruses *in vitro. Antimicrob. Agents Chemother.* **1988**, *32*, 906–911.

8. Hosoya, M.; Shigeta, S.; Ishii, T.; Suzuki, H.; De Clercq, E. Comparative inhibitory effects of various nucleoside and nonnucleoside analogues on replication of influenza types A and B *in vitro* and *in ovo*. *J. Infect. Dis.* **1993**, *168*, 641–646.

9. Shigeta, S. Chemotherapy for acute respiratory viral infections. *Shonika Rinsho* **1988**, *41*, 706–716. In Japanese.

10. Shigeta, S.; Mori, S.; Baba, M.; Ito, M.; Honzumi, K.; Nakamura, K.; Oshitani, H.; Numazaki, Y.; Matsuda, A.; Obara, T.; Shuto, S.; De Clercq, E. Antiviral activities of ribavirin, 5-ethynyl-1-β-D-ribofuranosylimidazole-4-carboxamide, and 6′-(R)-C-methylneplanocin A against several ortho- and paramyxoviruses. *Antimicrob. Agents Chemother.* **1992**, *36*, 435–439.

11. Shuto, S.; Obara, T.; Toriya, M.; Hosoya, M.; Snoeck, R.; Andrei, G.; Balzarini, J.; De Clercq, E. New neplanocin analogues. 1 Synthesis of 6′-modified neplanocin A derivatives as broad-spectrum antiviral agents. *J. Med. Chem.* **1992**, *35*, 324–331.

12. Kosugi, Y.; Saito, Y.; Mori, S.; Watanabe, J.; Baba, M.; Shigeta, S. Antiviral activities of mizoribine and other inocine monophosphate dehydrogenase inhibitors against several ortho- and paramyxoviruses. *Antiviral Chem. Chemother.* **1994**, *5*, 366–371.

13. Ito, M.; Baba, M.; Sato, A.; Pauwels, R.; De Clercq, E.; Shigeta, S. Inhibitory effect of dextran sulfate and heparin on the replication of human immunodeficiency virus (HIV) *in vitro*. *Antiviral Res.* **1987**, *7*, 361–367.

14. Baba, M.; Pauwels, R.; Balzarini, J.; Arnout, J.; Desmyter, J.; De Clercq, E. Mechanism of inhibitory effect of dextran sulfate and heparin on the replication of human immunodeficiency virus *in vitro*. *Proc. Natl. Acad. Sci. USA* **1988**, *85*, 6132–6136.

15. Hosoya, M.; Balzarini, J.; Shigeta, S.; De Clercq, E. Differential inhibitory effects of sulfated polysaccharides and polymers on the replication of various myxoviruses and retroviruses, depending on the comparison of the target amino acid sequences of the viral envelope glycoproteins. *Antimicrob. Agents Chemother.* **1991**, *35*, 2515–2520.

16. Hashimoto, K.; Kodama, E.; Mori, S.; Watanabe, J.; Baba, M.; Okutani, K.; Matsuda, M.; Shigeta, S. Antiviral activity of sulphated polysaccharides extracted from marine *Pseudomonas* and marine plant *Dinoflagellata* against human immunodeficiency viruses and other enveloped viruses. *Antiviral Chem. Chemother.* **1996**, *7*, 189–196.

17. Okutani, K.; Tandavaniji, S. Isolation and characterization of a fucosamine containing polysaccharides from a marine strain of *Psudomonas*. *Nippon Suisan Gakkaishi.* **1991**, *57*, 2151–2156.

18. Yamamoto, N.; Schols, D.; De Clercq, E.; Debyser, Z.; Pauwels, R.; Balzrini, J.; Nakashima, H.; Baba, M.; Hosoya, M.; Snoeck, R.; Neyts, J.; Andrei, G.; Murrer, R. A.; Theobald, B.; Bossard, G.; Henso, G.; Abrams, M.; Picker, D. Mechanism of anti-human immunodeficiency virus action

of polyoxometalates, a class of broad spectrum antiviral agents. *Mol. Pharmacol.* **1992**, *42*, 1109–1117.

19. Ikeda, S.; Neyts, J.; Yamamoto, N.; Burrer, B.; Theobald, B.; Bossard, G.; Henson, G.; Abrams, M.; De Clercq, E. *In vivo* activity of a novel series of polyoxosilicotungstates against human myxo-, herpes, and retroviruses. *Antiviral Chem. Chemother.* **1993**, *4*, 253–262.

20. Barnard, D.L.; Hill, C. L.; Gage, T.; Matheson, J. E.; Huffman, J. H.; Sidwell, R. W.; Otto, M. J.; Schinazi, R. F. Potent inhibition of respiratory syncytial virus by polyoxometalates of several structural classes. *Antiviral Res.* **1997**, *34*, 27–37.

21. Huffman, J. H.; Sidwell, R. W.; Barnard, D. L.; Morrison, A.; Otto, M. J.; Hill, C. L.; Schinazi, R. F. Influenza virus inhibitory effects of a series of germanium- and silicon-centered polyoxometalates. *Antiviral Chem. Chemother.* **1997**, *8*, 75–83.

22. Shigeta, S.; Mori, S.; Watanabe, J.; Baba, M.; Kehnkin, A. M.; Hill, C. L.; Shinazi, R. F. *In vitro* antimyxovirus and anti-human immunodeficiency virus activities of polyoxometalates. *Antiviral Chem. Chemother.* **1995**, *6*, 114–122.

23. Shigeta, S.; Mori, S.; Watanabe, J.; Yamase, T.; Schinazi, R. F. *In vitro* antimyxovirus activity and mechanism of anti-influenza virus activity of polyoxometalates PM-504 and PM-523. *Antiviral Chem. Chemother.* **1996**, *7*, 346–352.

24. Shigeta, S.; Mori, S.; Kodama, E.; Kodma, J.; Takahashi, K.; Yamase, T. Broad spectrum anti-RNA virus activities of titanium and vanadium substituted polyoxotungstates. *Antiviral Res.* **2003**, *58*, 265–271.

25. Shigeta, S.; Mori, S.; Yamase, T.; Yamamoto, N.; Yamamoto, N. Anti-RNA virus activity of polyoxometalates. *Biomed. Pharmacol.* **2006**, *60*, 211–219.

26. Hatta, T.; Nakagawa, Y.; Takai, K.; Nakada, S.; Yokota, T.; Takaku, H. Inhibition of influenza virus RNA polymerase and nucleoprotein gene expression by unmodified, phosphorothioated, and lipsomally encapsulated oligonucleotides. *Biochem. Biophys. Res. Commun.* **1996**, *223*, 341–346.

27. Abe, T.; Mizuta, T.; Hatta, T.; Miyano-Kurosaki, N.; Fujiwara, M.; Takai, K.; Shigeta, S.; Yokota, T.; Takaku, H. Antisense therapy of influenza. *Eur. J. Pharm. Sci.* **2001**, *13*, 61–69.

28. Hamazaki, H.; Aba, T.; Yamakawa, H.; Yokota, T.; Shigeta, S.; Tkaku, H. Inhibition of influenza virus replication in MDCK cells by circular dumbbell RNA/DNA chimeras with closed alkyl loop structures. *Helv. Chim. Acta* **2002**, *85*, 2183–2194.

29. Mizuta, T.; Fujiwara, M.; Hatta, T.; Abe, T.; Miyano-Kurosaki, N.; Shigeta, S.; Yokota, T.; Takaku, H. Antisense oligonucleotides directed against the

viral RNA polymerase gene enhance survival of mice infected with influenza A. *Nature Biothechnol.* **1999**, *17*, 583–587.

30. Torrence, R. F.; Maitra, R. K.; Lesiak, K.; Khamnei, S.; Zhou, A.; Silverman, R. H.; Targeting RNA for degradation with a (2′-5′) oligoadenylate-antisense chimera. *Proc. Natl. Acad. Sci. USA* **1993**, *90*, 1300–1304.

31. Leaman, D. W. 2-5A antisense treatment of respiratory syncytial virus. *Curr. Opin. Pharmacol.* **2005**, *5*, 502–507.

32. Cramer, H.; Okicki, J. R.; Kuang, M.; Zan, X. Targeted therapy of respiratory syncytial virus by antisense. *Nucleosides Nucleotides Nucleic Acid* **2005**, *24*, 497–501.

33. The Impact-RSV Study Group. Palivizmab, a humanized respiratory syncytial virus monoclonal antibody reduces hospitalization from respiratory syncytial virus infections in high risk infants. *Pediatrics.* **1998**, *102*, 531–537.

34. Kimura, K.; Mori, S.; Tomita, K.; Ohno, K.; Takahashi, K.; Shigeta, S.; Terada, M. Antiviral activity of NMSO3 against respiratory syncytial virus infection *in vitro* and *in vivo*. *Antiviral Res.* **2000**, *47*, 41–51.

35. Sudo, K.; Watanabe, W.; Konno, K.; Sato, R.; Kajiyashiki, T.; Shigeta, S.; Ykota, T. Efficacy of RD3-0028 aerosol treatment against respiratory syncytial virus infection in immunosuppressed mice. *Antimicrob. Agents Chemother.* **1999**, *43*, 752–757.

36. Douglas, J. L.; Panis, M. L.; Ho, E.; Lin, K. Y.; Krawczyk, S. H.; Grant, D. M.; Cai, R.; Swaminathan, S.; Cihlar, T. Inhibition of respiratory syncytial virus fusion by small molecule VP-14637 via specific interactions with F protein. *J. Virol.* **2003**, *77*, 5054–5064.

37. Wyde, P. R.; Laquerre, S.; Chetty, S. N.; Gilbert, B. E.; Nitz, T. J.; Pevear, D. C. Antiviral efficacy of VP14637 against respiratory syncytial virus *in vitro* and in cotton rats following delivery by small droplet aerosol. *Antiviral Res.* **2005**, *68*, 18–26.

38. Plemper, R. K.; Doyle, J.; Sun, A.; Prussia, A.; Cheng, L.-T.; Rota, P. A.; Liotta, D. C.; Synder, J. P.; Compans, R. W. Design of small-molecule entry inhibitor with activity against primary measles virus strains. *Antimicrob. Agents Chemother.* **2005**, *49*, 3755–3761.

39. Sun, A.; Prussia, A.; Zhan, W.; Murray, E. E.; Doyle, J.; Cheng, L.-T.; Yoon, J.-J.; Radchenko, E. V.; Palyulin, V. A.; Compans, R. W.; Liotta, D. C.; Plemper, R. K.; Snyder, J. P. Nonpeptide inhibitors of measles virus entry. *J. Med. Chem.* **2006**, *49*, 5080–5092.

40. Shigeta, S.; Mori, S.; Watanabe, J.; Soeda, S.; Takahashi, K; Yamase, T. Synergistic anti-influenza virus A (H1N1) activities of PM-523 (polyoxometalate) and ribavirin *in vitro* and *in vivo*. *Antimicrob. Agents Chemother.* **1997**, *41*, 1423–1427.

41. Shigeta, S.; Mori, S. Combination of ribavirin, interferons, thymosin α1 against RNA and DNA virus replications *in vitro*. The report to Schering Plough Co., unpublished data.

42. Takahashi, T.; Hosoya, M.; Kimura, K.; Ohno, K.; Mori, S.; Takahashi, K.; Shigeta, S. The cooperative effect of interferon α and ribavirin on subacute sclerosing panenecephalitis (SSPE) virus *in vitro* and *in vivo*. *Antiviral Res.* **1998**, *37*, 29–35.

43. Gotoh, B.; Komatsu, T.; Takeuchi, K.; Yokoo, J. Paramyxovirus accessory proteins as interferon antagonists. *Microbiol. Immunol.* **2001**, *45*, 787–800.

44. Andrejeva, J.; Childs, K. S.; Young, D. F.; Carlos, T. S.; Stock, N.; Goodbourn, S.; Randall, R. E. The V protein of paramyxoviruses bind the IFN-inducible RNA helicase, mda-5, and inhibit its activation of the IFN-β promoter. *Proc. Natl. Acad. Sci. USA* **2004**, *101*, 17264–17269.

5

CURRENT STATUS ON DEVELOPMENT OF NUCLEIC ACID-BASED ANTIVIRAL DRUGS AGAINST INFLUENZA VIRUS INFECTION

JONATHAN P. WONG AND MARY E. CHRISTOPHER

Chemical and Biological Defence Section, Defence R&D Canada–Suffield, Ralston, Alberta T1A 8K6, Canada

MURRAY CAIRNS

School of Biomedical Sciences, Faculty of Health, University of Newcastle, NSW 2308, Australia

L.-Q. SUN AND RODERIC M. K. DALE

Oligos Etc. Inc., Wilsonville, OR 97070

ANDRES M. SALAZAR

Oncovir Inc., Washington, DC 20008

INTRODUCTION

Seasonal and pandemic influenza viruses are highly contagious viruses that pose major threats to public health. The present global crisis posed by emergence of the avian H5N1 influenza virus provides testament to the challenge of defense against a deadly virus that is unpredictable and ever-changing. The world may be vulnerable to an influenza

Combating the Threat of Pandemic Influenza: Drug Discovery Approaches,
Edited by Paul F. Torrence
Copyright © 2007 by John Wiley & Sons, Inc.

pandemic by a highly transmissible strain of avian H5N1 influenza virus that, with a case fatality rate above 50%,[1] could potentially kill millions of people worldwide.

The availability of neuraminidase inhibitors and attenuated vaccines improves the ability to defend against influenza, but therapeutic benefits have been significantly limited by drug resistance and antigenic changes. To circumvent these changes, development of prophylactic and therapeutic strategies that are broad-spectrum and/or are less susceptible to the emergence of drug-resistant strains will significantly reduce the deadly impacts of influenza. Of particular importance are antiviral agents that can elicit long-lasting protective innate immune responses that are not directed against a specific range of viruses, and thus are less susceptible to the emergence of drug resistance.

Nucleic acid-based antiviral drugs have shown promising antiviral activities in animal studies and may represent a novel class of anti-influenza agents. These antiviral agents are versatile in their modes of action and can be generally classified into three categories: (1) immunomodulating nucleic acids, (2) catalytic ribozymes and DNAzymes, and (3) gene-silencing antisense ODNs and small interfering RNA (siRNA).

Nucleic acid-based immunomodulators are designed to stimulate the host's innate immunity to resist a number of viral infections. The ability of these drugs to elicit broad-spectrum antiviral immunity is of particular importance in the prevention and treatment of influenza infection. The enhancement of innate cellular immunity and antiviral resistance may offer the potential of protection against a number of seasonal and avian strains of influenza viruses, regardless of genetic mutation, reassortment, recombination, zoonotic origin, or drug resistance. Nucleic acid-based drugs currently in development that can stimulate the host's immune responses against viral infections include CpG containing ODNs[2] and double-stranded RNA such as poly ICLC.[3] These drugs are Toll-like receptor (TLR) agonists and are in various stages of clinical development.

Nucleic acids with enzyme-like catalytic activity, such as ribozymes (RNA) and DNAzymes (DNA), are exciting emerging antiviral agents. Ribozymes possess a unique RNA cleavage activity and can be designed to hybridize and cleave target viral mRNA molecules in a sequence-specific manner.[4] DNA enzymes, or DNAzymes, are capable of catalyzing the hydrolysis of mRNA at purine-pyrimidine junctions.[5] Catalytic ribozymes and DNAzymes have been explored for their applications against a number of clinically relevant human virus infections.[6]

Gene-silencing is a highly specific approach for inhibiting the expression of selected key proteins involved in disease initiation or progression. This innovative technology allows for the specific suppression of viral replication in the host by targeting key viral proteins required for the virus life cycle. Initially, it was speculated that the most effective mechanism for inhibiting viral RNA processing or translation was achieved through the use of a single-stranded RNA, such as anti-sense ODN, hybridizing to viral mRNA.[7] It is now known that post-transcriptional gene silencing using double-stranded siRNA can be a very potent alternate means to silence expression of viral proteins.[8]

The purpose of this review is to highlight the potential applications of the three major classes of nucleic acid-based antiviral agents, particularly against influenza virus infection. It will focus on mode of action, stability, chemistry, antiviral efficacy in *in vitro* tissue culture, and/or *in vivo* animal infection model systems. The antiviral application of siRNA for the prevention and treatment of influenza infection has been covered elsewhere in this special issue and will not be addressed here. This review will also cover the use of liposome drug delivery systems for nucleic acid-based antiviral drugs. Since nucleic acids, in general, are susceptible to nuclease degradation *in vivo*, the encapsulation of these drugs within, or complexed to, liposomes protect them against nuclease degradation *in vivo*. Furthermore, liposomes enhance both delivery to intracellular sites of infection and presentation to professional antigen presenting cells of the encapsulated nucleic acid. Liposome delivery of nucleic acids to sites of infection has been known to decrease drug toxicity and/or enhance antiviral activity.[9]

IMMUNOMODULATING NUCLEIC ACIDS AS ANTIVIRAL AGENTS

The development of a potent and broad-spectrum approach to elicit protective antiviral immunity against influenza viruses is fundamentally important in influenza prevention. Due to the ever-changing nature of influenza viruses, either by mutation, recombination, or reassortment, this nonspecific approach may offer protection against a number of influenza viruses, regardless of their genetic makeup, zoonotic origin, and resistance to anti-influenza drugs.

The ability of nucleic acids to activate both innate and adaptive immune responses is mediated through a signaling pathway involving TLRs found on dendritic cells (DCs), B-lymphocytes, and macrophages. The recognition of "non-self" nucleic acids by TLRs induces immuno-stimulatory responses as part of the host's first line of defense against invading pathogens.[10,11] There are two main types of nucleic acid-based TLR ligands that are known to induce antiviral immune responses that protect the host against viral diseases, including influenza.

Double-Stranded RNA

Poly ICLC. Poly ICLC, a synthetic, double-stranded polyriboinosinic-polyribocytidylic acid stabilized with poly-L-lysine carboxymethyl cellulose, is a potent immunomodulating agent.[3,12,13] Wong et al.[3] first reported that poly ICLC could elicit a prolonged antiviral effect in mice challenged with lethal influenza viral infection. In rodents and primates, poly ICLC has been shown to be effective in the protection against a number of other viral infections, including yellow fever,[14] Venezuelan equine encephalomyelitis,[15] Japanese encephalitis virus,[16] Rift Valley fever,[17] and rabies.[18] Recognition by and interaction with TLR-3[19] is responsible for the broad-spectrum antiviral immune response elicited by poly ICLC, which includes the production of interferons (IFN)-α, -β, and -γ.[13,18,20] This signaling pathway also accounts for stimulation of both innate and adaptive immune responses and activation of natural killer (NK) cells.[12]

Poly ICLC has been shown to be broadly effective against both seasonal and avian influenza viruses in animal efficacy studies.[3,9,21] When poly ICLC was used prophylactically to determine its efficacy in protecting mice against a respiratory challenge with a lethal challenge dose of mouse-adapted influenza A/PR/8/34 virus (H1N1), it was shown that pretreatment of mice with two intranasal (i.n.) doses of 1 mg/kg/dose was fully protective (100% survival rate), whereas all untreated control mice succumbed to the infection ($p < 0.01$ versus control). Mice pretreated with a single dose (1 mg/kg) of poly ICLC showed a slightly lower survival rate (80%) compared to those who received two doses of 500 µg/kg/dose (100% survival rate). Similarly, mice pretreated with a single 500 µg/kg/dose had a lower survival rate (60%) compared to mice pretreated with two 250 µg/kg doses. Poly ICLC was equally effective in the prophylactic protection against influenza A/Aichi/2 (H3N2). All mice pretreated with two i.n. doses of poly ICLC were protected against 10 LD$_{50}$ of influenza A/Aichi/2.[3,9] Compared to the prophylactic efficacy of mouse recombinant IFN-α, two i.n. doses (1 mg/kg/dose) of poly ICLC was found to be more efficacious than two i.n. doses (100,000 U/kg/dose) of IFN-α in the protection of mice against influenza A/PR/8 infection ($p < 0.05$).[3]

The window of protection provided by poly ICLC was determined by pretreating mice with two i.n. doses (1 mg/kg/dose) of poly ICLC 1–20 days prior to infection with 10 LD$_{50}$ of influenza virus. It was found that mice pretreated within 12 days of viral challenge were fully protected from infection.[3] The survival rates decreased to 80% and 40%, respectively, when pretreatment was given 14 and 16 days prior to viral challenge. Poly ICLC administered 20 days prior to infection provided no protection. Route of administration was important as mice treated with two intravenous (i.v.) doses (1 mg/kg/dose) of poly ICLC showed a small increase in survival (40%) compared to untreated control mice ($p = 0.064$), but less than when treated i.n. In general, poly ICLC was shown to be less effective when administered following influenza virus exposure. Post-exposure treatment of mice with a single 1 mg/kg/dose was found to be almost completely ineffective versus 80% survival when given prior to virus exposure.[3]

Utilization of a liposome drug delivery system for poly ICLC was found to significantly improve the antiviral and safety profiles in experimental animals.[9] Liposome encapsulation was found to prolong the poly ICLC-induced antiviral resistant state against influenza infection.[9] Mice receiving pretreatment with liposome-encapsulated poly ICLC within 21 days prior to virus challenge were fully protected. This represents an increase of greater than one week of extended protection compared to that provided by free unencapsulated poly ICLC. Depending on the route of administration, the toxicities of poly ICLC observed in mice were either significantly reduced or completely mitigated with liposome encapsulation. Intravenous administration of liposome-encapsulated poly ICLC abolished the hypothermia and body weight loss observed in mice treated with the same dosage of free unencapsulated poly ICLC.[9] It is unclear whether the significant reductions in poly ICLC toxicity provided by liposome encapsulation will also be observed in human patients. Such attenuation of toxic side effects in patients may result in increased drug tolerance and improved clinical outcomes.

Due to the promising antiviral activity of liposome-encapsulated poly ICLC observed against seasonal influenza A strains, a follow-up study was conducted in mice to evaluate whether liposome-encapsulated poly ICLC could exhibit antiviral activity against the highly pathogenic H5N1 avian influenza A virus. Preliminary results from this study suggest that two i.n. doses of liposome-encapsulated poly ICLC (1 mg/kg body weight) provided a high level of protection against a low-level (1 LD_{50}) challenge of H5N1 avian influenza virus.[21] In this study, 50% of untreated control mice died from the avian influenza infection, whereas all the liposome-encapsulated poly ICLC pretreated mice survived ($p < 0.05$). Currently, studies are underway to optimize the dosing regimen for liposome-encapsulated poly ICLC against a high (4–10 LD_{50}) challenge dose of avian influenza virus.

Poly I: Poly C12 U (Ampligen®). Another synthetic double-stranded RNA, poly I: poly C_{12} U (Ampligen®), with a mismatched nucleoside at position 12 has been shown to have both immunomodulating and antiviral activities against influenza infection.[22] In cell culture studies, Ampligen®, when used in combination with either oseltamivir or zanamivir, synergistically inhibited the cytopathic effect of an avian influenza A (H5N1) virus on infected MDCK cells.[22]

CpG Oligonucleotides

In 1995 Kreig et al.[23] reported that ODNs containing unmethylated (bacterial DNA-like) CpG motifs were able to induce murine B cells to proliferate and secrete immunoglobulin *in vitro* and *in vivo*. This discovery resulted in CpGs being classified as a new pathogen-associated molecular pattern (PAMP). PAMPs are conserved pathogen structures, such as bacterial lipoprotein and lipopolysaccharide, which elicit immunostimulatory responses. Responses to PAMPs are regulated through TLR proteins that bind specific classes of compounds. TLR-2 binds lipoproteins, TLR-4 binds lipopolysaccharide, and the response to CpG is regulated by TLR-9.[24,25] Early studies revealed a significant difference between human and murine cells in the optimal sequence context of the CpG motif.[26,27] The optimal murine CpG ODN motif (5'-CACGTT-3' flanked by two 5' purines and two 3' pyrimidines) is a weak adjuvant in human immune cells. After considerable study, an ODN containing repeats of the CpG motif (5'-GTCGTT-3') was found to be the optimal adjuvant for human, chimpanzee, and rhesus monkey leukocytes.[27] Sequence contexts of CpG motifs specific for NK-cell lytic activity and for stimulation of IFN-γ secretion have also been designed.[27]

CpG ODNs primarily stimulate B cells and DCs through the constitutively expressed TRL-9 receptor.[25] Human memory B cells (high TRL-9 expressing) but not naïve B cells (low TRL-9 expressing) are stimulated to proliferate and differentiate to immunoglobulin-secreting cells in response to CpG. Because of the low level of TRL-9 expression, the polyclonal response of naïve B cells is suppressed during the primary response.[28] DCs form a link between the innate and acquired immune systems. Stimulation of DCs shifts the balance from a Th-2 humoral response to a Th-1 cellular response. CpG motifs stimulate peripheral blood, but not monocyte-derived, DCs and thereby induce maturation, transiently increase antigen processing, and increase the half-life of peptide-MHC-II complexes, thus sustaining subsequent antigen presentation.[26,29] Th-2 humoral responses are overrepresented in the immune response of immature and aging animals. Treatment with CpG hastens maturation of DCs in immature mice and results in a recovery and enhancement of the Th-1 type response in aging mice.[30–32] If CpG stimulation of innate cellular immunity can also be observed in humans, it may be possible to use CpG as an adjuvant to expand the potency and efficacy of antiviral vaccines in the population that is most at risk and yet has the least effective immune response.

CpG as an Anti-influenza Adjuvant. Currently, CpG-induced activation of innate immunity is being investigated in a variety of models for protection against a diversity of pathogens and as a therapy for cancer and allergy.[25] In recent years, CpG ODNs adjuvant potential as an enhancer of antiviral vaccine efficacy, including vaccines against influenza A, have been studied in animal models. Mice primed with CpG ODN plus formalin-inactivated influenza virus vaccines were capable of producing virus-specific antibodies at levels seven times higher than mice administered vaccine without CpG.[33] A wide range of sites of administration including i.n., subcutaneous, oral, and intrarectal routes were compared in mice immunized with a killed influenza vaccine formulated with CpG ODN.[34] These studies revealed that mucosal delivery resulted in enhanced production of influenza-specific antibodies in the serum, saliva, and genital tract. Bare skin has also been used as a site of immunization with a synthetic peptide composed of a T-helper epitope of influenza hemagglutinin (HA), a CpG ODN, and cholera toxin.[35] Enhanced proliferation of virus-specific T cells and increased levels of IFN-γ were observed following immunization. Multilamellar liposome preparations of CpG ODNs and influenza subunit vaccine, alone or in combination, enhance vaccine potency and reduce the number of doses required for an effective immune response.[4] In mice, administration of co-encapsulated vaccine and CpG ODNs within liposomes was up to 30 times more effective 3–12 weeks post-vaccination in inducing serum and mucosal IgG2a and IgA and protecting against virus challenge than was observed in mice treated with nonencapsulated CpG ODN.[4]

CATALYTIC NUCLEIC ACIDS AS ANTIVIRAL AGENTS

Ribozymes

Ribozymes are catalytic RNA molecules that possess enzymatic cleavage and ligation activities driven by the free energy of Watson–Crick base pairing interactions.[36,37] In the 1980s, seven classes of naturally occurring ribozymes involved in RNA processing were discovered, including the hairpin,[37] hammerhead,[38] group I intron,[39] group II intron,[40] ribonuclease P,[41] hepatitis delta virus ribozyme,[42] and *Neurospora* VS RNA,[43] with each class representing a distinct catalytic mechanism.

Two classes of ribozymes, hairpin and hammerhead, have been extensively investigated because of their relative simplicity, small size, and the ability to alter sequences flanking the active site without loss of catalytic activity. The hammerhead ribozyme is derived from the satellite RNA strand (+) of the tobacco ringspot virus (TobSV) and its sequence consists of (i) a conserved 22-base catalytic region, (ii) base-pairing flanking arm sequences, and (iii) a recognition sequence on the target RNA (i.e., CUC).[44] Cleavage occurs 3' to the recognition sequence and results in a 2',3'-cyclic phosphate and a 5'-hydroxyl terminus on the 3' fragment (Fig. 5.1A). The catalytic moiety of hairpin ribozymes, which are formed by the (−) strand of the sTobSV, consist of a complex of four helices and five loop regions formed between the 50-base ribozyme and 14-base substrate sequence region (Fig. 5.1B). Cleavage occurs 5' to a bNGUC recognition sequence (where b is C, G, or U and N is any base).[45]

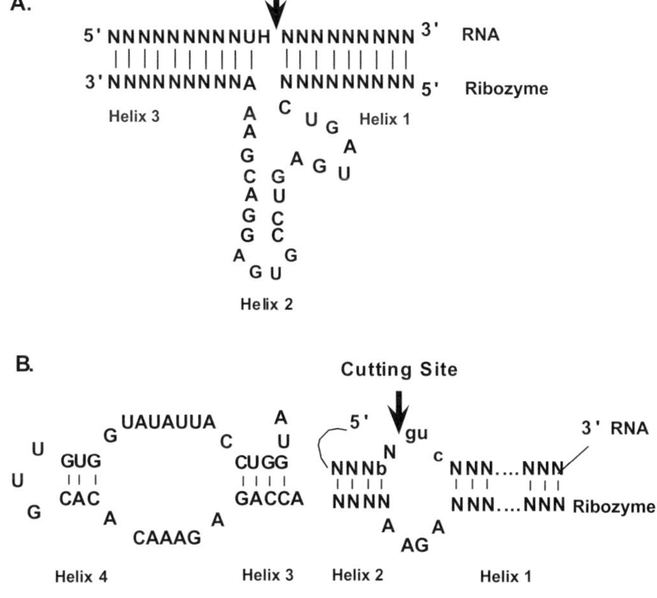

Fig. 5.1. Structures of (A) hammerhead ribozymes and (B) hairpin ribozymes.

Designing Antiviral Ribozymes. Extensive study of ribozyme-mediated catalysis has revealed that Michaelis–Menton kinetics can be used to describe the reaction where the enzyme (E) and substrate (S) assemble via Watson–Crick base pairing into an enzyme–substrate (E•S) complex. The E•S complex is converted to the 2′,3′-cyclic phosphate terminus (P1) and a 5′-hydroxyl terminus bound to the enzyme, followed by release of the products.[46] Under multiple turnover conditions (where the substrate is in excess of the enzyme) the k_{cat} or turnover number is used to determine the rate-limiting catalytic step for comparison of the relative efficiencies of ribozymes designed for a specific target. For example, extension of the binding arms of a hammerhead ribozyme increased Watson–Crick binding stability between enzyme and substrate with the effect of substantially decreasing k_{cat}.[47]

In nature, ribozymes are *cis*-cleaving, cutting RNA at intramolecular sites. However, by altering substrate recognition sequences, ribozymes have been altered to cleave a wide range of viral and other medically relevant target RNA molecules in *trans*.[48] Theoretically, a ribozyme containing any sequence recognition site could be designed; however, empirical *in vitro* studies have revealed basic rules of ribozyme design. Hammerhead ribozymes, for example, can cleave any 5′-NUH-3′, where N is any nucleotide, U is conserved, and H can be A, U, C, but not G with k_{cat} decreasing in the order AUC, GIC > GUA, AUA, CUC > AUU, UUC, UUA > GUU, CUA > UUU, CUU. This order of decreasing efficiency can, in general, be applied to levels of gene expression affected by ribozyme cleavage.[48]

In vitro studies of ribozymes with synthetic substrates have been invaluable in revealing the range and extent of cleavage activities; however, to be therapeutically relevant, consideration must be given to the native RNA substrate. Predicting the availability of the target site on the substrate RNA in the native *in vivo* state is a challenge common to all gene ablation agents. The native RNA substrate may have multitude secondary structures and be bound to a number of cellular proteins *in situ*, all of which may impair binding of the ribozyme to its predicted target site. A number of strategies have been utilized to reveal cleavage site accessibility including RNA secondary structure prediction programs or S1 nuclease and/or RNase mapping to probe the RNA secondary structure.[49] Because studies of synthetic RNA can be unreliable, empirical evaluation must be performed by creating a range of ribozymes in order to "walk" the target of interest and determine *in vivo* expression levels. Recent studies suggest using a combinatorial approach in order to more efficiently select a target site. A ribozyme library composed of a hammerhead ribozyme with random sequences in the binding arms can be screened using a RACE technique to identify active ribozymes that can subsequently be cloned.[50] Use of a similar approach with hairpin ribozymes suggests that activity-selected ribozymes have higher activity and cannot necessarily be predicted by computer-based substrate selection rules.[51]

Antiviral Ribozymes. Ribozymes (hammerhead, hairpin, and RNAse P) have been designed to cleave a number of viral targets in cell culture assays, including hepatitis B virus (HBV),[52] hepatitis C virus (HCV),[53] cytomegalovirus,[54] human immunodeficiency (HIV)-1,[55] human papillomavirus (HPV),[56] and influenza A.[57,58] Ribozymes (both hammerhead and RNAse P) directed against the polymerase (*PB1* and *PB2*) and nucleocapsid (*NP*) genes of influenza A have been shown to inhibit viral particle production and/or viral protein expression.[57–59] In virtually all cases, cells were transfected with plasmid or transduced with retrovirus or adenovirus vectors. Delivery in this manner resulted in endogenous expression of the ribozyme, potentially co-localizing it with the viral RNA target. This approach has been used in recent clinical trials of a *tat*-targeted anti-HIV ribozyme. Retroviral vectors were used to transduce patient derived CD34+ stem cells that were returned to the HIV-positive patient following expansion.[60] This form of *ex vivo* permanent transduction of the target host cell is ideally suited to treatment of a blood borne chronic viral infection but is unlikely to be practical for treatment of an acute infection with influenza virus.

Ribozyme ODNs, similar to antisense ODNs, have been synthesized and delivered exogenously; however, *in vivo* therapeutic applications are limited due to their biological lability. In order to minimize nuclease degradation, a range of chemical modifications have been employed. Typical ribonucleotide modifications include phosphorothioate (PS) linkages, 2′-*O*- substitutions (2′-*O*-methyl, 2′-*O*-allyl-, 2′-fluoro- and 2′-amino-), 3′-3′ inversions, or combinations of these.[61] Such modifications allow direct delivery (intravenous or direct tissue injection) of intact ribozymes and extend the biological half-life as much as 14,000-fold *in vivo*.[62,63] Recently, a modified hammerhead ribozyme directed against influenza A has been developed and patented, although no data describing its anti-influenza activity have yet been reported.[64]

DNAzymes

DNAzymes are RNA-cleaving catalytic DNA enzymes which, unlike ribozymes, are entirely synthetic and derived from a selection protocol developed to evolve DNA sequences capable of cleaving RNA[5]

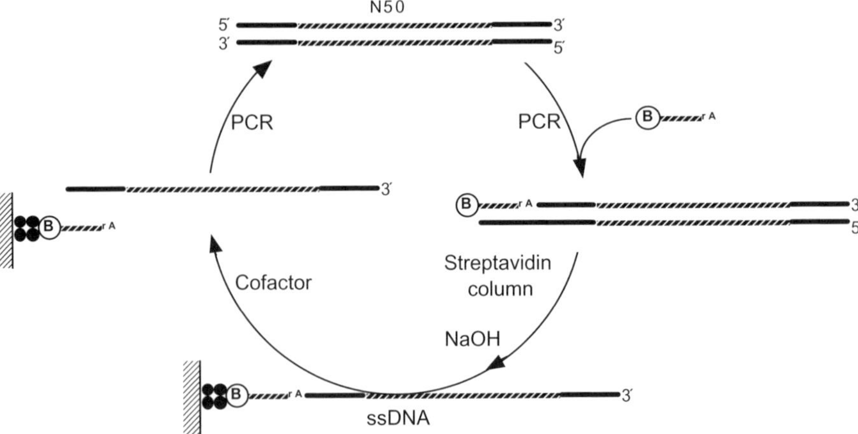

Fig. 5.2. A selection scheme for the evolution of RNA cleaving catalytic DNA. See text for detail. In this system a combinatorial library of different DNA sequences is generated by the synthesis of an oligonucleotide template with a 50 base (N50) stretch of random sequence (hatched lines). To enable amplification and reselection, each molecule from this diverse pool contains a fixed primer binding sequence at each end (black). Immobilization is achieved by tethering this assembly of potentially functional sequences through a biotinylated (B) RNA containing substrate (rA) to a solid streptavidin-coated support. After alkali denaturation (to strip away the template strand) the single-stranded residue is allowed to fold around its substrate linkage in the presence of suitable buffer and cofactors. The eluent of this washing (which contains catalytically active molecules) is then used as a PCR template for regenerating the assembly for a second round of selection. After multiple rounds of selection the relative abundance of each active molecule should be high enough to visualize the activity in a cleavage assay and clone the DNA for sequencing.

(Fig. 5.2). The "10–23" DNAzyme isolated by this *in vitro* selection protocol is a general-purpose enzyme capable of cleaving RNA at purine–pyrimidine junctions. The structure of the DNAzyme is reminiscent of the hammerhead ribozyme with a 16-mer 3'-AGCAAC-CATCGATCGG-5' catalytic core flanked by binding arms.[6] DNAzyme kinetic activity appears to be proportional to the degree of heteroduplex stability, wherein enzyme–substrate combinations with the lowest free energy of hybridization have the highest catalytic rate.[65] Extension of binding arm length and alteration of CG content generally increases catalytic efficiency and decreases K_m. Excessive heteroduplex binding efficiency, however, ultimately inhibits the release of cleaved substrate from the enzyme, thus reducing k_{cat}. Empirical studies have revealed that binding arm lengths of 8–9 bases yield the maximal overall efficiency.[66]

DNAZYME DESIGN

The ability to cleave at any purine-pyrimidine junction leaves open the possibility of a much wider target site range than that available to ribozymes. The design of an appropriate DNAzyme depends upon selecting a target site that has an appropriate free energy of hybridization and a location on the RNA that has not been rendered inaccessible by secondary or tertiary structure. A multiplex selection assay protocol based on primer extension and sequencing gel technology has been developed which allows the activity of a large number of DNAzymes to be observed simultaneously.[67] The wide range of potential target sites for DNAzymes relative to ribozymes does not come at the expense of specificity since 10–23 DNAzymes could discriminate between sequences that varied by as little as a single nucleotide.[68] Reactions between DNAzymes and matching substrate sequences were compared with reactions against unmatched substrates. In each case, only the perfectly matched type-specific DNAzymes were capable of achieving substantial cleavage of the corresponding substrates. This cleavage specificity has been used in the development of DNAzymes as clinical diagnostic reagents used for real-time PCR measurement of target RNA substrates.[69] This leaves open the exciting possibility of using DNAzymes as both a therapeutic and diagnostic tool against the same viral target.

DNAzymes, due to their synthetic nature, cannot be expressed intracellularly and therefore must be exogenously delivered. Although DNAzymes are inherently more stable than ribozymes, they must be modified to protect against nuclease degradation *in vivo*. To date, reported studies of DNAzyme activity have been limited to cell culture experiments and only a small range of nucleic acid modifications have been employed. A 3′ inversion modification has been shown to increase the half-life of a model DNAzyme from 2 hours (unmodified form) to 24 hours (3′ inversion modified form) when incubated in human serum.[70] Partial phosphorothioate modification (5′–3′ linkages on either binding arm) or 3′–3′ inversions on the 3′-terminus can also stabilize the DNAzyme in cell culture studies.[71] Comparison of the intracellular activity of phosphodiester and phosphorothioate or 2′-*O*-methyl modifications in the binding arms in the 10–23 DNAzyme have also been reported.[72] DNAzymes containing either of these modifications retained activity in mammalian cells longer than unmodified forms, with the 2′-*O*-methyl modification being the most stable.

The antiviral activity of the 10–23 DNAzyme has been examined against a range of viruses in cell culture experiments. Suppression of viral replication has been observed using DNAzymes directed against the HIV-1 *tat, rev,*[73] *gag,*[74] and *env*[75] genes, the HBV *X* gene,[76] and the HCV 5′-noncoding region.[77] In a study describing the antiviral activity of a 10–23 DNAzyme against the influenza A *PB2* gene, greater than 90% inhibition was observed.[78] While few potential gene targets for anti-influenza ribozyme or DNAzyme activity have been reported, a number of gene targets have been assessed using antisense technology. The antisense studies suggested that targeting the AUG codon for the *PB2* gene was more effective than targeting the AUG codons of the *PB1*, *NP*, and *PA* genes.[79] Interestingly, no studies to date have described selecting regions of the influenza genome that represent the most conserved sequences across all known virus subtypes. Such a strategy could produce a therapeutic enzyme less likely to be rendered ineffective by mutation.

ANTISENSE OLIGONUCLEOTIDES AS ANTIVIRAL AGENTS

Over two decades ago, Zamecnik and Stephenson[4,80] demonstrated that RNA translation, virus replication, and cell transformation of Rous sarcoma virus could be inhibited by a 13-mer deoxyribonucleotide that was complementary to the RSV repeat terminal sequence. This provided the first evidence that an antisense ODN could act as an antiviral agent. Studies of antisense ODNs over the past several years have demonstrated that the mechanisms of action are complex and may include steric hindrance of ribosomes, reverse transcriptase activity, increased target RNA susceptibility to RNAse H cleavage, blockage of viral binding, or enhanced immunostimulation via CpG motifs.[23,81–83] The susceptibility of phosphodiester ODNs to *in vivo* nuclease activity resulted in the development of a range of nuclease-resistant chemical modifications either to the phosphate backbone (i.e., phosphorothioate, phosphorodithioate, methyl phosphonate), to the 2′-position on the ribose sugar moiety (2′-*O*-methyl, 2′-methoxy ethyl), or to the oligonucleotide structure (3′-inversion).[83] Suitably modified antisense ODNs are designed for antiviral activity by targeting hybridization to an essential sequence such as the AUG start codon or by screening a range of antisense sequences in a walk of the viral genome. This can be achieved either in a comprehensive manner or aided by RNA secondary structure predicting programs to target regions lacking significant secondary structure. Typically, 5–30 antisense ODNs thus designed are tested for gene suppression using a range of criteria including *in vitro* translation inhibition, plaque assay, cell viability or proliferation, marker gene activity from cells transformed with viral constructs or antiviral activity *in vivo*.[81] Sequence specificity, a hallmark of antisense drug design, is evaluated using a range of control ODNs that may include random, sense, missense, or scrambled orientation sequences.[84]

The experimental usage of antisense ODNs against influenza virus infections have been reported in both *in vitro* tissue culture and *in vivo* animal infection model systems. The rational drug design for antisense ODNs against influenza has been focused on viral gene targets that are less prone to antigenic shift and/or drift. Therefore, the highly variable regions of mRNAs encoding HA and neuraminidase (NA) are usually not considered to be ideal gene targets. However, given the highly conserved regions of the polymerase (*PA, PB1, PB2*) and nucleoprotein (*NP*) genes, a number of potential broad-range antisense targets have been identified. Early work using MDCK cells demonstrated sequence-specific antiviral activity, although a specific effect on the target genes was not determined.[85,86] A transient influenza gene expression assay has been developed by sandwiching a chloramphenicol acetyltransferase (CAT) gene between the 5′ and 3′ terminal sequences of influenza A/PR/8/34 RNA segment 8. RNA from this expression vector was transfected into clone 76 cells, into which ODN was delivered using a cationic lipid complex.[87] Using either CAT expression or cell viability as a measure of antiviral activity, antisense ODN directed against *PB2* was consistently found to be the most potent inhibitor of influenza replication and gene expression.[87–89] *PB1*, *PB2*, and *PA* antisense ODNs were administered i.v. as a cationic lipid complex with Tfx-10 or DMRIE at twice daily intervals 1 day prior to infection and 4 days post-infection in a murine infection model with 100 LD_{50} of influenza A/PR/8/34.[79,90,91] *PB2* antisense ODN, which targeted the AUG region of *PB2*, consistently increased both the mean survival time and survival at day 14 post-infection (45%). Concomitant with increased survival was a decrease in *PB2* mRNA expression and viral titer in infected lungs 4 days after infection.

Antisense ODNs (15-mer) directed against a conserved region of the influenza A virus HA protein have also been shown to be effective in the post-exposure treatment of influenza A virus infection in mice.[21] In this study, both unencapsulated and liposome-encapsulated antisense ODNs, administered i.n., were completely effective in the treatment of mice against an otherwise lethal respiratory challenge. A significant therapeutic advantage was achieved with liposome encapsulation of the antisense ODNs as the dosage of antisense ODNs required to achieve complete protection was reduced by up to 80%.[92] The level of dose reduction was presumably due to protection of antisense ODNs against nuclease degradation in the body, as well as enhanced delivery of the antisense ODNs to intracellular sites of viral replication.

CONCLUSION

In light of increasing drug-resistance of influenza viruses to conventional antiviral drugs and the pandemic potential of avian H5N1 influenza virus, there is a critical need to develop new antiviral agents. Nucleic acid-based therapeutic drugs represent a promising new class of antiviral agents, offering significant therapeutic advantages over conventional antiviral drugs due to their versatility and specificity. This review has highlighted a range of applications for ODNs in antiviral therapy. Immunomodulating nucleic acids, catalytic nucleic acids, and antisense ODNs are three main classes of nucleic acid-based antiviral agents being evaluated in clinical studies. Double-stranded RNA (such as poly ICLC) and CpG ODNs may provide broad-spectrum protection against new and drug-resistant influenza virus variants by virtue of the enhancement of the host's innate and adaptive immune responses. DNAzymes and ribozymes are catalytic nucleic acids that cleave viral mRNAs, while antisense ODNs cause sequence-specific inhibition of viral gene expression. However, in order for these agents to meet therapeutic expectations, a number of issues will need to be addressed; these include the biological stability and safety of phosphorothioate and other chemically modified ODNs, as well as delivery and transport to intracellular sites of infection. Research and development efforts have been greatly aided by advances in synthetic medicinal chemistry which have resulted in the design of ODNs with improved stability and fewer side effects, some of which are currently being evaluated in clinical trials. Formulation improvements have also been made to enhance intracellular delivery of ODNs to sites where viruses replicate. Of particular interest is the use of novel liposome formulations that can protect ODNs from nuclease degradation and assist with target localization. Cationic and pH-sensitive liposomes are the formulations of choice for ODNs. Overcoming the challenges mentioned above will enable nucleic acid-based drugs to reach their full potential as antiviral therapeutics.

REFERENCES

1. World Health Organization. Cumulative number of confirmed human cases of avian influenza A/ (H5N1) reported to WHO. http://www.who.

int/csr/disease/avianinfluenza/country/cases_table_2007_01_12/en/index. html

2. Krieg, A. M. Mechanisms and applications of immune stimulatory CpG oligodeoxynucleotides. *Biochim. Biophys. Acta* **1999**, *1489*, 107–116.

3. Wong, J. P.; Saravolac, E. G.; Sabuda, D.; Levy, H. B.; Kende, M. Prophylactic and therapeutic efficacies of poly(IC.LC) against respiratory influenza A virus infection in mice. *Antimicrob. Agents Chemother.* **1995**, *39*, 2574–2576.

4. Haseloff, J.; Gerlach, W. L. Simple RNA enzymes with new and highly specific endoribonuclease activities. *Nature* **1988**, *334*, 585–591.

5. Santoro, S. W.; Joyce, G. F. A general purpose RNA-cleaving DNA enzyme. *Proc. Natl. Acad. Sci. USA* **1997**, *94*, 4262–4266.

6. Saravolac, E. G.; Sun, L.-Q.; Cairns, M. J.; Wong, J. P. Nucleic acid-based drugs as antiviral agents. *Recent Devel. Antiviral Res.* **2001**, *1*, 117–141.

7. Zamecnik, P. C.; Stephenson, M. L. Inhibition of Rous sarcoma virus replication and cell transformation by a specific oligodeoxynucleotide. *Proc. Natl. Acad. Sci. USA* **1978**, *75*, 280–284.

8. Haasnoot, P. C.; Cupac, D.; Berkhout, B. Inhibition of virus replication by RNA interference. *J. Biomed. Sci.* **2003**, *10*, 607–616.

9. Wong, J. P.; Yang, H.; Nagata, L.; Kende, M.; Levy, H.; Schnell, G.; Blasetti, K. Liposome-mediated immunotherapy against respiratory influenza virus infection using double-stranded RNA poly ICLC. *Vaccine* **1999**, *17*, 1788–1795.

10. McCluskie, M. J.; Weeratna, R. D. Novel adjuvant systems. *Curr. Drug Targets Infect. Disord.* **2001**, *1*, 263–271.

11. Vollmer, J.; Weeratna, R.; Payette, P.; Jurk, M.; Laucht, M.; Wader, T.; Tluk, S.; Liu, M.; Davis, H. L.; Krieg, A. M. Characterization of three CpG oligodeoxynucleotide classes with distinct immunostimulatory activities. *Eur. J. Immunol.* **2004**, *34*, 251–262.

12. Chirigos, M. A.; Welker, R.; Schlick, E.; Saito, T.; Ruffmann, R. Vaccine adjuvant effects and immune response to polymers MVE and poly ICLC. *Prog. Clin. Biol. Res.* **1984**, *161*, 467–479.

13. Levy, H. B.; Baer, G.; Baron, S.; Buckler, C. E.; Gibbs, C. J.; Iadarola, M. J.; London, W. T.; Rice, J. A modified polyriboinosinic–polyribocytidylic acid complex that induces interferon in primates. *J. Infect. Dis.* **1975**, *132*, 434–439.

14. Stephen, E. L.; Sammons, M. L.; Pannier, W. L.; Baron, S.; Spertzel, R. O.; Levy, H. B. Effect of a nuclease-resistant derivative of polyriboinosinic–polyribocytidylic acid complex on yellow fever in rhesus monkeys (*Macaca mulatta*). *J. Infect. Dis.* **1977**, *136*, 122–126.

15. Stephen, E. L; Hilmas, D. E.; Levy, H. B.; Spertzel, R. O. Protective and toxic effects of a nuclease-resistant derivative of polyriboinosinic–

polyribocytidylic acid on Venezuelan equine encephalomyelitis virus in rhesus monkeys. *J. Infect. Dis.* **1979**, *139*, 267–272.

16. Harrington, D. G.; Hilmas, D. E.; Elwell, M. R.; Whitmire, R. E.; Stephen, E. L. Intranasal infection of monkeys with Japanese encephalitis virus: Clinical response and treatment with a nuclease-resistant derivative of poly (I).poly (C). *Am. J. Trop. Med. Hyg.* **1977**, *26*, 1191–1198.

17. Kende, M. Prophylactic and therapeutic efficacy of poly (I,C)-LC against Rift Valley fever virus infection in mice. *J. Biol. Response Mod.* **1985**, *4*, 503–511.

18. Baer, G. M.; Shaddock, J. H.; Moore, S. A.; Yager, P. A.; Baron, S. S.; Levy, H. B. Successful prophylaxis against rabies in mice and Rhesus monkeys: The interferon system and vaccine. *J. Infect. Dis.* **1977**, *136*, 286–291.

19. Sivori, S.; Falco, M.; Della Chiesa, M.; Carlomagno, S.; Vitale, M.; Moretta, L.; Moretta, A. CpG and double-stranded RNA trigger human NK cells by Toll-like receptors: Induction of cytokine release and cytotoxicity against tumors and dendritic cells. *Proc. Natl. Acad. Sci. USA* **2004**, *101*, 10116–10121.

20. Levy, H. B.; Riley, F. L. In *Lymphokines*, Landy, M., Ed., Academic Press, Orlando, FL, **1983**, pp 302–322.

21. Wong, J. P.; Christopher, M. E.; Salazar, A. M.; Dale, R. M. K.; Sun, L.-Q.; Wang, M. Nucleic acid-based antiviral drugs against seasonal and avian influenza viruses. *Vaccine* **2007**, *25*, 3175–3178.

22. Mitchell, W.; Smee, D.; Strayer, D.; Carter, W. Synergistic inhibition of avian influenza virus (H5N1) by poly I: Poly C12U combined with oseltamivir or zanamivir. VIII International Symposium on Respiratory Viral Infections, 16–19 March 2006, Kohala Coast, Hawaii.

23. Krieg, A. M.; Yi, A. K.; Matson, S.; Waldschmidt, T. J.; Bishop, G. A.; Teasdale, R.; Koretzky, G. A.; Klinman, D. M. CpG motifs in bacterial DNA trigger direct B-cell activation. *Nature* **1995**, *374*, 546–549.

24. Hemmi, H.; Takeuchi, O.; Kawai, T.; Kaisho, T.; Sato, S.; Sanjo, H.; Matsumoto, M.; Hoshino, K.; Wagner, H.; Takeda, K.; Akira, S. A Toll-like receptor recognizes bacterial DNA. *Nature* **2000**, *408*, 740–745.

25. Krieg, A. M. CpG motifs in bacterial DNA and their immune effects. *Annu. Rev. Immunol.* **2002**, *20*, 709–760.

26. Hartmann, G.; Weiner, G. J.; Krieg, A. M. CpG DNA: A potent signal for growth, activation, and maturation of human dendritic cells. *Proc. Natl. Acad. Sci. USA* **1999**, *96*, 9305–9310.

27. Hartmann, G.; Weeratna, R. D.; Ballas, Z. K.; Payette, P.; Blackwell, S.; Suparto, I.; Rasmussen, W. L.; Waldschmidt, M.; Sajuthi, D.; Purcell, R. H.; Davis, H. L.; Krieg, A. M. Delineation of a CpG phosphorothioate oligodeoxynucleotide for activating primate immune responses *in vitro* and *in vivo*. *J. Immunol.* **2000**, *164*, 1617–1624.

28. Bernasconi, N. L.; Onai, N.; Lanzavecchia, A. A role for Toll-like receptors in acquired immunity: Up-regulation of TLR9 by BCR triggering in naïve B cells and constitutive expression in memory B cells. *Blood* **2003**, *101*, 4500–4504.

29. Askew, D.; Chu, R. S.; Krieg, A. M.; Harding, C. V. CpG DNA induces maturation of dendritic cells with distinct effects on nascent and recycling MHC-II antigen-processing mechanisms. *J. Immunol.* **2000**, *165*, 6889–6895.

30. Chu, R. S.; Targoni, O. S.; Krieg, A. M.; Lehmann, P. V.; Harding, C. V. CpG oligodeoxynucleotides act as adjuvants that switch on T helper 1 (Th1) immunity. *J. Exp. Med.* **1997**, *186*, 1623–1631.

31. Manning, B. M.; Enioutina, E. Y.; Visic, D. M.; Knudson, A. D.; Daynes. R. A. CpG DNA functions as an effective adjuvant for the induction of immune responses in aged mice. *Exp. Gerontol.* **2001**, *37*, 107–126.

32. Maletto, B.; Ropolo, A.; Moron, V.; Pistoresi-Palencia, M. C. CpG-DNA stimulates cellular and humoral immunity and promotes Th1 differentiation in aged BALB/c mice. *J. Leukoc. Biol.* **2002**, *72*, 447–454.

33. Moldoveanu, Z.; Love-Homan, L.; Huang, W. Q.; Krieg, A. M. CpG DNA, a novel immune enhancer for systemic and mucosal immunization with influenza virus. *Vaccine* **1998**, *16*, 1216–1224.

34. McCluskie, M. J.; Davis, H. L. Oral, intrarectal and intranasal immunizations using CpG and non-CpG oligodeoxynucleotides as adjuvants. *Vaccine* **2000**, *19*, 413–422.

35. Beignon, A. S.; Briand, J. P.; Muller, S.; Partidos, C. D. Immunization onto bare skin with synthetic peptides: immunomodulation with a CpG-containing oligodeoxynucleotide and effective priming of influenza virus-specific CD4+ T cells. *Immunology* **2002**, *105*, 204–212.

36. Joseph, A.; Louria-Hayon, I.; Plis-Finarov, A.; Zeira, E.; Zakay-Rones, Z.; Raz, E.; Hayashi, T.; Takabayashi, K.; Barenholz, Y.; Kedar, E. Liposomal immunostimulatory DNA sequences (ISS-ODN) and efficient parenteral and mucosal adjuvant for influenza and hepatitis B vaccines. *Vaccine* **2002**, *20*, 3342–3354.

37. Hampel, A.; Tritz, R. RNA catalytic properties of the minimum (–)sTRSV sequence. *Biochemistry* **1989**, *28*, 4929–4933.

38. Forster, A. C.; Symons, R. H. Self-cleavage of plus and minus RNAs of a virusoid and a structural model for the active sites. *Cell* **1987**, *49*, 211–220.

39. Kruger, K.; Grabowski, P. J.; Zaug, A. J.; Sands, J.; Gottschling, D. E.; Cech, T. R. Self-splicing RNA: Autoexcision and autocyclization of the ribosomal RNA intervening sequence of *Tetrahymena*. *Cell* **1982**, *31*, 147–157.

40. Peebles, C. L.; Perlman, P. S.; Mecklenburg, K. L.; Petrillo, M. L.; Tabor, J. H.; Jarrell, K. A.; Cheng H. L. A self-splicing RNA excises an intron lariat. *Cell* **1986**, *44*, 213–223.

41. Guerrier-Takada, C.; Gardiner, K.; Marsh, T.; Pace, N.; Altman, S. The RNA moiety of ribonuclease P is the catalytic subunit of the enzyme. *Cell* **1983**, *35*, 849–857.

42. Sharmeen, L.; Kuo, M. Y.; Dinter-Gottlieb, G.; Taylor, J. Antigenomic RNA of human hepatitis delta virus can undergo self-cleavage. *J. Virol.* **1988**, *62*, 2674–2679.

43. Saville, B. J.; Collins, R. A. A site-specific self-cleavage reaction performed by a novel RNA in *Neurospora* mitochondria. *Cell* **1990**, *61*, 685–696.

44. Saravolac, E. G.; Christopher, M. E.; Cairns, M. J.; Sun, L.-Q.; Dale, R. M. K.; Wong, J. P. Recent developments in influenza chemotherapy: Are answers in the viral genome? *Recent Dev. Antiviral Res.* **2003**, *2*, 1–27.

45. Symons, R. H. Ribozymes. *Curr. Opin. Struct. Biol.* **1994**, *4*, 322–330.

46. Fedor, M. J.; Uhlenbeck, O. C. Substrate sequence effects on "hammerhead" RNA catalytic efficiency. *Proc. Natl. Acad. Sci. USA* **1990**, *87*, 1668–1672.

47. Hertel, K. J.; Herschlag, D.; Uhlenbeck, O. C. A kinetic and thermodynamic framework for the hammerhead ribozyme reaction. *Biochemistry* **1994**, *33*, 3374–3385.

48. Sun, L.-Q.; Cairns, M. J.; Saravolac, E. G.; Baker, A.; Gerlach, W. L. Catalytic nucleic acids: from lab to application. *Pharmacol. Rev.* **2000**, *52*, 325–347.

49. Knapp, G. Enzymatic approaches to probing of RNA secondary and tertiary structure. *Methods Enzymol.* **1989**, *180*, 192–212.

50. Lieber, A.; Strauss, M. Selection of efficient cleavage sites in target RNAs by using a ribozyme expression library. *Mol. Cell Biol.* **1995**, *15*, 540–551.

51. Yu, Q.; Pecchia, D. B.; Kingsley, S. L.; Heckman, J. E.; Burke, J. M. Cleavage of highly structured viral RNA molecules by combinatorial libraries of hairpin ribozymes. The most effective ribozymes are not predicted by substrate selection rules. *J. Biol. Chem.* **1998**, *273*, 23524–23533.

52. Welch, P. J.; Tritz, R.; Yei, S.; Barber, J.; Yu, M. Intracellular application of hairpin ribozyme genes against hepatitis B virus. *Gene Ther.* **1997**, *4*, 736–743.

53. Welch, P. J.; Tritz, R.; Yei, S.; Leavitt, M.; Yu, M.; Barber, J. A potential therapeutic application of hairpin ribozymes: *In vitro* and *in vivo* studies of gene therapy for hepatitis C virus infection. *Gene Ther.* **1996**, *3*, 994–1001.

54. Trang, P.; Lee, M.; Nepomuceno, E.; Kim, J.; Zhu, H.; Liu, F. Effective inhibition of human cytomegalovirus gene expression and replication by a ribozyme derived from the catalytic RNA subunit of RNase P from Escherichia coli. *Proc. Natl. Acad. Sci. USA* **2000**, *97*, 5812–5817.

55. Sun, L. Q.; Pyati, J.; Smythe, J.; Wang, L.; Macpherson, J.; Gerlach, W.; Symonds, G. Resistance to human immunodeficiency virus type 1 infection conferred by transduction of human peripheral blood lymphocytes with

ribozyme, antisense, or polymeric trans-activation response element constructs. *Proc. Natl. Acad. Sci. USA* **1995**, *92*, 7272–7276.

56. Liu, D. Z.; Jin, Y. X.; Hou, H.; Huang, Y. Z.; Yang, G. C.; Xu, Q. Preparation and identification of activity of anti-HPV-6b/11E1 universal ribozyme—Rz1198 *in vitro. Asian J. Androl.* **1999**, *1*, 195–201.

57. Tang, X. B.; Hobom, G.; Luo, D. Ribozyme mediated destruction of influenza A virus *in vitro* and *in vivo. J. Med. Virol.* **1994**, *42*, 385–395.

58. Lazarev, V. N.; Shmarov, M. M.; Zakhartchouk, A. N.; Yurov, G. K.; Misurina, O. U.; Akopian, T. A.; Grinenko, N. F.; Grodnitskaya, N. G.; Kaverin, N. V.; Naroditsky, B. S. Inhibition of influenza A virus reproduction by a ribozyme targeted against PB1 mRNA. *Antiviral Res.* **1999**, *42*, 47–57.

59. Plehn-Dujowich, D.; Altman, S. Effective inhibition of influenza virus production in cultured cells by external guide sequences and ribonuclease P. *Proc. Natl. Acad. Sci. USA* **1998**, *95*, 7327–7332.

60. Amado, R. G.; Mitsuyasu, R. T.; Symonds, G.; Rosenblatt, J. D.; Zack, J.; Sun, L. Q.; Miller, M.; Ely, J.; Gerlach, W. A phase I trial of autologous CD34+ hematopoietic progenitor cells transduced with an anti-HIV ribozyme. *Hum. Gene Ther.* **1999**, *10*, 2255–2270.

61. Beigelman, L.; McSwiggen, J. A.; Draper, K. G.; Gonzalez, C.; Jensen, K.; Karpeisky, A. M.; Modak, A. S.; Matulic-Adamic, J.; DiRenzo, A. B.; Haeberli, P.; Sweedler, D.; Tracz, D.; Grimm, S.; Wincott, F. E.; Thackray, V. G.; Usman, N. Chemical modification of hammerhead ribozymes. Catalytic activity and nuclease resistance. *J. Biol. Chem.* **1995**, *270*, 25702–25708.

62. Desjardins, J. P.; Sproat, B. S.; Beijer, B.; Blaschke, M.; Dunkel, M.; Gerdes, W.; Ludwig, J.; Reither, V.; Rupp, T.; Iverson, P. L. Pharmacokinetics of a synthetic, chemically modified hammerhead ribozyme against the rat cytochrome P-450 3A2 mRNA after single intravenous injections. *J. Pharmacol. Exp. Ther.* **1996**, *278*, 1419–1427.

63. Sioud, M.; Sorensen, D. R. A nuclease-resistant protein kinase C alpha ribozyme blocks glioma cell growth. *Nat. Biotechnol.* **1998**, *16*, 556–561.

64. Draper, K. G. Method and reagent for inhibiting influenza virus replication. **2001**, US Patent No. 6,258,585.

65. Sugimoto, N.; Nakano, S.; Katoh, M.; Matsumura, A.; Nakamuta, H.; Ohmichi, T.; Yoneyama, M.; Sasaki, M. Thermodynamic parameters to predict stability of RNA/DNA hybrid duplexes. *Biochemistry* **1995**, *34*, 11211–11216.

66. Santoro, S. W.; Joyce, G. F. Mechanism and utility of an RNA-cleaving DNA enzyme. *Biochemistry* **1998**, *37*, 13330–13342.

67. Cairns, M. J.; Hopkins, T. M.; Witherington, C.; Wang, L.; Sun, L. Q. Target site selection for an RNA-cleaving catalytic DNA. *Nat. Biotechnol.* **1999**, *17*, 480–486.

68. Cairns, M. J.; King, A.; Sun, L. Q. Nucleic acid mutation analysis using catalytic DNA. *Nucleic Acids Res.* **2000**, *28*, E9.

69. Todd, A. V.; Fuery, C. J.; Impey, H. L.; Applegate, T. L.; Haughton, M. A. DzyNA-PCR: Use of DNAzymes to detect and quantify nucleic acid sequences in a real-time fluorescent format. *Clin. Chem.* **2000**, *46*, 625–630.

70. Sun, L. Q.; Cairns, M. J.; Gerlach, W. L.; Witherington, C.; Wang, L.; King, A. Suppression of smooth muscle cell proliferation by a c-myc RNA-cleaving deoxyribozyme. *J. Biol. Chem.* **1999**, *274*, 17236–17241.

71. Dass, C. R.; Saravolac, E. G.; Li, Y.; Sun, L. Q. Cellular uptake, distribution, and stability of 10–23 deoxyribozymes. *Antisense Nucleic Acid Drug Dev.* **2002**, *12*, 289–299.

72. Warashina, M.; Kuwabara, T.; Nakamatsu, Y.; Taira, R. Extremely high and specific activity of DNA enzymes in cells with a Philadelphia chromosome. *Chem. Biol.* **1999**, *6*, 237–250.

73. Unwalla, H.; Banerjea, A. C. Novel mono- and di-DNA-enzymes targeted to cleave TAT or TAT-REV RNA inhibit HIV-1 gene expression. *Antiviral Res.* **2001**, *51*, 127–139.

74. Sriram, B.; Banerjea, A. C. *In vitro*-selected RNA cleaving DNA enzymes from a combinatorial library are potent inhibitors of HIV-1 gene expression. *Biochem. J.* **2000**, *352*, 667–673.

75. Zhang, X.; Xu, Y.; Ling, H.; Hattori, T. Inhibition of infection of incoming HIV-1 virus by RNA-cleaving DNA enzyme. *FEBS Lett.* **1999**, *458*, 151–156.

76. Goila, R.; Banerjea, A. C. Inhibition of hepatitis B virus X gene expression by novel DNA enzymes. *Biochem. J.* **2001**, *353*, 701–708.

77. Oketani, M.; Asahina, Y.; Yu, C. H.; Wu, G. Y. Inhibition of hepatitis C virus-directed gene expression by a DNA ribonuclease. *J. Hepatol.* **1999**, *31*, 628–634.

78. Toyoda T.; Imamura, Y.; Takaku, H.; Kashiwagi, T.; Hara, K.; Iwahashi, J.; Ohtsu, Y.; Tsumura, N.; Kato, H.; Hamada, N. Inhibition of influenza virus replication in cultured cells by RNA-cleaving DNA enzyme. *FEBS Lett.* **2000**, *481*, 113–116.

79. Abe, T.; Mizuta T.; Hatta T.; Miyano-Kurosaki, N.; Fujiwara, M.; Takai, K.; Shigeta, S.; Yokota, T.; Takaku, H. Antisense therapy of influenza. *Eur. J. Pharm. Sci.* **2001**, *13*, 61–69.

80. Stephenson, M. L.; Zamecnik, P. C. Inhibition of Rous sarcoma viral RNA translation by a specific oligodeoxyribonucleotide. *Proc. Natl. Acad. Sci. USA* **1978**, *75*, 285–288.

81. Alama, A.; Barbieri, F.; Cagnoli, M.; Schettini, G. Antisense oligonucleotides as therapeutic agents. *Pharmacol. Res.* **1997**, *36*, 171–178.

82. Crooke, S. T. Molecular mechanisms of antisense drugs: RNase H. *Antisense Nucleic Acid Drug Dev.* **1998**, *8*, 133–134.

83. Juliano, R. L.; Alahari, S.; Yoo, H.; Kole, R.; Cho, M. Antisense pharmacodynamics: Critical issues in the transport and delivery of antisense oligonucleotides. *Pharm. Res.* **1999**, *16*, 494–502.

84. Stein, C. A. How to design an antisense oligodeoxynucleotide experiment: A consensus approach. *Antisense Nucleic Acid Drug Dev*. **1998**, *8*, 129–132.

85. Zerial, A.; Thuong, N. T.; Helene, C. Selective inhibition of the cytopathic effect of type A influenza viruses by oligodeoxynucleotides covalently linked to an intercalating agent. *Nucleic Acids Res*. **1987**, *15*, 9909–9919.

86. Leiter, J. M.; Agrawal, S.; Palese, P.; Zamecnik, P. C. Inhibition of influenza virus replication by phosphorothioate oligodeoxynucleotides. *Proc. Natl. Acad. Sci. USA* **1990**, *87*, 3430–3434.

87. Hatta, T.; Nakagawa, Y.; Takai, K.; Nakada, S.; Yokota, T.; Takaku, H. Inhibition of influenza virus RNA polymerase and nucleoprotein genes expression by unmodified, phosphorothioated, and liposomally encapsulated oligodeoxynucleotides. *Biochem. Biophys. Res. Commun*. **1996**, *223*, 341–346.

88. Hatta, T.; Takai, K.; Nakada, S.; Yokota, T.; Takaku, H. Specific inhibition of influenza virus RNA polymerase and nucleoprotein genes expression by liposomally endocapsulated antisense phosphorothioate oligonucleotides: Penetration and localization of oligonucleotides in clone 76 cells. *Biochem. Biophys. Res. Commun*. **1997**, *232*, 545–549.

89. Abe, T.; Hatta, T.; Takai, K.; Nakashima, H.; Yokota, T.; Takaku, H. Inhibition of influenza virus replication by phosphorothioate and liposomally endocapsulated oligonucleotides. *Nucleosides Nucleotides* **1998**, *17*, 471–478.

90. Mizuta, T.; Fujiwara, M.; Hatta, T.; Abe, T.; Miyano-Kurosaki, N.; Shigeta, S.; Yokota, T.; Takaku, H. Antisense oligonucleotides directed against the viral RNA polymerase gene enhance survival of mice infected with influenza A. *Nat. Biotechnol*. **1999**, *17*, 583–587.

91. Mizuta, T.; Fujiwara, M.; Abe, T.; Miyano-Kurosaki, N.; Yokota, T.; Shigeta, S.; Takaku, H. Inhibitory effects of an antisense oligonucleotide in an experimentally infected mouse model of influenza A virus. *Biochem. Biophys. Res. Commun*. **2000**, *279*, 158–161.

92. Wong, J. P. H.; Nagata, L. P. Therapy of respiratory influenza virus infection using free and liposome-encapsulated ribonucleotides. **2003**, US Patent No. 6,544,958.

6

ANTIVIRAL RNA INTERFERENCE STRATEGIES TARGETING INFLUENZA VIRUS AND OTHER RESPIRATORY VIRUSES

JOOST HAASNOOT AND BEN BERKHOUT

Laboratory of Experimental Virology, Department of Medical Microbiology, Center for Infection and Immunity Amsterdam (CINIMA), Academic Medical Center of the University of Amsterdam, Meibergdreef 15, 1105 AZ Amsterdam, The Netherlands

INTRODUCTION

Viral respiratory tract infections contribute significantly to illness, hospitalisation, and death of young, elderly, and immunocompromised individuals. In most cases, vaccines and antiviral drugs give only limited protection. In particular, viruses such as influenza A virus are a serious health threat for which new antiviral vaccines and treatments need to be developed. A possible addition to the antiviral arsenal is RNA-interference (RNAi)-based therapeutics. Ever since its discovery, RNAi has been considered a potentially powerful new tool to combat viruses. These "great expectations" were recently underscored by awarding the 2006 Noble prize for physiology and medicine to Andrew Fire and Graig Mellow for their pioneering work on the description and mechanism of RNAi. Their finding that double-stranded RNA (dsRNA) triggered sequence-specific gene silencing in *Caenorhabditis elegans* is now

Combating the Threat of Pandemic Influenza: Drug Discovery Approaches,
Edited by Paul F. Torrence

at the basis of the development of several RNAi therapeutics.[1] The applications range from compounds for the treatment of virus infections or genetic diseases to cosmetic compounds as in Sirna's hair removal program (http://www.sirna.com). Currently, several RNAi-based therapeutics are being tested in clinical trials. Both Acuity Pharmaceuticals and Sirna began testing siRNAs in humans as an alternative treatment for the wet form of age-related macular degeneration (AMD). In April 2006, Alnylam presented phase I clinical data on an siRNA-based drug against respiratory syncytial virus (RSV) (http://www.alnylam.com).

RNAi-mediated inhibition has been reported for a large variety of viruses. These include important human pathogens such as human immunodeficiency virus type 1 (HIV-1), hepatitis C virus (HCV), dengue virus, poliovirus, hepatitis D virus (HDV), hepatitis B virus (HBV), herpes simplex virus type-1, human papillomavirus, JC virus, Epstein–Barr virus, and cytomegalovirus (CMV).[2] Important respiratory viruses for which RNAi-mediated inhibition has been reported include severe acute respiratory syndrome coronavirus (SARS-CoV), NL63 coronavirus (NL63-CoV), influenza A virus, parainfluenza virus (PIV), RSV, and human rhinovirus-16 (HRV-16). The results for all respiratory viruses are summarized in Table 6.1—except for SARS and other coronavirus studies, which are summarized in Table 6.2. Animal respiratory viruses are also included in Table 6.1: porcine reproductive and respiratory syndrome virus (PRRSV) and avian metapneumovirus (aMPV). Although profound inhibition of virus replication has been reported *in vitro* and *in vivo*, it has become clear that several problems need to be resolved before RNAi therapeutics will reach the clinic. Important concerns include virus escape from RNAi, possible off-target effects of RNAi treatment, and the delivery of the RNAi-inducer to the right target cell.

Respiratory viruses appear to be ideal targets for the development of RNAi-therapeutics because the upper airways and lungs are relatively easy to reach target tissues. In this review, we provide an overview of RNAi studies on influenza and other respiratory viruses and discuss the possibility to develop RNAi-based antiviral therapies.

MECHANISM OF RNA INTERFERENCE

RNAi is a conserved sequence-specific gene silencing mechanism in eukaryotic cells that is induced by dsRNA. It plays a pivotal role in the regulation of cellular gene expression via microRNAs (miRNAs). These

TABLE 6.1. RNAi-Mediated Inhibition of Influenza Virus and Other Respiratory Viruses

Virus	Targeted Gene	RNAi Inducer	Cell Type	Fold Inhibition of Virus Replication	Reference
Influenza A virus	PB1, PB2, PA, NP, M, NS	siRNA	MDCK, chicken embryos	200	30
	NP, PA	siRNA	Mice	56	32
	NP, PA, PB1	siRNA, shRNA[a]	Mice, Vero	~10	31
	M	shRNA[a]	MDCK	~5	68
PIV	P	siRNA	A549, mice	~100	34
RSV	P, F	siRNA	A549	~10	33
	P	siRNA	A549, mice	~5000	34
	NS1	shRNA	A549, Vero, mice	~100	35
	P	siRNA	Mice	~100	72
EV71	VP1, 3D	shRNA	Hela, Vero	5–10	37
HRV-16	5′-UTR, vp4, vp2, vp3, vp1, 2A, 2C, 3A, 3C, 3D	siRNA	Hela	~10–20	69
PRRSV	GP5, N	shRNA	MARC	~1000	75
	N	shRNA	MARC	~10	76
	ORF7	shRNA[b]	MARC	~681	74
aMPV	P	siRNA	Vero	~8	73

All siRNAs were chemically synthesized and transfected into cells unless indicated otherwise. ShRNAs were intracellularly expressed from transfected plasmids under the control a pol III promoter (H1 or U6). Stable expression of shRNAs was obtained using a lentiviral vector ([a]) or a baculovirus vector ([b]). The fold inhibition of virus production represents the result obtained with the most efficient si or shRNA.

TABLE 6.2. RNAi-Mediated Inhibition of Human Coronaviruses

Virus	Target Gene	RNAi Inducer	Cell Type	Fold Inhibition of Virus Replication	Reference
SARS-CoV	Pol	shRNA	Vero	5	38
	Pol	shRNA	Vero-E6, 293, Hela	16	37
	Pol	siRNA	FRhk-4	7–14	36
	Spike	shRNA	293T, Vero-E6	~10	39
	5′-UTR, TRS, Spike, 3′-UTR	siRNA	Vero-E6	~10	41
	E, N	shRNA[a]	293T, COS7	ND	35
	5′-UTR	shRNA	Vero-E6	>10	70
	Spike, NSP12	siRNA	Rhesus macaque	~2[b]	42
	Spike	siRNA	293T	ND	71
	7a/7b, 3a/3b, S	shRNA[c]	Vero-E6	>10	77
HCoV-NL63	Spike	siRNA	LLC-Mk2	>10	43

See Table 6.1 for details. ([a]) Stable expression using an adenovirus vector, ([b]) Inhibition of virus infected cell count in lung tissue. ([c]) Stable expression via selection using antibiotics. (ND) not done.

miRNAs represent a family of highly structured small noncoding RNAs that negatively regulate gene expression at the post-transcriptional level.[3] They are expressed as primary miRNAs (pri-miRNAs) and processed by the proteins Drosha and Dicer into, respectively, a ~70-nucleotide (nt) stem-loop precursor miRNA (pre-miRNA) and the mature miRNA of 21–25 nt. One strand of the mature miRNA, the antisense or guide strand, is loaded in the RNA-induced silencing complex (RISC). This guide strand targets RISC to the mRNA, where the complex hybridizes to (partially) complementary sequences, triggering mRNA cleavage or translational inhibition. RNAi is also believed to be involved in inhibition of viruses and silencing of transposable elements by generation of virus-specific small interfering RNAs (siRNAs, 21-nt dsRNA). Similar to miRNAs, these siRNAs are loaded into RISC and target viral RNAs for destruction or translational repression.[4] Although the antiviral function of RNAi is well established in plants, insects, and nematodes, it is still unclear whether RNAi has a similar role in mammals.[5–7]

The standard method to induce RNAi against viruses in mammalian cells is via transfection of synthetic siRNAs corresponding to viral sequences before or after a viral challenge. These siRNA duplexes are generally 21 nt long with 2-nt 3′ overhangs and are modeled after the natural Dicer cleavage products. Once the antisense strand of the antiviral siRNA is loaded into RISC, the complex will target the viral RNAs in a sequence-specific manner. Alternatively, transient transfection of plasmids that express antiviral short hairpin RNAs (shRNAs) is also commonly used to induce RNAi. These shRNAs are typically 19–29 base pairs long with a small apical loop and a 3′-terminal UU overhang. ShRNAs are usually expressed in the nucleus under control of a polymerase III promoter, are translocated to the cytoplasm by Exportin-5, and are further processed by Dicer in the cytoplasm into functional siRNAs. The first vectors for the expression of functional shRNA were described in 2002.[8,9] Several modifications of this system have been reported. For example, the enhancer from the CMV immediate-early promoter (a Pol II unit) can enhance the expression of siRNA from a Pol III unit.[10] The two human Pol III promoters that have been most widely are the U6 and H1 promoters that naturally drive expression of respectively a snRNA and the RNA component of the RNase P complex. More efficient siRNA expression was reported for a modified tRNA^{met} promoter (MTD unit).[11] Other improvements include the design of a doxycycline-regulated H1 promoter that allows the inducible knockdown of gene expression by siRNAs.[12] Recently, inhibition by shRNA-induced RNAi has also been significantly improved by using shRNA that more closely resemble miRNAs. These second-generation shRNAs (shRNA-mirs) are designed using the increased knowledge of RNAi biochemistry and miRNA biogenesis. shRNA-mirs are expressed as larger transcripts and contain bulged nucleotides and large loops as present in pri- or pre-miRNAs.[13–15] Strategies to express multivalent shRNA constructs have also been described,[16,17] which seems very important to avoid the danger of viral escape.[18]

Transient transfection of siRNAs or shRNA expression plasmids results in potent, albeit temporary, inhibition of virus replication. In order to obtain long-term virus suppression, researchers have turned to a combined RNAi/gene therapy approach. In this approach, lenti-, retro-, or adeno-associated virus (AAV) vectors are used to stably transduce cells with constructs expressing shRNA, resulting in viral resistance. Such gene therapy strategies in which cells are stably transduced to express antiviral siRNAs are presumably the best way to counter chronic virus infections such as HIV-1, HCV, and HSV. In contrast, viruses causing more acute temporary infections, including all respiratory viruses, might be candidates for transient treatment with synthetic siRNAs. Another possibility is to use nonpathogenic, but replicating, viruses as a vector to express siRNAs against other pathogenic viruses.[19]

INFLUENZA VIRUS

Worldwide, an estimated half million deaths per year are attributed to influenza virus infections, and there is the continuous threat of the emergence of a novel pandemic strain. Due to limitations of anti-influenza vaccines and drugs, there is an urgent need for novel strategies to inhibit influenza virus. Influenza A viruses are members of the family of Orthomyxoviridae, which are enveloped viruses containing a segmented genome of eight strands of minus-strand RNA.[20] The gene segments encode 10 viral proteins: a nucleoprotein (NP), three subunits of the viral polymerase (PB1, PB2, and PA), two glycoproteins [hemagglutinin (HA) and neuramidase (NA)], a matrix protein (M1), a membrane protein (M2), and two nonstructural proteins (NS1 and NS2). Influenza virus infects epithelial cells in the upper airways and lungs. In healthy individuals the virus is cleared in seven days. In young, elderly, and immunocompromized individuals, influenza virus infection might lead to more serious disease progression (pneumonia) and in some cases death. Influenza virus replication takes place in the cell nucleus, where the viral RNAs (vRNA) are transcribed by the viral polymerase into mRNAs for viral protein synthesis. Besides production of viral mRNAs, transcription of the genomic RNAs also results in the synthesis of complementary plus-strand RNA templates (cRNA) for synthesis of new vRNAs.[20]

Influenza viruses are notorious for their genetic diversity. The main reasons for this are the error-prone RNA polymerase, which lacks proofreading activity, and the fact that the virus has a segmented RNA genome. The major viral antigens HA and NA display high sequence variation that causes the virus to rapidly escape protective immune responses (antigenetic drift). A great concern is the emergence of new virus strains when influenza viruses from different species end up in the same host and eventually the same cell. If this happens, reassortment of the genomic RNA segments may lead to new virus strains against which humans have no protective immune response (antigenetic shift).[21] Two major pandemics caused by the 1957 Asian flu virus and the 1968 Hong Kong flu virus originate from the process of gene reassortment between human and avian influenza strains.[22–24] The highly virulent influenza strain causing the 1918 pandemic with an estimated 20–40 million deaths was previously also believed to have emerged after reassortment. However, high sequence similarity between the 1918 virus and avian influenza viruses suggest that the virus originated from an avian influenza virus that became adapted to humans.[25] Currently, reassortment of human and avian influenza strains and direct infection of humans with avian influenza viruses are considered serious threats. During recent outbreaks of avian influenza virus in Hong Kong and the Netherlands, several human cases were reported.[26–29] It therefore appears only a matter of time before reassortment and/or adaptation will lead to the emergence of a highly virulent influenza A strain.

There are currently, two licensed vaccines for human influenza virus in the United States.[26] One is based on inactivated virus, the other is a live-attenuated virus vaccine. Each year an international surveillance team coordinated by the WHO determines the components of the inactivated vaccine. Thus, the vaccine is generally designed against the virus strain that is expected to become the most prevalent during the next season. However, different virus strains—against which the vaccine is ineffective—may emerge rapidly. FluMist is a cold-adapted live-attenuated virus vaccine that was licensed in 2003. This virus is able to replicate at a low level in the upper airways, but is restricted in the lung due to the higher temperature. An important criterion for use of this vaccine is that the patient should have a fully functional immune system. This is often not the case for elderly people. RNAi therapeutics could therefore be particularly beneficial for the elderly and otherwise immunocompromised persons. However, it is currently unknown whether RNAi responses require a functional immune system.

RNA-INTERFERENCE-MEDIATED INHIBITION OF INFLUENZA A VIRUS

To obtain broad protection against different strains of influenza, it is essential to target RNAi against highly conserved viral sequences. The RNA encoding the main viral antigens HA and NA are no suitable targets because these proteins exist, respectively, as 15 and 9 different serotypes, with a large degree of sequence diversity. Instead, conserved regions in the NP, PA, PB1, PB2, M, and NS genes provide candidate targets for RNAi (Table 6.1). In their initial study, Ge et al.[30] tested 20 different siRNAs against sequences that were conserved in virus strains from human, chicken, duck, horse, and swine. Influenza production in MDCK cells and embryonated chicken eggs was strongly inhibited. siRNAs against NP and PA were found to be highly effective because they not only target the specific mRNAs for degradation, but also block the accumulation of all other viral RNAs.[30] These siRNAs also profoundly inhibited virus replication *in vivo*. Lung virus titers were significantly reduced in infected mice when siRNAs were administered through hydrodynamic intravenous injection.[31] Similarly, virus titers were reduced when mice were given DNA vectors intravenously or intranasally that express antiviral shRNAs.[31] Interestingly, reduced virus-induced mortality was observed in mice that were targeted with siRNAs after virus infection. This result supports the idea that siRNAs could act both as a prophylactic and in treatment of established infections. For delivery of the siRNAs and a lentiviral vector expressing shRNAs, polyethyleneimine (PEI) was used intravenously or intratracheally.[31] PEI is a cationic polymer that has been used to deliver DNA into lung cells. In a similar study, siRNAs against NP and PA sequences also protected mice against a lethal influenza virus challenge.[32] Moreover, siRNA treatment resulted in a broad protection against the pathogenic avian influenza A viruses of the H5 and H7 subtypes. In this study, the anti-influenza siRNAs were delivered intranasally with the cationic transfection reagent Oligofectamine.[32]

RNA-INTERFERENCE-MEDIATED INHIBITION OF RSV

RSV was the first human pathogenic virus for which RNAi-mediated inhibition was reported.[33] This virus belongs to the Paramyxoviridae and is an enveloped, nonsegmented, negative-stranded RNA virus. RSV is a major cause of respiratory illnesses in both the upper and lower respiratory tract, typically leading to cold-like symptoms that in some cases—especially in very young children—lead to more serious illness such as bronchiolitis and pneumonia. Currently, no vaccine is approved and RSV infection in young children accounts for more than 100.000 hospitalizations per year in the United States. In their initial report, Bitko and Baric described a 10-fold inhibition of RSV replication *in vitro* using nanomolar concentrations of synthetic siRNAs that target sequences encoding the viral polymerase subunit P and the fusion protein F.[33] Similar to influenza virus, replication of RSV and also human parainfluenza virus (PIV) could be blocked in mice by synthetic siRNAs[34] (Table 6.1). This therapy is effective both with and without the use of transfection reagents. Besides synthetic siRNAs, also intranasal administration of plasmids expressing shRNA against RSV resulted in a significant decrease of viral titers.[35] Treatment with siRNAs was effective both before and after infection with RSV. These findings suggest that low dosages of inhaled or intravenously administered siRNAs or shRNA-encoding plasmids may provide an easy and efficient basis for prophylaxis and antiviral therapy against respiratory viruses in human populations.

In April 2006, Alnylam presented the results of a phase I clinical trial with its leading siRNA drug candidate ALN-RSV01 (http://www. alnylam.com/). ALN-RSV01 is being evaluated for the treatment of RSV infection and is the first RNAi therapeutic in human clinical development for an infectious disease. The drug was found to be safe and well-tolerated when administered intranasally in two phase I clinical studies. A total of 101 subjects were enrolled in the trials, 65 of which were exposed to the drug that was given in single or multiple doses in a nasal spray. Alnylam expects to initiate phase II clinical trials in naturally infected RSV patients in the first half of 2007. Phase I human clinical trials are underway to test the nebulizer systems for aerosol delivery of siRNAs to the lungs.

INHIBITION OF HUMAN CORONAVIRUSES BY RNA INTERFERENCE

Since it became clear that the outbreak of SARS in 2003 was caused by the virus currently known as SARS-CoV, researchers have tried to find cures for this new human pathogen. Because SARS is a disease of the upper airways and lungs, it could be relatively easy to administer therapeutic siRNAs. As mentioned above, replication of influenza virus, RSV and PIV in the lungs of mice can be inhibited by intravenous or intranasal administration of siRNAs/shRNAs.[31,32,34,35] Following a similar route, siRNAs against SARS-CoV might be effective as new antiviral therapeutics. Both shRNAs and siRNAs could efficiently block SARS-CoV replication in cell culture infections[36-41] (Table 6.2). The main viral target in these studies is the polymerase gene, although also other regions such as the 5′ and 3′ untranslated regions (UTRs), the spike protein gene, and the transcriptional regulator sequence (TRS) have been targeted successfully.[39] Potent siRNA inhibitors against the SARS-CoV spike and pol genes were further tested for efficacy and safety in a rhesus macaque SARS model. The siRNAs were administered intranasally as prophylactic, concurrent, or early post-exposure treatments.[42] Similar to studies in mice with anti-RSV siRNAs, these treatments with anti-SARS siRNAs showed both prophylactic and therapeutic effects. siRNA treatment showed a significant reduction in SARS-like symptoms, viral RNA levels, and lung histopathology.

Antiviral RNAi strategies were also tested against the recently discovered human coronavirus, NL63-CoV.[43,44] This virus is associated with acute respiratory illness in young children, elderly, and immunocompromised persons, and it was recently linked more specifically to croup.[45] siRNAs targeting the spike sequences significantly inhibited virus replication at 3–5 nM concentration [43] (Table 6.2).

VIRUS ESCAPE FROM RNA INTERFERENCE

Potent inhibition of virus replication can be obtained by transient transfection of synthetic siRNAs or intracellular expression of shRNAs. However, the use of these approaches appears to be limited due to the rapid emergence of virus escape variants. RNAi escape variants may contain point mutations or deletions within the siRNA target sequences. So far, escape from RNAi has been reported for HIV-1, poliovirus, hepatitis A virus, HBV, and HCV.[46–52]

Studying anti-HIV RNAi approaches, Boden et al.[46] expressed shRNA against the HIV-1 tat gene in an adeno-associated virus (AAV) vector with an H1-promoter. Potent inhibition was scored, but an escape virus variant appeared in prolonged cultures. Similar results were described by Das et al.[47] using a retroviral vector with an H1 unit expressing an siRNA against sequences in the nef gene. The latter study described seven independent HIV-1 escape variants. Point mutation, double-point mutations, and partial or complete deletion of the target sequence all lead to RNAi-resistant escape variants. These results convincingly demonstrate that inhibition was potent and sequence-specific, but also that viruses are able to escape from the inhibitory action of a single siRNA.

We recently discovered an alternative resistance mechanism that is not triggered by mutation of the target sequence. Instead, a mutation in the flanking HIV-1 sequences was selected, which was subsequently shown to induce a conformational change within the target sequence such that it is protected from RISC-attack.[49] This finding indicates that it will not be very straightforward to predict viral escape routes.

A deletion-based resistance mechanism seems impossible in case essential viral genes or critical sequence motifs are targeted. Thus, one should preferentially target essential sequences that are well-conserved among virus isolates.[17] Interesting targets with relatively little mutational freedom are overlapping reading frames. Ideally, one should target multiple of these essential and well-conserved viral sequences. Such combination siRNA therapy mimics the successful strategy to combat HIV-1 with multiple antiviral drugs and should avoid the evolution of escape variants. We calculated that with four effective siRNAs, the chance of HIV-1 escape drops to 2.1×10^{-14}.[18] In practice, this means that viral escape is impossible as long as viral suppression is nearly complete. Efficient expression systems should be developed for multiple shRNAs[17] or long hairpin inhibitors (lhRNA) that generate multiple siRNAs.[53]

An alternative antiviral strategy is to target host-encoded functions that are important for viral replication, but not essential for survival of the host cell.[4] For HIV-1, such targets include the mRNAs for the CCR5 or CXCR4 co-receptors. Importantly, an inactivating mutation in the CCR5 gene is known to be compatible with normal life, indicating that it plays no essential role in human physiology.[54,55] A 63% and 48% reduction in CXCR4 and CCR5 expression resulted in a modest two- to three-fold decrease of HIV-1 entry.[56] When a lentivirus-based vector system was used to introduce shRNAs against CCR5 into peripheral blood T lymphocytes, expression of CCR5 on the cell surface was reduced 10-fold, resulting in a three- to seven-fold decrease in the number of infected cells.[57] In comparison to direct HIV-1 RNA targeting, the indirect silencing of viral receptors appears less effective in reducing virus production. A major advantage of host factor silencing is the possibility that viral escape may not occur, although that should be verified experimentally.

SIDE EFFECTS

Although RNAi may be considered a highly specific tool to knockdown genes, recent findings show that high expression of siRNA/shRNAs may induce interferon responses and other unwanted toxic side effects.[58,59] It was found that transcripts containing partial complementarity with an siRNA can also be targeted for RNAi-mediated knockdown.[60–62] Such off-target effects can have an impact on cell viability.[59,61] High expression of shRNAs also interferes with cellular miRNA processing and function. Exportin 5, which is required for nuclear export and stability of miRNAs, was found to be a limiting factor in the RNAi pathway that could be saturated by exogenous shRNAs. Fatal off-target effects were observed in mice that were treated with an AAV8 vector for high expression of shRNAs in the liver.[63] This study showed that there is an shRNA threshold for toxicity. Therefore, low expression of highly active shRNAs is essential for the development of safe RNAi therapeutics. Inducible promoters could be used to regulate shRNA expression to avoid off-target effects. In case of synthetic siRNAs, it was reported that chemical modification of the siRNAs can reduce toxicity.[61] Moreover, a strong correlation was found between the presence of the UGGC sequence motif and toxicity.[61] To avoid toxic off-target effects of antiviral RNAi therapeutics, viruses should ideally be targeted transiently, locally, and with a low dosage. This could be realized for acute respiratory viral infections, but treatment of chronic viral infections may require a durable gene therapy approach.

Delivery of the siRNAs into the right target cells will also limit the impact of potential off-target effects. Some recent progress has been reported using nanoparticles loaded with siRNAs. These particles, preferably ranging between 25 and 40 nm in diameter, can be used to load high concentrations of siRNAs into a protected environment. Most interesting is the fact that the nanoparticles can be targeted to specific cells by decorating their surface with ligands that target specific cell-surface receptors. For example, ligands such as transferrin, Her2 antibodies, folate, and integrin-targeting peptide have been successfully used to target siRNAs to cells bearing the corresponding receptors.[64–67] These results look promising and will contribute to the further development of safe and efficient siRNA delivery systems.

CONCLUSIONS

Many laboratories and pharmaceutical companies have recently focused on the development of RNAi-based therapeutics. As a result, RNAi has moved in a short time from an obscure phenomenon in plants and *C. elegans* to therapeutic compounds that are being tested in clinical trials. It has become clear that RNAi therapy might not be as straightforward as initially hoped. However, the results from *in vitro* studies and animal models show that RNAi therapeutics can be highly effective at a low dosage, which makes them outstanding candidates for future clinical use. Further optimization of the RNAi inducers and delivery tools/vectors is expected in the near future. Respiratory illnesses such as asthma and infection with respiratory viruses will be among the first to be targeted with RNAi-based therapeutics.

ACKNOWLEDGMENTS

We thank Lia van der Hoek for critical reading of the manuscript. RNAi research in the Berkhout lab is sponsored by ZonMw (VICI grant) and by Senter-Novem (TS grant together with Viruvation BV).

REFERENCES

1. Fire, A.; Xu, S.; Montgomery, M. K.; Kostas, S. A.; Driver, S. E.; Mello, C. C. Potent and specific genetic interference by double-stranded RNA in *Caenorhabditis elegans*. *Nature* **1998**, *391*, 806–811.

2. Haasnoot, P. C. J.; Berkhout, B. RNA interference: Its use as antiviral therapy. In *Handbook of Experimental Pharmacology*, Springer-Verlag, Berlin, **2006**, pp. 117–150.

3. Bartel, D. P. MicroRNAs: genomics, biogenesis, mechanism, and function. *Cell* **2004**, *116*, 281–297.

4. Haasnoot, P. C. J.; Cupac, D.; Berkhout, B. Inhibition of virus replication by RNA interference. *J. Biomed. Sci.* **2003**, *10*, 607–616.

5. Bennasser, Y.; Le, S. Y.; Benkirane, M.; Jeang, K. T. Evidence that HIV-1 encodes an siRNA and a suppressor of RNA silencing. *Immunity* **2005**, *22*, 607–619.

6. Cullen, B. R. Is RNA interference involved in intrinsic antiviral immunity in mammals? *Nat. Immunol.* **2006**, *7*, 563–567.

7. Berkhout, B.; Haasnoot, J. The interplay between virus infection and the cellular RNA interference machinery. *FEBS Lett.* **2006**, *580*, 2896–2902.

8. Paddison, P. J.; Caudy, A. A.; Bernstein, E.; Hannon, G. J.; Conklin, D. S. Short hairpin RNAs (shRNAs) induce sequence-specific silencing in mammalian cells. *Genes Dev.* **2002**, *16*, 948–958.

9. Brummelkamp, T. R.; Bernards, R.; Agami, R. A system for stable expression of short interfering RNAs in mammalian cells. *Science* **2002**, *296*, 550–553.

10. Xia, X. G.; Zhou, H.; Ding, H.; Affar, E. B.; Shi, Y.; Xu, Z. An enhanced U6 promoter for synthesis of short hairpin RNA. *Nucleic Acids Res.* **2003**, *31*, e100.

11. Boden, D.; Pusch, O.; Lee, F.; Tucker, L.; Shank, P. R.; Ramratnam, B. Promoter choice affects the potency of HIV-1 specific RNA interference. *Nucleic Acids Res.* **2003**, *31*, 5033–5038.

12. van de Wetering, M.; Oving, I.; Muncan, V.; Pon Fong, M. T.; Brantjes, H.; Van Leenen, D.; Holstege, F. C.; Brummelkamp, T. R.; Agami, R.; Clevers, H. Specific inhibition of gene expression using a stably integrated, inducible small-interfering-RNA vector. *EMBO Rep.* **2003**, *4*, 609–615.

13. Boden, D.; Pusch, O.; Silbermann, R.; Lee, F.; Tucker, L.; Ramratnam, B. Enhanced gene silencing of HIV-1 specific siRNA using microRNA designed hairpins. *Nucleic Acids Res.* **2004**, *32*, 1154–1158.

14. Du, G.; Yonekubo, J.; Zeng, Y.; Osisami, M.; Frohman, M. A. Design of expression vectors for RNA interference based on miRNAs and RNA splicing. *FEBS J.* **2006**, *273*, 5421–5427.

15. Silva, J. M.; Li, M. Z.; Chang, K.; Ge, W.; Golding, M. C.; Rickles, R. J.; Siolas, D.; Hu, G.; Paddison, P. J.; Schlabach, M. R.; Sheth, N.; Bradshaw, J.;

Burchard, J.; Kulkarni, A.; Cavet, G.; Sachidanandam, R.; McCombie, W. R.; Cleary, M. A.; Elledge, S. J.; Hannon, G. J. Second-generation shRNA libraries covering the mouse and human genomes. *Nat. Genet.* **2005**, *37*, 1281–1288.

16. Anderson, J.; Banerjea, A.; Akkina, R. Bispecific short hairpin siRNA constructs targeted to CD4, CXCR4, and CCR5 confer HIV-1 resistance. *Oligonucleotides.* **2003**, *13*, 303–312.

17. Ter Brake, O.; Konstantinova, P.; Ceylan, M.; Berkhout, B. Silencing of HIV-1 with RNA Interference: a multiple shRNA approach. *Mol. Ther.* **2006**, *14*, 883–892.

18. Berkhout, B. RNA interference as an antiviral approach: targeting HIV-1. *Curr. Opin. Mol. Ther.* **2004**, *6*, 141–145.

19. Westerhout, E. M.; Vink, M.; Haasnoot, P. C.; Das, A. T.; Berkhout, B. A conditionally replicating HIV-based vector that stably expresses an antiviral shRNA against HIV-1 replication. *Mol. Ther.* **2006**, *14*, 268–275.

20. Steinhauer, D. A.; Skehel, J. J. Genetics of influenza viruses. *Annu. Rev. Genet.* **2002**, *36*, 305–332.

21. Young, J. F.; Palese, P. Evolution of human influenza A viruses in nature: Recombination contributes to genetic variation of H1N1 strains. *Proc. Natl. Acad. Sci. USA* **1979**, *76*, 6547–6551.

22. Kawaoka, Y.; Krauss, S.; Webster, R. G. Avian-to-human transmission of the PB1 gene of influenza A viruses in the 1957 and 1968 pandemics. *J. Virol.* **1989**, *63*, 4603–4608.

23. Schafer, J. R.; Kawaoka, Y.; Bean, W. J.; Suss, J.; Senne, D.; Webster, R. G. Origin of the pandemic 1957 H2 influenza A virus and the persistence of its possible progenitors in the avian reservoir. *Virology* **1993**, *194*, 781–788.

24. Webster, R. G.; Sharp, G. B.; Claas, E. C. Interspecies transmission of influenza viruses. *Am. J. Respir. Crit. Care Med.* **1995**, *152*, S25–S30.

25. Taubenberger, J. K.; Reid, A. H.; Lourens, R. M.; Wang, R.; Jin, G.; Fanning, T. G. Characterization of the 1918 influenza virus polymerase genes. *Nature* **2005**, *437*, 889–893.

26. Gillim-Ross, L.; Subbarao, K. Emerging respiratory viruses: Challenges and vaccine strategies. *Clin. Microbiol. Rev.* **2006**, *19*, 614–636.

27. Claas, E. C.; de Jong, J. C.; van Beek, R.; Rimmelzwaan, G. F.; Osterhaus, A. D. Human influenza virus A/HongKong/156/97 (H5N1) infection. *Vaccine* **1998**, *16*, 977–978.

28. Fouchier, R. A.; Schneeberger, P. M.; Rozendaal, F. W.; Broekman, J. M.; Kemink, S. A.; Munster, V.; Kuiken, T.; Rimmelzwaan, G. F.; Schutten, M.; van Doornum, G. J.; Koch, G.; Bosman, A.; Koopmans, M.; Osterhaus, A. D. Avian influenza A virus (H7N7) associated with human conjunctivitis and a fatal case of acute respiratory distress syndrome. *Proc. Natl. Acad. Sci. USA* **2004**, *101*, 1356–1361.

29. Subbarao, K.; Klimov, A.; Katz, J.; Regnery, H.; Lim, W.; Hall, H.; Perdue, M.; Swayne, D.; Bender, C.; Huang, J.; Hemphill, M.; Rowe, T.; Shaw, M.; Xu, X.; Fukuda, K.; Cox, N. Characterization of an avian influenza A (H5N1) virus isolated from a child with a fatal respiratory illness. *Science* **1998**, *279*, 393–396.

30. Ge, Q.; McManus, M. T.; Nguyen, T.; Shen, C. H.; Sharp, P. A.; Eisen, H. N.; Chen, J. RNA interference of influenza virus production by directly targeting mRNA for degradation and indirectly inhibiting all viral RNA transcription. *Proc. Natl. Acad. Sci. USA* **2003**, *100*, 2718–2723.

31. Ge, Q.; Filip, L.; Bai, A.; Nguyen, T.; Eisen, H. N.; Chen, J. Inhibition of influenza virus production in virus-infected mice by RNA interference. *Proc. Natl. Acad. Sci. USA* **2004**, *101*, 8676–8681.

32. Tompkins, S. M.; Lo, C. Y.; Tumpey, T. M.; Epstein, S. L. Protection against lethal influenza virus challenge by RNA interference *in vivo. Proc. Natl. Acad. Sci. USA* **2004**, *101*, 8682–8686.

33. Bitko, V.; Barik, S. Phenotypic silencing of cytoplasmic genes using sequence-specific double-stranded short interfering RNA and its application in the reverse genetics of wild type negative-strand RNA viruses. *BMC Microbiol.* **2001**, *1*, 34.

34. Bitko, V.; Musiyenko, A.; Shulyayeva, O.; Barik, S. Inhibition of respiratory viruses by nasally administered siRNA. *Nat. Med.* **2005**, *11*, 50–55.

35. Zhang, W.; Yang, H.; Kong, X.; Mohapatra, S.; Juan-Vergara, H. S.; Hellermann, G.; Behera, S.; Singam, R.; Lockey, R. F.; Mohapatra, S. S. Inhibition of respiratory syncytial virus infection with intranasal siRNA nanoparticles targeting the viral NS1 gene. *Nat. Med.* **2005**, *11*, 56–62.

36. He, M. L.; Zheng, B.; Peng, Y.; Peiris, J. S.; Poon, L. L.; Yuen, K. Y.; Lin, M. C.; Kung, H. F.; Guan, Y. Inhibition of SARS-associated coronavirus infection and replication by RNA interference. *JAMA* **2003**, *290*, 2665–2666.

37. Lu, A.; Zhang, H.; Zhang, X.; Wang, H.; Hu, Q.; Shen, L.; Schaffhausen, B. S.; Hou, W.; Li, L. Attenuation of SARS coronavirus by a short hairpin RNA expression plasmid targeting RNA-dependent RNA polymerase. *Virology* **2004**, *324*, 84–89.

38. Wang, Z.; Ren, L.; Zhao, X.; Hung, T.; Meng, A.; Wang, J.; Chen, Y. G. Inhibition of severe acute respiratory syndrome virus replication by small interfering RNAs in mammalian cells. *J. Virol.* **2004**, *78*, 7523–7527.

39. Zhang, Y.; Li, T.; Fu, L.; Yu, C.; Li, Y.; Xu, X.; Wang, Y.; Ning, H.; Zhang, S.; Chen, W.; Babiuk, L. A.; Chang, Z. Silencing SARS-CoV Spike protein expression in cultured cells by RNA interference. *FEBS Lett.* **2004**, *560*, 141–146.

40. Ni, B.; Shi, X.; Li, Y.; Gao, W.; Wang, X.; Wu, Y. Inhibition of replication and infection of severe acute respiratory syndrome-associated coronavirus with plasmid-mediated interference RNA. *Antivir. Ther.* **2005**, *10*, 527–533.

41. Wu, C. J.; Huang, H. W.; Liu, C. Y.; Hong, C. F.; Chan, Y. L. Inhibition of SARS-CoV replication by siRNA. *Antiviral Res.* **2005**, *65*, 45–48.

42. Li, B. J.; Tang, Q.; Cheng, D.; Qin, C.; Xie, F. Y.; Wei, Q.; Xu, J.; Liu, Y.; Zheng, B. J.; Woodle, M. C.; Zhong, N.; Lu, P. Y. Using siRNA in prophylactic and therapeutic regimens against SARS coronavirus in Rhesus macaque. *Nat. Med.* **2005**, *11*, 944–951.

43. Pyrc, K.; Bosch, B. J.; Berkhout, B.; Jebbink, M. F.; Dijkman, R.; Rottier, P.; van der Hoek, L. Inhibition of HCoV-NL63 infection at early stages of the replication cycle. *Antimicrob. Agents Chemother.* **2006**, *50*, 2000–2008.

44. van der Hoek L.; Pyrc, K.; Jebbink, M. F.; Vermeulen-Oost, W.; Berkhout, R. J.; Wolthers, K. C.; Wertheim-van Dillen, P. M.; Kaandorp, J.; Spaargaren, J.; Berkhout, B. Identification of a new human coronavirus. *Nat. Med.* **2004**, *10*, 368–373.

45. van der Hoek L.; Sure, K.; Ihorst, G.; Stang, A.; Pyrc, K.; Jebbink, M. F.; Petersen, G.; Forster, J.; Berkhout, B.; Uberla, K. Croup is associated with the novel coronavirus NL63. *PLoS. Med.* **2005**, *2*, e240.

46. Boden, D.; Pusch, O.; Lee, F.; Tucker, L.; Ramratnam, B. Human immuno-deficiency virus type 1 escape from RNA interference. *J. Virol.* **2003**, *77*, 11531–11535.

47. Das, A. T.; Brummelkamp, T. R.; Westerhout, E. M.; Vink, M.; Madiredjo, M.; Bernards, R.; Berkhout, B. Human immunodeficiency virus type 1 escapes from RNA interference-mediated inhibition. *J. Virol.* **2004**, *78*, 2601–2605.

48. Gitlin, L.; Stone, J. K.; Andino, R. Poliovirus escape from RNA interference: Short interfering RNA-target recognition and implications for therapeutic approaches. *J. Virol.* **2005**, *79*, 1027–1035.

49. Westerhout, E. M.; Ooms, M.; Vink, M.; Das, A. T.; Berkhout, B. HIV-1 can escape from RNA interference by evolving an alternative structure in its RNA genome. *Nucleic Acids Res.* **2005**, *33*, 796–804.

50. Wilson, J. A.; Richardson, C. D. Hepatitis C virus replicons escape RNA interference induced by a short interfering RNA directed against the NS5b coding region. *J. Virol.* **2005**, *79*, 7050–7058.

51. Kusov, Y.; Kanda, T.; Palmenberg, A.; Sgro, J. Y.; Gauss-Muller, V. Silencing of hepatitis A virus infection by small interfering RNAs. *J. Virol.* **2006**, *80*, 5599–5610.

52. Wu, H. L.; Huang, L. R.; Huang, C. C.; Lai, H. L.; Liu, C. J.; Huang, Y. T.; Hsu, Y. W.; Lu, C. Y.; Chen, D. S.; Chen, P. J. RNA interference-mediated control of hepatitis B virus and emergence of resistant mutant. *Gastroenterology* **2005**, *128*, 708–716.

53. Konstantinova, P.; de Vries, W.; Haasnoot, J.; Ter Brake, O.; De Haan, P.; Berkhout, B. Inhibition of human immunodeficiency virus type 1 by RNA interference using long-hairpin RNA. *Gene Ther.* **2006**, *13*, 1403–1413.

54. Liu, R.; Paxton, W. A.; Choe, S.; Ceradini, D.; Martin, S. R.; Horuk, R.; MacDonald, M. E.; Stuhlmann, H.; Koup, R. A.; Landau, N. R. Homozygous defect in HIV-1 coreceptor accounts for resistance of some multiply-exposed individuals to HIV-1 infection. *Cell* **1996**, *86*, 367–377.

55. Samson, M.; Libert, F.; Doranz, B. J.; Rucker, J.; Liesnard, C.; Farber, C.-M.; Saragosti, S.; Lapoumeroulie, C.; Cognaux, J.; Forceille, C.; Muyldermans, G.; Verhofstede, C.; Burtonboy, G.; Georges, M.; Imai, T.; Rana, S.; Yi, Y.; Smyth, R. J.; Collman, R. G.; Doms, R. W.; Vassart, G.; Parmentier, M. Resistance to HIV-1 infection in caucasian individuals bearing mutant alleles of the CCR-5 chemokine receptor gene. *Nature* **1996**, *382*, 722–725.

56. Martinez, M. A.; Gutierrez, A.; Armand-Ugon, M.; Blanco, J.; Parera, M.; Gomez, J.; Clotet, B.; Este, J. A. Suppression of chemokine receptor expression by RNA interference allows for inhibition of HIV-1 replication. *AIDS* **2002**, *16*, 2385–2390.

57. Qin, X. F.; An, D. S.; Chen, I. S. Y.; Baltimore, D. Inhibiting HIV-1 infection in human T cells by lentiviral-mediated delivery of small interfering RNA against CCR5. *Proc. Natl. Acad. Sci. USA* **2003**, *100*, 183–188.

58. Bridge, A. J.; Pebernard, S.; Ducraux, A.; Nicoulaz, A. L.; Iggo, R. Induction of an interferon response by RNAi vectors in mammalian cells. *Nat. Genet.* **2003**, *34*, 263–264.

59. Jackson, A. L.; Linsley, P. S. Noise amidst the silence: Off-target effects of siRNAs? *Trends Genet.* **2004**, *20*, 521–524.

60. Birmingham, A.; Anderson, E. M.; Reynolds, A.; Ilsley-Tyree, D.; Leake, D.; Fedorov, Y.; Baskerville, S.; Maksimova, E.; Robinson, K.; Karpilow, J.; Marshall, W. S.; Khvorova, A. 3′ UTR seed matches, but not overall identity, are associated with RNAi off-targets. *Nat. Methods* **2006**, *3*, 199–204.

61. Fedorov, Y.; Anderson, E. M.; Birmingham, A.; Reynolds, A.; Karpilow, J.; Robinson, K.; Leake, D.; Marshall, W. S.; Khvorova, A. Off-target effects by siRNA can induce toxic phenotype. *RNA* **2006**, *12*, 1188–1196.

62. Jackson, A. L.; Bartz, S. R.; Schelter, J.; Kobayashi, S. V.; Burchard, J.; Mao, M.; Li, B.; Cavet, G.; Linsley, P. S. Expression profiling reveals off-target gene regulation by RNAi. *Nat. Biotechnol.* **2003**, *21*, 635–637.

63. Grimm, D.; Streetz, K. L.; Jopling, C. L.; Storm, T. A.; Pandey, K.; Davis, C. R.; Marion, P.; Salazar, F.; Kay, M. A. Fatality in mice due to oversaturation of cellular microRNA/short hairpin RNA pathways. *Nature* **2006**, *441*, 537–541.

64. Guo, S.; Huang, F.; Guo, P. Construction of folate-conjugated pRNA of bacteriophage phi29 DNA packaging motor for delivery of chimeric siRNA to nasopharyngeal carcinoma cells. *Gene Ther.* **2006**, *13*, 814–820.

65. Hu-Lieskovan, S.; Heidel, J. D.; Bartlett, D. W.; Davis, M. E.; Triche, T. J. Sequence-specific knockdown of EWS-FLI1 by targeted, nonviral delivery

of small interfering RNA inhibits tumor growth in a murine model of metastatic Ewing's sarcoma. *Cancer Res.* **2005**, *65*, 8984–8992.

66. Schiffelers, R. M.; Ansari, A.; Xu, J.; Zhou, Q.; Tang, Q.; Storm, G.; Molema, G.; Lu, P. Y.; Scaria, P. V.; Woodle, M. C. Cancer siRNA therapy by tumor selective delivery with ligand-targeted sterically stabilized nanoparticle. *Nucleic Acids Res.* **2004**, *32*, e149.

67. Tan, W. B.; Jiang, S.; Zhang, Y. Quantum-dot based nanoparticles for targeted silencing of HER2/neu gene via RNA interference. *Biomaterials* **2007**, *28*, 1565–1571.

68. Hui, E. K.; Yap, E. M.; An, D. S.; Chen, I. S.; Nayak, D. P. Inhibition of influenza virus matrix (M1) protein expression and virus replication by U6 promoter-driven and lentivirus-mediated delivery of siRNA. *J. Gen. Virol.* **2004**, *85*, 1877–1884.

69. Phipps, K. M.; Martinez, A.; Lu, J.; Heinz, B. A.; Zhao, G. Small interfering RNA molecules as potential anti-human rhinovirus agents: *In vitro* potency, specificity, and mechanism. *Antiviral Res.* **2004**, *61*, 49–55.

70. Li, T.; Zhang, Y.; Fu, L.; Yu, C.; Li, X.; Li, Y.; Zhang, X.; Rong, Z.; Wang, Y.; Ning, H.; Liang, R.; Chen, W.; Babiuk, L. A.; Chang, Z. siRNA targeting the leader sequence of SARS-CoV inhibits virus replication. *Gene Ther.* **2005**, *12*, 751–761.

71. Qin, Z. L.; Zhao, P.; Zhang, X. L.; Yu, J. G.; Cao, M. M.; Zhao, L. J.; Luan, J.; Qi, Z. T. Silencing of SARS-CoV spike gene by small interfering RNA in HEK 293T cells. *Biochem Biophys. Res. Commun.* **2004**, *324*, 1186–1193.

72. Bitko, V.; Musiyenko, A.; Barik, S. Viral infection of the lungs through the eye. *J. Virol.* **2007**, *81*, 783–790.

73. Munir, S.; Kaur, K.; Kapur, V. Avian metapneumovirus phosphoprotein targeted RNA interference silences the expression of viral proteins and inhibits virus replication. *Antiviral Res.* **2006**, *69*, 46–51.

74. He, Y. X.; Hua, R. H.; Zhou, Y. J.; Qiu, H. J.; Tong, G. Z. Interference of porcine reproductive and respiratory syndrome virus replication on MARC-145 cells using DNA-based short interfering RNAs. *Antiviral Res.* **2006**.

75. Huang, J.; Jiang, P.; Li, Y.; Xu, J.; Jiang, W.; Wang, X. Inhibition of porcine reproductive and respiratory syndrome virus replication by short hairpin RNA in MARC-145 cells. *Vet. Microbiol.* **2006**, *115*, 302–310.

76. Lu, L.; Ho, Y.; Kwang, J. Suppression of porcine arterivirus replication by baculovirus-delivered shRNA targeting nucleoprotein. Biochem Biophys. *Res. Commun.* **2006**, *340*, 1178–1183.

77. Akerstrom, S.; Mirazimi, A.; Tan, Y. J. Inhibition of SARS-CoV replication cycle by small interference RNAs silencing specific SARS proteins, 7a/7b, 3a/3b and S. *Antiviral Res.* **2007**, *73*, 219–227.

7

PROMISING ANTIVIRAL GLYCO-MOLECULES FROM AN EDIBLE ALGA

TOSHIMITSU HAYASHI, KYOKO HAYASHI, KENJI KANEKIYO, YUKO OHTA AND JUNG-BUM LEE

Graduate School of Medicine and Pharmaceutical Sciences, University of Toyama, Toyama 930-0194, Japan,

MINORU HASHIMOTO AND TAKAHISA NAKANO

Riken Vitamin Co., Ltd., Chiyoda-ku, Tokyo 101-8370, Japan

INTRODUCTION

For a long time, influenza has continued to be a significant public health concern, since annual epidemics by the pathogen is responsible for serious morbidity and mortality.[1] Highly pathogenic avian influenza virus H5N1, in particular, has recently become of major concern after it was documented to cause severe respiratory disease and death in humans.[2–4] Therefore, much attention has been given to the development of antiviral agents for the treatment of the infectious disease by influenza A virus (IFV). Since the clinical efficacy of two neuraminidase (NA) inhibitors, oral oseltamivir[5,6] and inhaled zanamivir[7–9], has been recently reported, the hope that chemotherapy with these drugs may provide a means for effective containment of influenza has been provided. However, Kiso et al.[10] have reported more recently that oseltamivir-resistant mutants were detected in children being treated with the drug more frequently than previously reported.[11–13] In immunocompromised hosts, the emergence of resistance to NA inhibitors was also observed.[14,15]

In order to overcome the disadvantages of oseltamivir for treating IFV infections, other drug candidates with anti-IFV activity and mechanism of action different from that of oseltamivir are needed. Sulfated polysaccharides should be one of the candidates because these compounds such as dextran sulfate have been found to inhibit the replication of IFV *in vitro*.[16,17] Recently, we have reported on structural characterization and antiviral activities of fucoidan, a sulfated polysaccharide isolated from an edible alga (*Undaria pinnatifida*).[18] The fucoidan was composed of fucose and galactose with an approximately ratio of 1.0:1.1, and its apparent molecular weight is 9000. The compound showed selective *in vitro* antiviral activity against IFV replication. In general, sulfated polysaccharides are also known to have the immunomodulating activity.[19–23] These effects of sulfated polysaccharides might be favorable to the suppression of IFV replication in the body. Therefore, we have been assessing the efficacy of the fucoidan from *U. pinnatifida* by determining virus yields and virus-specific antibodies in IFV-infected mice.

Combination chemotherapy with synergistically active antiviral agents that have different targets from each other for viral replication may offer several advantages over single agent therapy, such as greater potency, superior clinical efficacy, reduction of toxicity and side effects due to the reduction of the drug dosage needed, suppression of the emergency of drug-resistant viruses, and greater cost effectiveness. With this in mind, several reports address the anti-IFV drug combinations— for example, amantadine or rimantadine with ribavirin,[24,25] rimantadine with aprotinin,[26] ribavirin with an NA inhibitor (RWJ-270201),[27,28] and NA inhibitors with rimantadine.[29] So far, there is only one report on the synergistic anti-IFV effect of oseltamivir, where the combination of oseltamivir carboxylate and rimantadine, an M2 ion blocker, was found to show synergism *in vitro*.[29] In this context, we have also evaluated the combination of the fucoidan and oseltamivir in suppressing IFV replication.

IN VITRO ANTI-INFLUENZA VIRUS ACTIVITY OF FUCOIDAN

Antiviral Activity of Fucoidan

The fucoidan was assessed for its anti-IFV (A/NWS/33 strain, H1N1) potency. The 50% inhibitory concentration of the fucoidan for virus replication (IC_{50}) was 15 µg/ml when determined by plaque yield reduction assay. The 50% inhibitory concentration of the fucoidan for host cell (MDCK cell) growth (CC_{50}) was >2000 µg/ml. Thus, the resulting selectivity index (CC_{50}/IC_{50}) was more than 130, indicating that the fucoidan has potent antiviral activity against IFV.

Antiviral Target of Fucoidan

To determine the stage of viral replication which is the most sensitive to the fucoidan, antiviral time-of-addition experiments were performed. The fucoidan (100 µg/ml) or oseltamivir (5 µM) was added to cells infected with IFV at 1 plaque-forming unit (PFU) per cell at different time points. As shown in Fig. 7.1, the fucoidan acted most effectively when added during viral infection and throughout the incubation for 24 hr thereafter. Oseltamivir showed potent inhibition of viral replication when added by 3 hr after infection. A delay of addition of oseltamivir at 6 hr post-infection led to only a little reduction in activity, while the fucoidan showed only weak activity in this time point of addition. The presence of the fucoidan in viral infection with cells produced approximately 40% reduction of virus yield, while

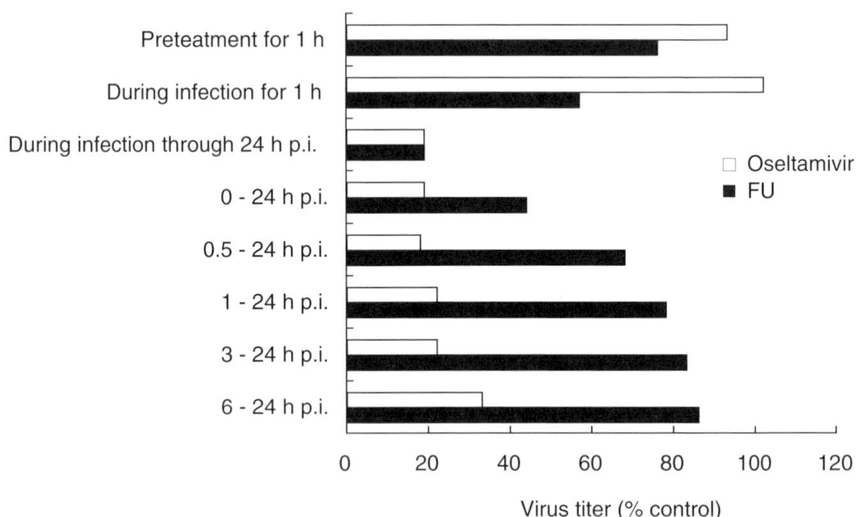

Fig. 7.1. Time-of-addition experiments comparing the antiviral activity of fucoidan (FU) to that of oseltamivir. FU (100 µg/ml) or oseltamivir (5 µM) was added to cells infected with influenza A/NWS/33 (H1N1) virus at the indicated time points. Inhibition of viral replication was determined by plaque yield reduction assays in MDCK cells on samples taken at 24 hr post-infection (p.i.). Data are presented as the mean of duplicate assays.

the presence of oseltamivir during infection had no effect on viral replication.

Fucoidans are sulfated polysaccharides isolated from several brown algae[18,19,30] and show antiviral activity.[31] The mechanism of anti-influenza virus action of sulfated polysaccharides was reported to be the inhibition of the fusion between the viral envelope and host cell membrane.[16,32] In accord with this finding, the most sensitive stage of influenza virus replication to the fucoidan derived from *Undaria pinnatifida* was the early replication stage including virus attachment and internalization to host cells as shown by time-of-addition experiments. In other experiments, the effects of the fucoidan on virus attachment and penetration to host cells were evaluated. The fucoidan inhibited the binding of IFV to MDCK cells at 10 and 100 µg/ml by approximately 15% and 30%, respectively. Virus penetration into host cells occurs immediately after virus attachment. The fucoidan also inhibited this step of viral replication at 10 and 100 µg/ml by approximately 25% and 40%, respectively. These results mean that the fucoidan is different in anti-influenza virus targets from oseltamivir, which is an inhibitor of influenza virus neuraminidase.

EFFECTS OF FUCOIDAN ON IMMUNE SYSTEM

Effect of Fucoidan on the Function of Macrophages

When invaded the human body, viruses are encountered by the host immune responses, which can be typically subdivided into nonspecific and specific immunity. One of the former is supported by macrophages. Macrophages have a phagocytic ability that contributes to eliminate virus from the circulation after a blood-borne infection. Their scavenger function serves as an early reduction of the virus load. When this function of macrophages was evaluated by the method of latex bead endocytosis, the fucoidan was shown to stimulate the phagocytic activity of macrophages in *in vitro* conditions. Another function of macrophages in virus infection is the production of nitric oxide (NO). NO is involved nonspecifically in immunological defense, and its overproduction, mainly by inducible NO synthase (iNOS), has been reported in infectious events of viruses including IFV, herpes simplex virus, rabies virus, and coxsackievirus.[33–36] When the effect of the fucoidan on *in vitro* production of NO_2^-, which is known to be an oxidized metabolite of NO, was investigated, there was no significant enhancement or suppression of NO production. These results suggest that the fucoidan might cause at least no NOS inhibition.

Effect of Fucoidan on Natural Killer Cell-Mediated Cytotoxicity

In the state of virus infections, natural killer (NK) cells provide an early line of host defense before antigen-specific immune responses develop, and they play a role in recovery from these infectious diseases.[37–39] The immunosuppressed state, which mimics the decline of the immune function due to age, stress, or medical interventions such as surgical operation, radiotherapy or chemotherapy, can be experimentally produced in the animals and human by the treatment with some anticancer drugs, including mitomycin C and 5-fluorouracil (5-FU).[40–45] When BALB/c mice were treated with 5-FU, the anticancer drug caused the reduction of NK activity as reported previously.[42,45,46] Interestingly, oral administration of the fucoidan from *U. pinnatifida* showed selective augmentation of NK activity only in such an immunosuppressed state of 5-FU-injected mice, since the same treatment with the fucoidan exerted no significant change in NK activity in the animals without 5-FU injection where the normal level of NK activity was maintained.

Effect of Fucoidan on Blast Formation of B Cells

When the population of B cells derived from the spleen of BALB/c mice was cultured in the presence of the fucoidan, a higher proportion of large B cells could be observed as compared with that of no treatment control. This result implies that the fucoidan might induce the differentiation of B cells—that is B cell blastogenesis. Therefore, the fucoidan was expected to promote the maturation of B cells that might result in the stimulation of antibody-secreting activity. This concept might be supported by the elevated production of neutralizing antibodies that recognize the surface antigens on virus particles as described later.

IN VITRO EFFECTS OF THE COMBINATION OF FUCOIDAN AND OSELTAMIVIR

From the fact that the fucoidan and oseltamivir have different targets of viral replication from each other as shown in the section entitled "*In Vitro* Anti-Influenza Virus Activity of Fucoidan," it could be expected that favorable antiviral interaction might exist between the two compounds. Thus, the antiviral effects of the fucoidan and oseltamivir alone and in combinations were evaluated in MDCK cell cultures by virus yield reduction assay. Six different concentrations of the fucoi-

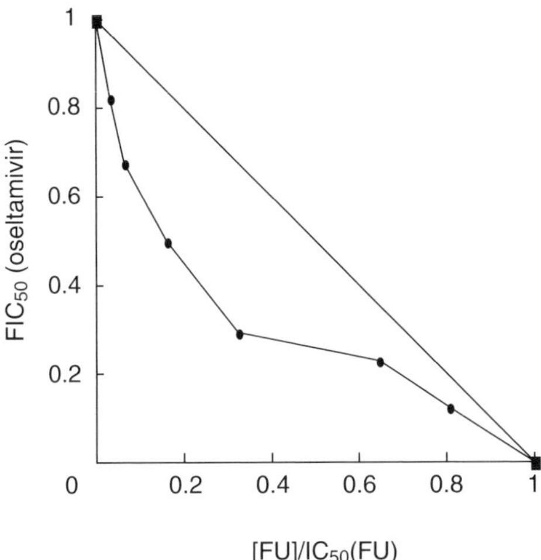

Fig. 7.2. *In vitro* interaction between oseltamivir and fucoidan (FU). FU (2–50 µg/ml) was combined with oseltamivir (0.5–200 nM) against influenza A virus. Virus yield was determined by plaque assay. The drug interaction was evaluated by isobologram.

dan (2–50 µg/ml) or oseltamivir (0.5–200 nM) were tested. The drug combinations produced greater antiviral effects than did each drug alone. For example, the combination of 10 µg/ml fucoidan, which was only slightly effective by itself, with oseltamivir resulted in approximately 50% reduction of IC$_{50}$ value of the NA inhibitor itself. The overall interaction between the fucoidan and oseltamivir was found to be synergistic as evaluated by isobologram[47] in which the x and y axes showed the ratio of the concentrations in µg/ml of FU and IC$_{50}$ values of FU, and FIC$_{50}$s of oseltamivir, respectively (Fig. 7.2). There was no enhancement of cytotoxicity in these drug combinations (data not shown).

IN VIVO EFFECTS OF FUCOIDAN IN INFLUENZA VIRUS-INFECTED ANIMALS

Effects of Oral Treatment with Fucoidan on Mortality of Mice Inoculated with Influenza Virus

To determine the ability of the fucoidan to prevent the death in mice infected with influenza virus, A/NWS/33 virus was inoculated intranasally at 1×10^6 PFU per animal. The fucoidan was administered perorally at a dose of 5 mg/day three times daily (every 8 hr) for 10 consecutive days beginning immediately after viral inoculation. At this dose, no toxicity was observed. In the placebo (distilled water) group, seven of 19 mice died during 4–10 days post-infection, the mortality being 37%. In fucoidan-treated group, however, no death was observed in 14 mice (data not shown).

Effects of Fucoidan on Virus Production in Mice Inoculated with Influenza Virus

Mouse model of nasal infection was used for determination of *in vivo* activity of the fucoidan against influenza virus. Mice were intranasally inoculated with a sublethal dose of A/NWS/33 virus fluid containing 1×10^5 PFU per animal. Twenty-five mice per drug treatment group were included in the experiments, and no death was observed at this viral challenge dose throughout the experiments. The fucoidan and oseltamivir were orally administered alone or in combinations at a daily dose of 5 mg or 0.1 mg, respectively, twice a day (every 12 hr) for seven consecutive days beginning just after viral inoculation. The fucoidan was administered ad libitum from drinking water during days 8–21 after inoculation.

The daily virus titers in the lung of mice treated with each drug or in combinations are shown in Fig. 7.3. Treatment with fucoidan alone produced no marked inhibition of viral replication on day 1 of the infection, but it did inhibit viral replication at later assay times of days 2, 3, 4, 5, and 7, virus titer being reduced to 63 ($p < 0.05$), 50, 70, 50 ($p < 0.05$) and 58%, respectively, as compared with no drug control. Oseltamivir treatment lessened virus titers on days 1, 2, 3, 4, 5, and 7 to 30 ($p < 0.01$), 24 ($p < 0.05$), 8.5 ($p < 0.001$), 12 ($p < 0.05$) and 13%, respectively, as compared with no drug control. The combination of fucoidan and oseltamivir yielded significant reduction in lung titers throughout the assay times. It is noteworthy that on days 3 ($p < 0.01$) and 4 ($p < 0.001$), significant inhibition of viral replication in lung was observed in the combination group as compared with oseltamivir alone.

Effects of Fucoidan on the Production of Influenza Virus-Specific and Neutralizing Antibodies in Mucosa

Antibody responses were compared after infection with influenza virus among the groups of fucoidan-, oseltamivir-, and fucoidan plus oseltamivir-treated mice. The titers of mucosal neutralizing antibody were determined by plaque reduction assay of diluted bronchoalveolar fluid (BALF) and expressed as the highest dilution of BALF that reduced the plaque numbers by 50% as compared with that of control without BALF. The levels of the antibody were always higher in

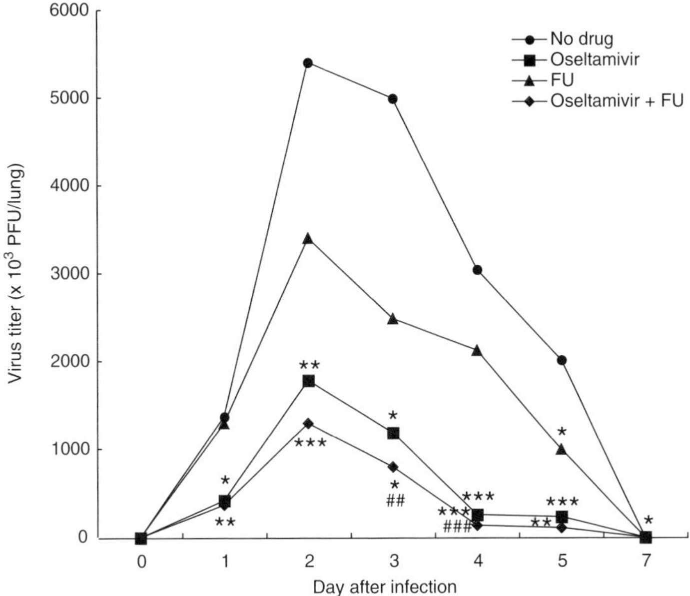

Fig. 7.3. Effects of peroral treatment with fucoidan (FU) (5 mg/day) and oseltamivir (0.1 mg/day) alone or in combinations on daily virus titers in the lung of mice infected with influenza A virus. Treatment of mice ($n = 3$) was twice a day beginning just after virus inoculation. *Significant reduction ($p < 0.05$) as compared with no drug control; **significant reduction ($p < 0.01$) as compared with no drug control; ***significant reduction ($p < 0.001$) as compared with no drug control; ##significant reduction ($p < 0.01$) as compared with oseltamivir alone; ###significant reduction ($p < 0.001$) as compared with oseltamivir alone.

fucoidan-treated animals than those in no drug control, showing significant increase ($p < 0.05$) at day 7 (Fig. 7.4). In contrast, oseltamivir depressed the antibody responses at days 14 ($p < 0.05$) and 21. The combination of fucoidan and oseltamivir did not significantly decrease the levels of neutralizing antibody throughout the evaluation period of 21 days as compared with no drug control, although the average titers in this group did not rise as high as those in control group after 2 and 3 weeks of infection.

The magnitude of virus-specific IgA antibody in BALF after infection was determined by an ELISA assay. The fucoidan increased IgA production throughout the period of 21 days after infection, leading to significant increase ($p < 0.05$) at day 21 (Fig. 7.5). There was no significant difference in IgA levels between control and oseltamivir or fucoidan plus oseltamivir groups.

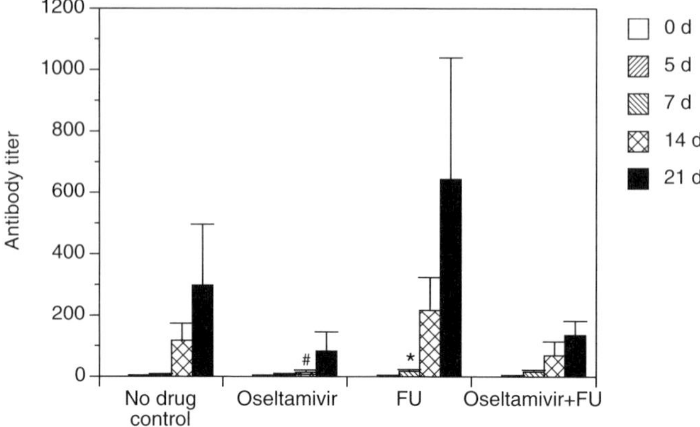

Fig. 7.4. Effects of peroral treatment with fucoidan (FU) and oseltamivir alone or in combinations on the production of neutralizing antibody in the mucosa of mice infected with influenza A virus. Treatment was done as described in Fig. 7.3. *Significant increase ($p < 0.05$) as compared with no drug control; #significant reduction ($p < 0.05$) as compared with no drug control.

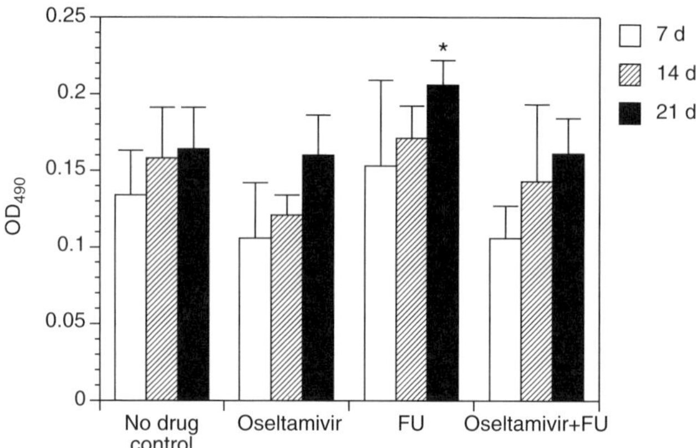

Fig. 7.5. Effects of peroral treatment with fucoidan (FU) and oseltamivir alone or in combinations on the production of influenza virus-specific IgA in the mucosa of mice infected with influenza A virus. Treatment was done as described in Fig. 7.3. *Significant increase ($p < 0.05$) as compared with no drug control.

Effects of Fucoidan on the Production of Influenza Virus-Specific and Neutralizing Antibodies in Sera

To test whether the fucoidan stimulates systemic immunoresponses by oral administration, the levels of neutralizing antibody IgM and IgG in sera of mice were determined. Fucoidan group had higher neutralizing titers than control group at earlier phase of viral infection, with 1.4-,

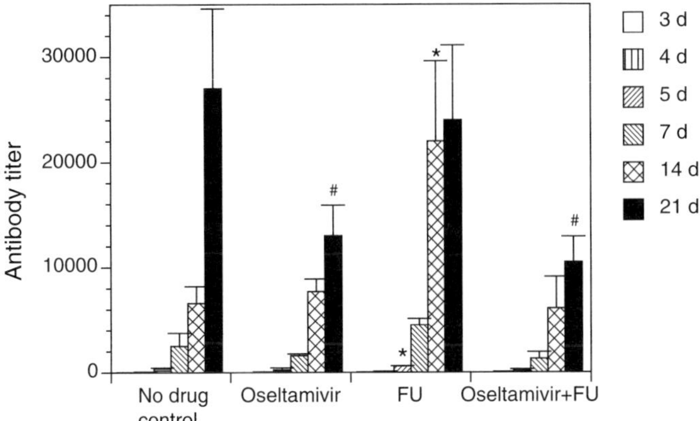

Fig. 7.6. Effects of peroral treatment with fucoidan (FU) and oseltamivir alone or in combinations on the production of neutralizing antibody in the sera of mice infected with influenza A virus. Treatment was done as described in Fig. 7.3. *Significant increase ($p < 0.05$) as compared with no drug control; #significant reduction ($p < 0.05$) as compared with no drug control.

1.2-, 1.6- ($p < 0.01$), 1.8- and 2.1-fold ($p < 0.01$) higher titers at days 3, 4, 5, 7, and 14 (Fig. 7.6). Both oseltamivir alone and combination of oseltamivir and fucoidan groups showed no significant change in neutralizing antibody titers by 14 days after viral inoculation, but showed significant reduction ($p < 0.05$) in the titers at day 21.

The levels of IFV-specific IgM were also affected by drug administration. Fucoidan group had a tendency to increase the IgM production as compared with control group, showing a significant increase ($p < 0.05$) in IgM level at day 5 (Fig. 7.7). IgM production in both oseltamivir alone and the combination of fucoidan and oseltamivir groups was significantly less than that in control group ($p < 0.05$) at day 5. Higher levels of IgM were seen in the combination group as compared with oseltamivir alone group after 1 week of viral inoculation.

The levels of virus-specific IgG in sera increased rapidly from day 7 (Fig. 7.8). The fucoidan showed no significant change in IgG production as compared with no drug control during 3 weeks after viral inoculation. Oseltamivir treatment, however, suppressed the IgG production throughout the observation period of 3 weeks, reducing the levels of IgG significantly at day 7 ($p < 0.01$). The combination of oseltamivir and fucoidan significantly lowered the IgG production at day 3 ($p < 0.05$). There was no significant difference in IgG production between oseltamivir alone and the drug combination groups.

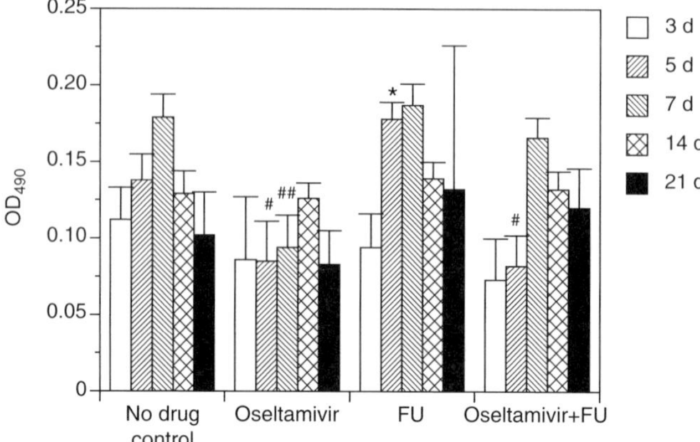

Fig. 7.7. Effects of peroral treatment with fucoidan (FU) and oseltamivir alone or in combinations on the production of influenza virus-specific IgM in the sera of mice infected with influenza A virus. Treatment was done as described in Fig. 7.3. *Significant increase ($p < 0.05$) as compared with no drug control; [#]significant reduction ($p < 0.05$) as compared with no drug control; [##]significant reduction ($p < 0.01$) as compared with no drug control.

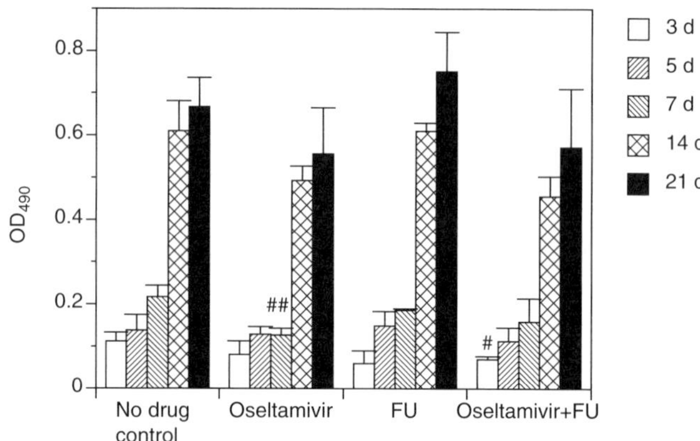

Fig. 7.8. Effects of peroral treatment with fucoidan (FU) and oseltamivir alone or in combinations on the production of influenza virus-specific IgG in the sera of mice infected with influenza A virus. Treatment was done as described in Fig. 7.3. [#]Significant reduction ($p < 0.05$) as compared with no drug control; [##]significant reduction ($p < 0.01$) as compared with no drug control.

Summary of the Effects of Fucoidan on *In Vivo* Immune Responses

It is important to induce mucosal immunity since influenza virus particles enter their host through a mucosal surface. Oseltamivir reduced mucosal immunoresponces as the virus yield in the mucosa decreased when determined by the levels of virus-specific IgA and neutralizing antibody in bronchoalveolar lavage fluid. Here, the fucoidan was unique in reducing virus yield in the mucosa with stimulating mucosal immunoresponses. Neutralizing antibody recognizes the surface antigens present on virus particles or virus-infected cells.[48,49] While oseltamivir produced significantly lower titers of neutralizing antibody in sera than did the placebo treatment, the fucoidan significantly promoted its production in sera. This might mean that hosts treated with oseltamivir alone would remain less protected against re-infection with the same influenza virus. Significant increase in virus-specific IgM production in sera of fucoidan-treated mice at the acute phase of influenza virus infection (5 days post-infection) might play a role at least in part in the reduction of virus yield. Based on the findings that the fucoidan is different from oseltamivir in antiviral targets and immunoresponses in host, we also evaluated the combined effects of the two compounds on *in vivo* influenza virus replication. This combination treatment markedly reduced virus yields in mice as compared with the yields obtained after treatment with either single compound.

SUMMARY AND CONCLUSIONS

From sporophyll of an edible alga *Undaria pinnatifida*, fucoidan, a sulfated polysaccharide, was isolated and evaluated *in vitro* and *in vivo* as an inhibitor of influenza A virus replication. The fucoidan showed *in vitro* antiviral activity with selectivity index of more than 130. In the time-of-addition experiments, the most sensitive stage of viral replication to the fucoidan was shown to be earlier than that to a neuraminidase inhibitor oseltamivir. The binding of the virus to host cells and the penetration into host cells were inhibited by the fucoidan. *In vitro* experiments demonstrated that the fucoidan plus oseltamivir synergistically reduced virus yields at low concentrations of each compound. Virus-infected BALB/c mice were treated with oral fucoidan at 5 mg/day combined with oral oseltamivir at 0.1 mg/day, or used alone. The fucoidan prevented mortality, reduced virus yields in the lung, and significantly increased neutralizing antibody levels in the mucosa and the blood in the acute phase of infection. In contrast, oseltamivir treatment markedly suppressed the production of neutralizing antibody. The combination of the fucoidan and oseltamivir inhibited the virus replication in the lung significantly compared to oseltamivir alone, and it increased neutralizing antibody in the mucosa and IgM in the sera. The fucoidan is worthy of further exploration for its potential of single use or combination therapy with neuraminidase inhibitors in the treatment of influenza.

REFERENCES

1. Lui, K. J.; Kendal, A. P. Impact of influenza epidemics on mortality in the United States from October 1972 to May 1985. *Am. J. Public Health* **1987**, *77*, 712–176.

2. Yuen, K. Y.; Chan, P. K.; Peiris, M.; Tsang, D. N.; Que, T. L.; Shortridge, K. F.; Cheung, P. T.; To, W. K.; Ho, E. T.; Sung, R.; Cheng, A. F. Clinical features and rapid viral diagnosis of human disease associated with avian influenza A H5N1 virus. *Lancet* **1998**, *351*, 467–471.

3. Subbarao, K.; Klimov, A.; Katz, J.; Regnery, H.; Lim, W.; Hall, H.; Perdue, M.; Swayne, D.; Bender, C.; Huang, J.; Hemphil, M.; Rowe, T.; Shaw, M.; Xu, X.; Fukuda, K.; Cox, N. Characterization of an avian influenza A (H5N1) virus isolated from a child with a fetal respiratory illness. *Science* **1998**, *279*, 393–396.

4. Claas, E. C.; Osterhaus, A. D.; van Beek, R.; De Jong, J. C.; Rimmelzwaan, G. F.; Senne, D. A.; Krauss, S.; Shortridge, K. F.; Webster, R. G. Human influenza A H5N1 virus related to a highly pathogenic avian influenza virus. *Lancet* **1998**, *351*, 472–477.

5. Hayden, F. G.; Treanor, J. J.; Fritz, R. S.; Lobo, M.; Betts, R. F.; Miller, M.; Kinnersley, N.; Mills, R. G.; Ward, P.; Straus, S. E. Use of the oral NA inhibitor oseltamivir in experimental human influenza: Randomized controlled trials for prevention and treatment. *JAMA* **1999**, *282*, 1240–1246.

6. Nicholson, K. G.; Aoki, F. Y.; Osterhaus, A. D.; Trottier, S.; Carewicz, O.; Mercier, C. H.; Rode, A.; Kinnersley, N.; Ward, P. Efficacy and safety of oseltamivir in treatment of acute influenza: A randomised controlled trial. *Lancet* **2000**, *355*, 1845–1850.

7. Hayden, F. G.; Osterhaus, A. D.; Treanor, J. J.; Fleming, D. M.; Aoki, F. Y.; Nicholson, K. G.; Bohnen, A. M.; Hirst, H. M.; Keene, O.; Wightman, K. Efficacy and safety of the neuraminidase inhibitor zanamivir in the treatment of influenza virus infection. *N. Engl. J. Med.* **1997**, *337*, 874–880.

8. Mist Study Group. Randomized trial of efficacy and safety of inhaled zanamivir in treatment of influenza A and B virus infections. *Lancet* **1998**, *352*, 1877–1881.

9. Monto, A. S.; Fleming, D. M.; Henry, D.; de Groot, R.; Makela, M.; Klein, T.; Eliott, M.; Keene, O. N.; Man, C. Y. Efficacy and safety of the neuraminidase inhibitor zanamivir in the treatment of influenza A and B virus infections. *J. Infect. Dis.* **1999**, *180*, 254–261.

10. Kiso, M.; Mitamura, K.; Sakai-Tagawa, Y.; Shiraishi, K.; Kawakami, C.; Kimura, K.; Hayden, F. G.; Sugaya, N.; Kawaoka, Y. Resistant influenza A

viruses in children treated with oseltamivir: Descriptive study. *Lancet* **2004**, *264*, 759–765.

11. Zambon, M.; Hayden, F. G. Position statement: Global neuraminidase inhibitor susceptibility network. *Antiviral Res.* **2001**, *49*, 147–156.

12. Hayden, F. G. Perspectives on antiviral use during pandemic influenza. *Phil. Trans. R. Soc. Lond.* **2001**, *356*, 1877–1884.

13. Gubareva, L. V.; Kaiser, L.; Metrosovich, M. N.; Soo-Hoo, Y.; Hayden, F. G. Selection of influenza virus mutants in experimentally infected volunteers treated with oseltamivir. *J. Infect. Dis.* **2001**, *183*, 523–531.

14. Ison, M. G.; Gubareva, L. V.; Atmar, R. L.; Treanor, J.; Hayden, F. G. Recovery of drug-resistant influenza virus from immunocompromised patients: A case series. *J. Infect. Dis.* **2006**, *193*, 760–764.

15. Ison, M. G.; Mishin, V. P.; Braciale, T. J.; Hayden, F. G.; Gubareva, L. V. Comparative activities of oseltamivir and A-322278 in immunocmpetent and immunocompromised murine models of influenza virus infection. *J. Infect. Dis.* **2006**, *193*, 765–772.

16. Hosoya, M.; Balzarini, J.; Shigeta, S.; De Clercq, E. Differential inhibitory effects of sulfated polysaccharides and polymers on the replication of various myxoviruses and retroviruses, depending on the composition of the target amino acid sequences of the viral envelope glycoproteins. *Antimicrob. Agents Chemother.* **1991**, *35*, 2515–2520.

17. Hosoya, M.; Shigeta, S.; Ishii, T.; Suzuki, H.; De Clercq, E. Comparative inhibitory effects of various nucleoside and nonnucleoside analogues on replication of influenza virus types A and B *in vitro* and *in ovo*. *J. Infect. Dis.* **1993**, *168*, 641–646.

18. Lee, J. B.; Hayashi, K.; Hashimoto, M.; Nakano, T.; Hayashi, T. Novel antiviral fucoidan from sporophyll of *Undaria pinnatifia* (Mekabu). *Chem. Pharm. Bull.* **2004**, *52*, 1091–1094.

19. Itoh, H.; Noda, H.; Amano, H.; Zuaug, C.; Mizuno, T.; Ito, H. Antitumor activity and immunological properties of marine algal polysaccharides, especially fucoidan, prepared from *Sargassum thunbergii* of Phaeophyceae. *Anticancer Res.* **1993**, *13*, 2045–2052.

20. Itoh, H.; Noda, H.; Amano, H.; Itoh, H. Immunological analysis of inhibition of lung metastases by fucoidan (GIV-A) prepared from brown seaweed *Sargassum thunbergii. Anticancer Res.* **1995**, *15*, 1937–1948.

21. Okai, Y.; Higashi-Okai, K.; Ishizuka, S.; Ohtani, K.; Matzui-Yuasa, I.; Yamashita, U. Possible immunomodulating activities in an extract of edible brown alga, *Hijikia fusiforme* (Hijiki). *J. Sci. Food. Agric.* **1998**, *76*, 56–62.

22. Shan, B. E.; Yoshida, Y.; Kuroda, E.; Yamashita, U. Immunomodulating activity of seaweed extract on human lymphocytes *in vitro*. *Int. J. Immunopharmacol.* **1999**, *21*, 59–70.

23. Liu, J. N.; Yoshida, Y.; Wang, M. Q.; Okai, Y.; Yamashita, U. B cell stimulating activity of seaweed extracts. *Int. J. Immunopharmacol.* **1997**, *19*, 135–142.

24. Wilson, S. Z.; Knight, V.; Wyde, P. R.; Drake, S.; Couch, R. B. Amantadine and ribavirin aerosol treatment of influenza A and B infection in mice. *Antimicrob. Agents Chemother.* **1980**, *17*, 642–648.

25. Hayden, F. G. Combinations of antiviral agents for treatment of influenza virus infections. *J. Antimicrob. Chemother.* **1986**, *18* (Suppl. B), 77–83.

26. Zhirnov, O. P. High protection of animals lethally infected with influenza virus by aprotinin-rimantadine combination. *J. Med. Virol.* **1987**, *21*, 161–167.

27. Sidwell, R. W.; Smee, D. F.; Huffman, J. H.; Barnard, D. L.; Bailey, K. W.; Morrey, J. D.; Babu, Y. S. *In vivo* influenza virus-inhibitory effects of the cyclopentane neuraminidase inhibitor RWJ-270201. *Antimicrob. Agents Chemother.* **2001**, *45*, 749–757.

28. Smee, D. F.; Bailey, K. W.; Morrison, A. C.; Sidwell, R. W. Combination treatment of influenza A virus infections in cell culture and in mice with the cyclopentane neuraminidase inhibitor RWJ-270201 and ribavirin. *Chemother.* **2002**, *48*, 88–93.

29. Govorkova, E. A.; Fang, H. B.; Tan, M.; Webster, R. G. Neuraminidase inhibitor-rimantadine combinations exert additive and synergistic anti-influenza virus effects in MDCK cells. *Antimicrob. Agents Chemother.* **2004**, *48*, 4855–4863.

30. Sugawara, I.; Ishizaka, S. Polysaccharides with sulfate groups are human T-cell mitogens and murine polyclonal B-cell activators (PBAs). *Cellular Immunol.* **1982**, *74*, 162–171.

31. Baba, M.; Snoeck, R.; Pauwels, R.; De Clercq, E. Sulfated polysaccharides are potent and selective inhibitors of various enveloped viruses, including herpes simplex virus, cytomegalvirus, vesicular stomatitis virus, and human immunodeficiency virus. *Antimicrob. Agents Chemother.* **1988**, *32*, 1742–1745.

32. Lüscher-Mattli, M.; Gluck, R. Dextran sulfate inhibits the fusion of influenza virus with model membranes, and suppresses influenza virus replication *in vivo*. *Antiviral Res.* **1990**, *14*, 39–50.

33. Akaike, T.; Weihe, E.; Schaefer, M.; Fu, Z. F.; Zheng, Y. M.; Vogel, W.; Schmidt, H.; Koprowski, H. Effect of neurotropic virus infection on neuronal and inducible nitric oxide synthase activity in rat brain. *J. Neurovirol.* **1995**, *1*, 118–125.

34. Akaike, T.; Noguchi, Y.; Ijiri, S.; Setoguchi, K.; Suga, M.; Zeng, Y. M.; Dietzscold, B.; Maeda, H. Pathogenesis of influenza virus-induced pneumonia involvement of both nitric oxide and oxygen radicals. *Proc. Natl. Acad. Sci. USA* **1996**, *93*, 2448–2453.

35. Mikami, S.; Kawashima, S.; Kanazawa, K.; Hirata, K.; Katayama, Y.; Hotta, H.; Hayashi, Y.; Ito, H.; Yokoyama, M. Expression of nitric oxide synthase in a murine model of viral myocarditis induced by coxsackievirus B3. *Biochem. Biophys. Res. Commun.* **1996**, *220*, 983–989.

36. Fujii, S.; Akaike, T.; Maeda, H. Role of nitric oxide in pathogenesis of herpes simplex virus encephalitis in rats. *Virology* **1999**, *256*, 203–212.

37. Bukowski, L. K.; Woda, B. A.; Habu, S.; Okumura, K.; Welsh, R. M. Natural killer cell depletion enhances virus synthesis and virus-induced hepatitis *in vivo*. *J. Immunol.* **1983**, *131*, 1531–1538.

38. Habu, S.; Akamatsu, I.; Tamaoki, N.; Okumura, K. *In vivo* significance of NK cells on resistance against virus (HSV-1) infections in mice. *J. Immunol.* **1984**, *133*, 2743–2747.

39. Roger-Zisman, B.; Quan, P. C.; Rosner, M.; Moller, J. R.; Bloom, B. R. Role of NK cells in protection of mice against herpes simplex virus-1 infection. *J. Immunol.* **1987**, *138*, 884–888.

40. March, J. C. The effects of cancer chemotherapeutic agents on normal hematopoietic precursor cells. *Cancer Res.* **1976**, *19*, 135–142.

41. Shih, W. W.; Baumhefner, R. W.; Tourtellotte, W. W.; Haskell, C. M.; Korn, E. L.; Fahey, J. L. Difference in effect of single immunosuppressive agents (cyclophosphamide, CCNU, 5-FU) on peripheral blood immune cell parameters and central nervous system immunoglobulin synthesis rate in patients with multiple sclerosis. *Clin. Exp. Immunol.* **1983**, *53*, 122–132.

42. Umeda, Y.; Sakamoto, A.; Nakamura, J.; Ishitsuka, H.; Yagi, Y. Thymosin alpha 1 restores NK-cell activity and prevents tumor progression in mice immunosuppressed by cytostatics or X-rays. *Cancer Immunol. Immunother.* **1983**, *15*, 78–83.

43. Rasi, G.; Silecchis, G.; Sinibaldi-Vallebona, P.; Spaziani, E.; Pierimaechi, P.; Sivilia, M.; Tremeterra, S.; Garaci, E. Anti-tumor effect of combined treatment with thymosin alpha 1 and inteleukin-2 after 5-fluorouracil in liver metastases from colorectal cancer in rats. *Internat. J. Cancer* **1994**, *57*, 701–705.

44. Rafique, M.; Adachi, W. Effects of intraportal administration of chemoimmunotherapeutic agents on natural killer cell activity in the rat liver. *J. Surgical Oncol.* **1995**, *60*, 154–159.

45. Kido, T.; Mori, K.; Daikuhara, H.; Tuchiya, H.; Ishige, A.; Sasaki, H. The protective effect of Hochu-ekki-to (TJ-41), a Japanese herbal medicine, against HSV-1 infection in mytomycin C-treated mice. *Anticancer Res.* **2000**, *20*, 4109–4114.

46. Ochiai, H.; Niwayama, S.; Masuyama, K. Inhibition of experimental pulmonary metastasis in mice by β-cyclodextrin-benzaldehyde. *J. Cancer Res. Clin. Oncol.* **1986**, *112*, 216–220.

47. Elion, G. B.; Singer, S.; Hitchings, G. H. Antagonists of nucleic acid derivatives. VIII. Synergism in combinations of biologically related antimetabolites. *J. Biol. Chem.* **1954**, *208*, 477–488.

48. Epstein, S. L.; Misplon, J. A.; Lawson, C. M.; Subbara, E. K.; Connors, M.; Murphy, B. R. Beta 2-microglobulin-deficient mice can be protected against influenza A injection by vaccination with vaccinia-influenza recombinants

expressing hemagglutinin and neuraminidase. *J. Immunol.* **1993**, *150*, 5484–5493.

49. Tao, T.; Davoodi, F.; Cho, C. J.; Skiadopoulos, M. H.; Durbin, A. P.; Colins, P. L.; Murphy, B. R. A live attenuated recombinant chimeric parainfluenza virus (PIV) candidate vaccine containing the hemagglutinin-neuraminidase and fusion glycoproteins of PIV1 even in animals immune to PIV3. *Vaccine* **2000**, *18*, 1359–1366.

<h1>8</h1>

RATIONAL DESIGN OF AN ANTI-ADHESION DRUG FOR INFLUENZA

NICOLAI V. BOVIN AND ALEXANDRA S. GAMBARYAN
Shemyakin Institute of Bioorganic Chemistry RAS, 117997, Moscow, Russia

INTRODUCTION

Carbohydrate chains on human cells are primary receptors for many microorganisms. The corresponding lectin of a microorganism ensures the specific carbohydrate–protein binding and could be the target for therapeutic intervention. Anti-adhesion therapy means inhibition or complete blocking of lectin-mediated adhesion (Fig. 8.1), without killing of the pathogen.[1] Antibiotics and conventional antivirals exert strong evolution pressure on pathogens, thus increasing the probability that resistance will develop. In contrast, an anti-adhesion strategy could minimize or even avoid mutational escape or development of strains resistant to the therapeutic.[2] Another evident advantage of anti-adhesion strategy is well-known structure of carbohydrate receptors and three-dimensional organization of many lectins—potential targets for rational drug design that allows us to avoid the time-consuming high-throughput screening stages and thus to accelerate drug discovery process. The idea of inhibition of viral attachment to the host cell arose just after first experiments demonstrating the potency of synthetic sialooligosaccharides as targets for influenza virus hemagglutinin, in 1971.[3] Later, anti-adhesion therapy was discussed mostly in context of

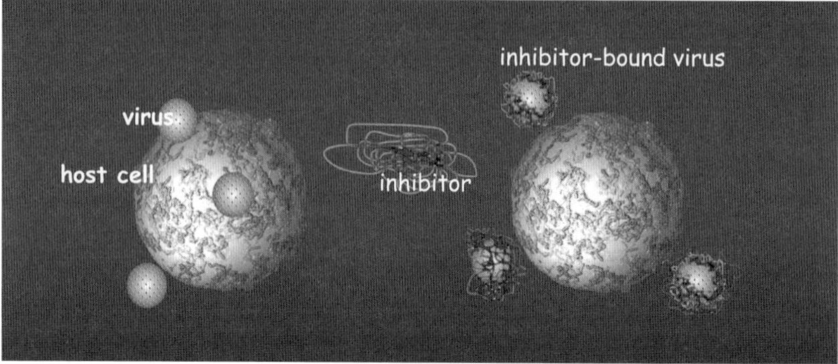

Fig. 8.1. Anti-adhesion principle. Oligosaccharide (OS) of host cell serves as receptor for virus. Natural mucin or synthetic bulky conjugate of this OS able to attain high-affinity binding to virus particle and to inhibit virus-to-cell binding, thus blocking infectivity. See color insert.

anti-bacterials. Last decade was the time for experimental evaluation of this idea, including clinical trials. However, there are still no anti-adhesion drugs on the shelves of drug stores. The reason is the belief that soluble oligosaccharide drugs are incapable of effective competition with the same oligosaccharides on the cell surface. Lectin on the microorganism surface is interacting with the target cell multipointly with high affinity, whereas a small-molecule free oligosaccharide binds to the same lectin in a monovalent manner and therefore with low affinity.[4] To be a good anti-adhesion drug, a blocker must be more affine toward pathogen as compared to the natural receptor on the cell surface. Therefore, the first key problem of anti-adhesion design is crucial improvement of oligosaccharide affinity.

The second key problem is diversity of pathogen strains binding specificity. Indeed, if H1, H3, H5, and B influenza viruses recognize different oligosaccharides, one should design several drug variants, thereby killing all the advantages of the anti-adhesion strategy. Fortunately, all H1, H3, and B human strains recognize the same target, trisaccharide 6′SLN, whereas the solution of the first-mentioned problem remains to be more intriguing.

TARGET OLIGOSACCHARIDE FOR DESIGNING THE ANTI-INFLUENZA THERAPEUTIC

The choice of 6′SLN trisaccharide as a drug candidate is based on (a) investigation of carbohydrate specificity of numerous virus strains and (b) occurrence of sialylated carbohydrate chains in the composition of respiratory glycoproteins. The detailed reasoning of this choice is discussed in the section entitled "Complementary Material", along with our thoughts on why glycomimetics could not replace 6'SLN. Here we explain our choice in brief.

Influenza virus infection is initiated by specific interactions between viral HA and host cell-surface receptors.[5–7] Terminal sialic acid residue of sialoglycoconjugates is known to be the minimum binding determinant of these receptors. Virus binding also depends on the type of the Neu5Ac linkage to penultimate galactose and on the structure of the more distant parts of the sialyl oligosaccharides.[8–11] According to the well-established simplification, human viruses bind to fragment Neu5Acα2–6Gal, whereas avian strains bind to Neu5Acα2–3Gal. More recent data[9] indicate that the next residue of the carbohydrate chain, namely GlcNAc, also has a significant role in reception, that is, the shared receptor for all human influenza viruses is trisaccharide Neu5Acα2–6Galβ1–4GlcNAc (6'SLN). Interestingly, 6'SL differing from 6'SLN by just one small NHAc group, is a poor receptor for modern H1 and H3 human strains (Fig. 8.2), and this preference of 6'SLN versus 6'SL tended to be more pronounced during last decade. At the same time, B strains do not differentiate 6'SLN and 6'SL. This unexplained conservatism of human HA toward 6'SLN looks irrational, especially in the light of avian viruses unpretentiousness (see

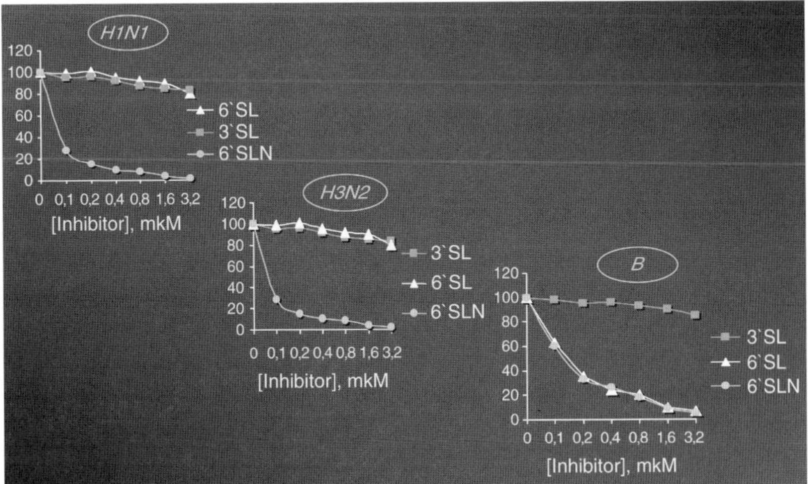

Fig. 8.2. High specificity of modern human H1, H3, and B influenza viruses toward trisaccharide 6'SLN. Solid-phase assay (FBI) in inhibitory mode, polyacrylamide (30 kDa) conjugates of 6'SLN, 6'SL, and 3'SLN as inhibitors. Similar results were observed with all other modern isolates propagated in MDCK or Vero cell culture. See color insert.

section entitled "Compementary Material" and Ref. 12). Nevertheless, narrow specificity of modern human strains ascertains to be well-documented, and the selection of 6'SLN trisaccharide as the ligand for the design of therapeutic blocker is apparent.

OLIGOSACCHARIDE/POLYMER CONJUGATES FOR MODELING ANTI-INFLUENZA DRUG

As mentioned above, the high-activity blocker has to be multivalent. An evident and simplest way to multivalency is conjugation of oligosaccharide with soluble polymer. Indeed, we demonstrated, *in vitro* and *in vivo*, the efficiency of polyacrylamide-conjugated oligosaccharides as influenza virus blockers. Realizing that therapeutics on the base of PAA and other true polymers do not have real chances to gain FDA approval (due to their production and composition inconsistency as well as high risk of side effects), we have been working with PAA glycoconjugates as a convenient model for comparison of monomeric versus multivalent blockers. PAA glycoconjugates showed ability to hamper cell culture infection. In the *in vitro* inhibition assay (FBI assay,[13] when the drug candidate competes with fetuin-peroxidase for binding to virus coated onto plate) a high-molecular-weight polymer, 6'SLN-PAA, was at least five orders of magnitude more potent than the monomer. Both FBI assay and experiments on the infectivity inhibition test (MDCK cells) demonstrated high potency of 6'SLN-PAA as blocker for all modern human H1, H3, and B strains. Next, the mouse model was approved for testing of influenza virus blockers *in vivo* (see legend to Fig. 8.3; Ref. 14); for this a human H1 (without any passage in chicken embryo) virus was adapted to mice by continuous re-infection. Importantly, receptor specificities of initial and adapted viruses, namely, high binding to 6'SLN and absence of binding to 3'SLN, were identical. Figure 8.3 demonstrates the pronounced therapeutic effect of 6'SLN-PAA, whereas infection of mice without the blocker caused 90% mortality. Notably, the therapeutic dose calculated for human body weight seems to be reasonable for intranasal administration.

SELF-ASSEMBLED GLYCOPEPTIDES AS PRACTICAL DRUG CANDIDATE

How can we preserve outstanding blocking potency of high-molecular-weight polymers and at the same time avoid generic drawbacks (see

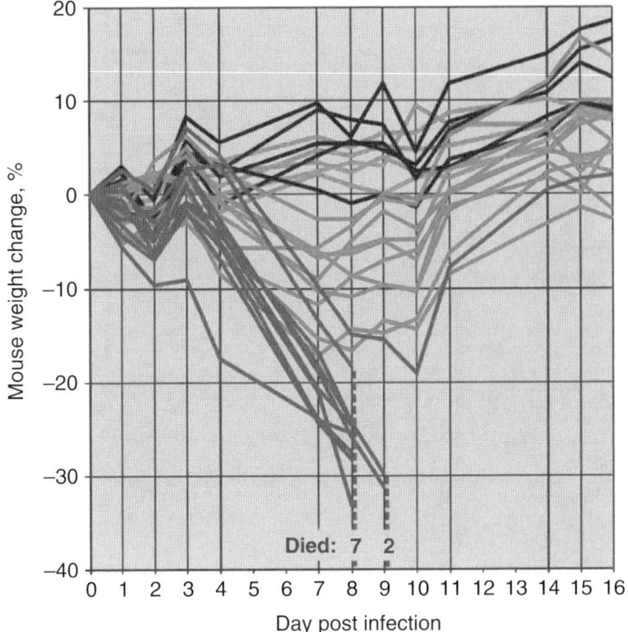

Fig. 8.3. Weight dynamics and survival of A/Sn mice from noninfected control group treated with placebo (blue); noninfected control group treated with 6′-SLN-PAA (cyan); and virus-infected mice treated either with placebo (red, 10 mice) or 6′-SLN-PAA (green). On days 2–5 after infection (10^3 IU of virus), mice were treated by 10-min exposures with 6′-SLN-PAA in aerosol form every 2 hr with 10-hr night break. The preparation dose (for each administration) was ~1 nmol by sialic acid per mouse. *P*-value for WL difference between the two control groups and between the two infected groups was 0.528 and <0.001, respectively. (Adapted from Ref. 14.) See color insert.

above) of true polymers? We have launched two approaches to overcome this problem. One of them is based on rational design of relatively small tri- and tetrantennary blockers optimized for trivalent binding (see below), and the second one exploits the idea of supramolecular assemblies instead of true polymers[15] (see Fig. 8.4). Supramolecular polymers (we use the term *tectomer*) do not have the inconsistency problem; clearance of glycopeptide tectomers from the organism seems to follow standard metabolic pathways because the tectomers are constructed from oligoglycine and mammalian monosaccharides. Actually, compounds of this class demonstrated the absence of acute toxicity in mice.

The main requirement for design of the self-assembling molecules as potential therapeutics was the absence of hydrophobicity, thus avoiding any nonspecific interaction with the cell membrane—even weak

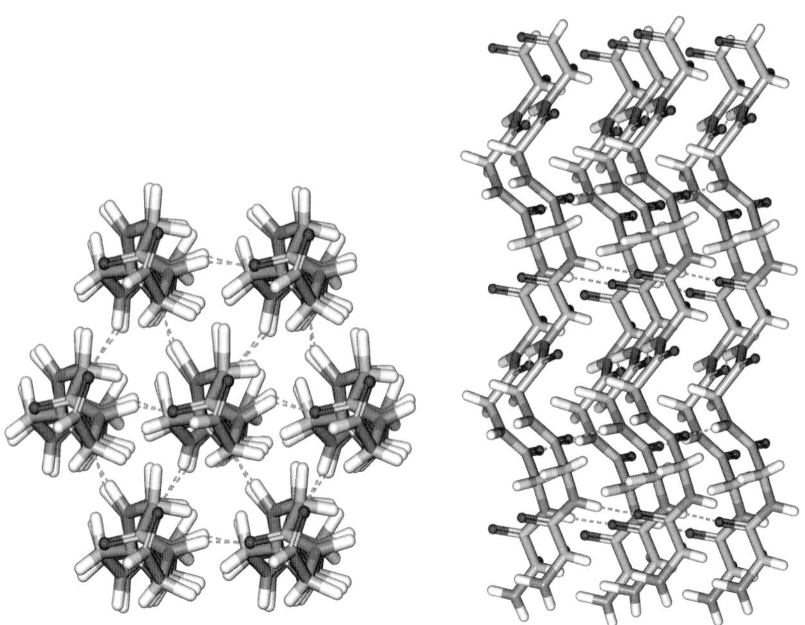

Fig. 8.4. Supramolecular organisation of monomeric glycopeptides into one-molecule-thick tectomer. Glycopeptides consist of two parts: A saccharide is capable of binding to viral lectin, whereas peptide is capable of self-assembling due to formation of multiple hydrogen bonds of polyglycine II type (see Fig. 8.5).

hydrophobicity at the monomer level could result in multiplied non-specific binding at the multivalent level. Therefore, liposomes, micelles, and all other entities based on the hydrophobic principle of assembling were excluded from consideration. Due to similar reasons, charge-based interaction also did not fit the background criteria. In contrast, hydrogen bonding in pure form, not contaminated with hydrophobic and charge constituents, is expected to be an ideal driving force for this purpose. Ironically, practically all known hydrogen-bonded supramolecular assemblies are formed either in organic solvents or in solid phase but not in water.[16–19] An additional problem at the designing stage was the requirement of chemical simplicity. Nevertheless, peptide molecules corresponding to all the mentioned criteria have been designed, namely tri- and tetraantennary (see Fig. 8.5) oligoglycines. The so-called polyglycine II secondary structure of peptide chains is distinct from canonical α-helix and β-sheet; the conformation of the polypeptide chain is 3_1 helix ($\phi = -76.9°$, $\psi = 145.3°$) where all the NH and CO groups form highly cooperative intermolecular hydrogen bonds with the six parallel or antiparallel surrounding chains (see Fig. 8.5).

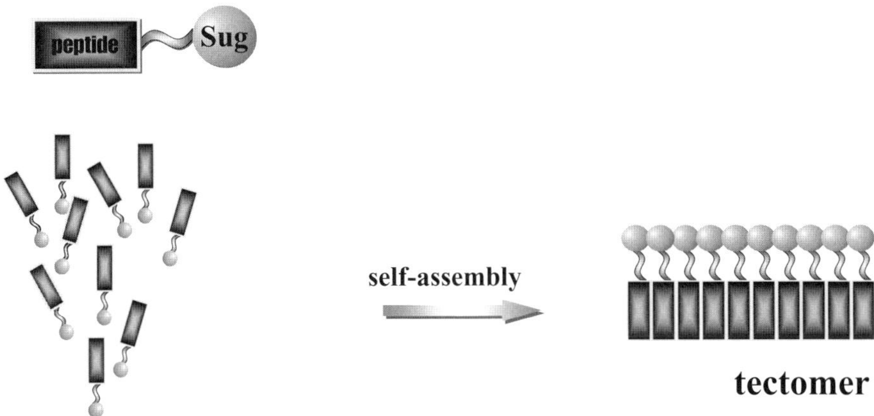

Fig. 8.5. Structure of polyglycine II, top view (left) and side view (right), Gly$_7$ fragments of polyglycine chains is presented. Hydrogen bonds between chains are shown.

The distance of 5 Å between two polypeptides is so small that any substituent in the CH_2 group kills the polyglycine II structure this means that only polymers of NH_2CH_2COOH itself or, generally, of $NH_2(CH_2)_nCOOH$ are capable of forming this secondary structure. Polyglycine II was found in several crystalline substances such as glycine polymer,[20] bolaamphiphils,[21] and nylons.[22] In contrast to the cited examples, we have succeeded in finding short (heptamers) peptides capable of forming stable polyglycine II structure in water media. The first reported example was a series of tetraantennary oligoglycines without substituents or with pendant SA residues. The polyglycine II structure of the tectomers is apparent from Raman spectra; the spectrum profiles of both water-soluble peptide and glycopeptide tectomers comprise a banding pattern with the position and relative intensity consistent with polyglycine II spatial organization. The tectomers were investigated by AFM and EM methods,[15] indicating that they were shaped as thin, flat sheets; the experimentally determined thickness of the core glycopeptide tectomer $[Gly_7\text{-}NHCH_2]_4C$ was ~45 Å. A number of more simple oligoglycines, namely tri-, di- and even mono-antennary ones, also demonstrated the ability to form polyglycine II structures.[23] The unusual stability of tectomers in aqueous media is explained by the participation of all CO and NH glycine groups in H-bonding, and thus the exclusion of any H-bond interactions with water inside the body of two-dimensional crystal, where all except peripheral chains are hidden by each other.

As expected, the attachment of 6′SLN to the polyglycine II tectomer led to a high potency blocker for the influenza virus. The nonassembling glycopeptides of a general formula [6'SLN-linker-Gly$_n$-NHCH$_2$]$_4$C ($n = 1 \div 6$) did not show a substantial increase in activity relative to monovalent 6'SLN. However, the corresponding Gly$_7$ and more continuous analogues demonstrated antiviral potency by at least three orders of magnitude higher. Notably, the observed anti-influenza activity of the tectomers approached that of the 6'SLN derivatives of true polymers.

VIRUS-PROMOTED ASSEMBLY INSTEAD OF SELF-ASSEMBLY

While the above-presented results have focused on the activity of pre-formed tectomers, a more promising way is believed to be a prodrug strategy, when tectomer is formed *only in the presence of virus* (see Fig. 8.6). If so, the drug formulation (prodrug) is a relatively small molecule having, in contrast to high-molecular-weight compounds, unequivocal chemical structure and acceptable diffusion properties. From the per-

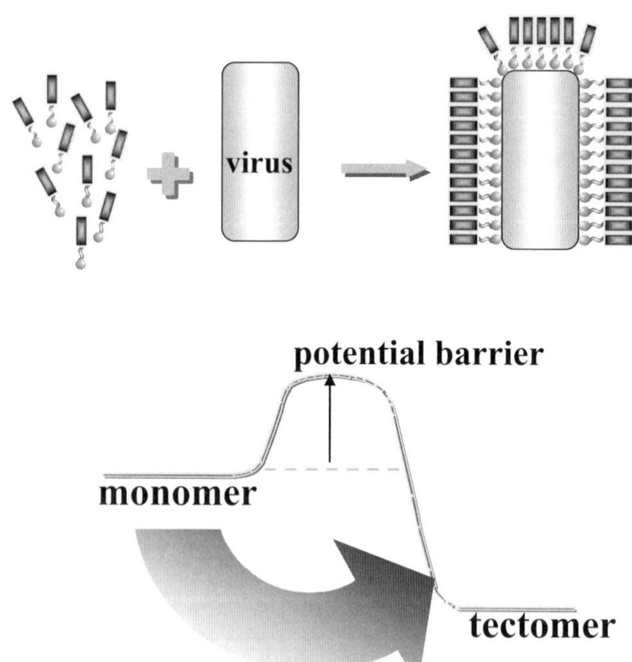

Fig. 8.6. Principle of virus-promoted assembly. In contrast to the above-described molecules (see Fig. 8.5), here glycopeptides are not able to assemble simultaneously.

spective of antiviral therapy, the assembly of small molecules into a tectomer directly on a virion has clear advantages as compared to the administration of the same but preformed tectomer.

Experimental approval of this concept was performed. Four moles of Neu5Ac were coupled to tetraantennary oligoglycine peptide in the presence of LiBr (see section entitled "Complementary Material"). The synthesis in the presence of LiBr enables the achievement of 100% substitution by Neu5Ac; glycopeptide obtained in these conditions is incapable of *spontaneous* assembling into tectomer due to mutual spatial hindrance and charge of neighbor Neu5Ac residues in composition of tectomer to be formed. Potential barrier (see Fig. 8.6) of the aggregation is too high for a spontaneous step-by-step process; however, such glycopeptides are finally capable of forming tectomer in the presence of the virus particle. Virus plays a role of priming: HA trimers are densely situated on a virion and thus serve as a scaffold, which locally concentrates the monomers and stabilizes tectomer germs (process similar to crystallization). Thus, the driving force of virus promotion seems to be (a) double cooperativity of glycopeptide assembly on the one hand and (b) their binding to a pattern of hemagglutinins on a viral surface on the other hand. Actually, we observed a dynamic mixture of monomeric form and small aggregates; probably, such pretectomers are oligovalently adsorbed onto a virion surface followed by maturation and further growth processes. Importantly, this virus-promoted assembly is ligand-specific; in the same conditions an analogue with a corrupted saccharide (β- instead of α-) demonstrated no aggregation when contacted with the virus particle. One can suppose an alternative mechanism: Viral neuraminidase splits off one "extra" Neu5Ac residue from tetra-substituted molecule; after that the tri-substituted version becomes capable of assembling simultaneously. However, the presence of a neuraminidase inhibitor, 4-amino-4-deoxy-Neu5Ac2en, does not affect the phenomenon; thus the virus-promoted assembly cannot be explained by neuraminidase participation.

Thus, the microorganism-promoted self-assembly of prodrug is a novel paradigm offering to surmount much better the general problem of design of anti-adhesion therapeutics.

"TETRAHEDRONS": SMALL NONASSEMBLING GLYCOPEPTIDES

Another group of potent influenza virus blockers was synthesized, with small molecules bearing three or four copies of 6'SLN spatially organized by optimal way. Several groups reported synthesis of clusters or star-like molecules with SA as ligand[24–27]; however, only a limited number of them demonstrated enhanced activity compared to monomeric sialosides. Key points in rational design of such molecules are optimal distance between the ligands and their correct spatial organization. We assumed that clusters with tetrahedral display of 6′SLN (Fig. 8.7) would be especially potent for influenza virus inhibitors. First, their symmetry is suitable for trivalent binding. Second, the tetrahedron has four equivalent planes for trivalent contact with HA. Third, symmetrical tetrahedron is preferable due to the dynamics of interaction: Being bound with HA by the first of 6′SLN residues, it can easily adjust itself for the other two 6′SLN/HA interactions. In a rigid tetrahedron the distance between ligands could be regulated in a custom fashion and thus optimized for binding to multivalent protein. Influenza virus HA is homotrimer with intra-CBS distance of ~50 Å,[28] whereas an average inter-CBS distance (for neighbor trimers) is ~100 Å.[29,30] We supposed that formally tetrahedral molecules (Fig. 8.7) with the distances between two 6′SLN residues of 50–100 Å should be strong HA blockers. Indeed, *sym* tetra-sialosides of general formula $[\text{Neu5Ac-sp-AC}_n\text{-NHCH}_2]_4\text{C}$ (sp is spacer-arm, AC is aminocaproic residue) with *n* value equal 5–6

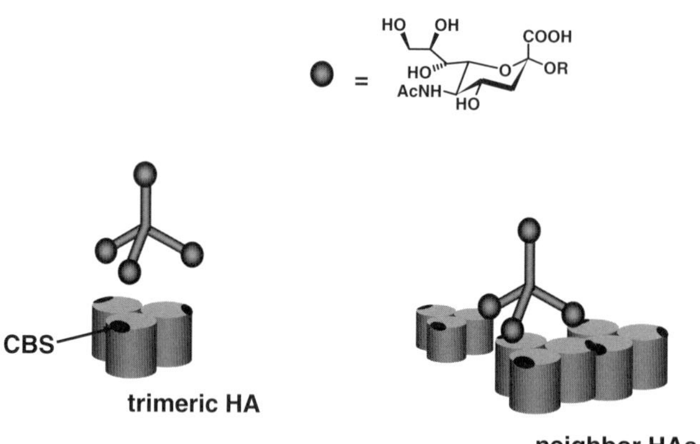

Fig. 8.7. Rationales for designing tetravalent nonassembling influenza blockers. Optimal length of antennae in combination with general rigidity of the molecule provides a convenience for trivalent binding to viral hemagglutinin. Two possible modes of docking are shown. First, intra-trimer binding (left): HA is a symmetrical trimer, CBS are located at the end of each HA subunit, and distance between CBS is ~50 Å. Second, inter-trimer binding (right): HA trimers are evenly distributed on the viral membrane with the center distance of ~100 Å. Sialic acid is shown as a ligand for simplicity.

(i.e., when the theoretical distance between two SA residues fits the required interval 50–100 Å) were three orders of magnitude more potent comparing to monomeric Neu5Ac-sp, whereas all shorter compounds ($n = 1$–4) demonstrated activity equal to the monomer.[31]

Lead optimization resulted in similar *sym* molecules where (i) relatively hydrophobic (risk of side effects!) AC residues were substituted for hydrophilic ones, (ii) Neu5Ac was substituted for 6′SLN, and (iii) the molecule as a whole was organized in a rigid manner allowing the saccharide ligands to occupy peripheral, maximally distanced positions from each other. As a result, this last generation of nonassembling molecules demonstrated high antiviral potency—as compared with self-assembled glycopeptides—in FBI assay, cell culture assay, and *in vivo*, especially against H1 and H3 strains.

ADMINISTRATION, CLEARANCE, STABILITY

In contrast to many other preparations, anti-adhesion drugs act outside the cell and, correspondingly, should not penetrate into it. Ultimately, low-molecular-weight, highly restricted hydrophobic–hydrophilic balance and other strict requirements that have become dogmas and stereotypes in drug discovery should not be taken into consideration in this case. Thus, the relatively high molecular weight (about several thousand daltons) and high hydrophilicity (correspondingly, the inability to cross plasmatic membrane) of the sialylated peptides plays a positive rather than negative role when acting outside the cell.

A limited group of respiratory epithelium cells is the target for common (H1, H3, B) influenza viruses in humans. Evidently, the drug should be delivered precisely there, locally, whereas systemic administration of the drug seems to be at least wasteful. Unfortunately, pharmaceutical bosses still believe that a pill is more convenient for a consumer than a spray. This is confirmed by recent statistics of sales of neuraminidase inhibitors: Relenza used as spray has been brought to market earlier than Tamiflu (pills), and Relenza is more preferable with respect to appearance of drug-resistant strains; nevertheless, its sales are one order of magnitude lower. We believe that now is the time to overcome this stereotype, and consumers should be educated that a locally administered drug is much better than pills from the point of view of human ecology. Happily, sprays and similar dosing delivery devices have been technically developed and are more widespread nowadays.

COMPARISON OF SYNTHETIC BLOCKERS WITH NATURAL MUCINS

Containment and prevention of influenza by an anti-adhesion mechanism is used by Nature: Well-known mucins are the innate therapeutics preventing numerous infectious diseases, including influenza. However, why do mucins not always execute this function and how did we become confident that synthetic preparation can be more efficient than analogous "drug" polished by evolution? To answer this question, we have compared anti-influenza virus potency of synthetic and natural sialosides[14]: The values of dissociation constants for human tracheal and nasal mucins and polymer 6′SLN-PAA are given in Table 8.1. Affinity of mucins, with respect to total concentration of sialic acid, is rather high and is comparable to that of 6′SLN-PAA. Notably, mucin concentration in human respiratory epithelium corresponds to approximately 100 K_d, which should be enough for strong competition with cellular receptors and thus prevention of the infection. If so, use of synthetic sialylglycopolymers does not seem promising. However, as all we know, in the course of natural infection the virus is able to efficiently overcome the mucin barrier causing disease. The same is true also for viral infection in cell culture (Table 8.1). In contrast, the synthetic inhibitor 6′SLN-PAA strongly suppressed the infection of MDCK cells under the same experimental conditions and capable of preventing infection in mice (see above). This marked difference between the synthetic inhibitor and the natural mucins in cell culture and *in vivo* could first be explained by higher stability of 6′SLN-PAA to cleavage by proteases: proteolytic digestion decreases multivalency and thus antiviral potency of mucins *in vivo*. Second, "rational" Nature utilizes mucins as universal therapeutic against numerous carbohydrate-recognizing pathogens, and the molecule contains big variety of OSs types and thus a limited number of copies of each particular type. Much higher content

TABLE 8.1. DissociationConstants (K_d, μM Sia) of Virus Complexes with Human Mucins and Sialopolymer (FBI assay), and Concentration of 90% Neutralization (IC$_{90\%}$, μM Sia) of Virus Infectivity, A/NIB23/89M (H1N1) Strain

Inhibitors	K_d	IC$_{90\%}$
Human tracheal mucin	0.1	>10
Human nasal mucin	0.2	>10
6′SLN-PAA	0.01	0.05

of 6'SLN (and therefore higher multivalency) in the composition of 6'SLN-PAA, as compared to the natural mucin, is believed to explain the high potency of the synthetic blocker. Will this obvious advantage of a true polymer be retained in the case of tectomers? Most probably, yes, because common proteases hardly cleave oligoglycine fragments. Moreover, oligoglycines are so tightly packed in the formed tectomer that the enzyme can reach them only from periphery of the tectomer, that is, slowly. Preliminary tests demonstrate that tectomers resemble true polymers rather than mucins by their activity *in vivo.*

One more mechanism sharply decreasing the potency of sialosides-blockers is viral neuraminidase action. This can be crucial in the case of mucins where the density of 6'SLN residues is low. We expected that neuraminidase action would not be so critical for synthetic blockers with high density of the receptor trisaccharide. The results of cell culture and murine model tests lived up to our expectations. The study of kinetics of oligosaccharide desialylation by influenza viruses demonstrated[32] that all viruses cleaved 2–6 sialosides much slower than 2–3 ones, whereas neuraminidase from human viruses was inferior to avian viruses enzyme, which is by all means a factor assisting the application of the blockers based on natural trisaccharide 6'SLN. This is another argument against necessity of the search for molecules-mimetics stable to NA action.

COMPLEMENTARY MATERIAL

1. Change of Receptor Specificity During Adaptation of Influenza Virus to a New Host

Waterfowl birds, first of all wild ducks, are primary hosts of influenza viruses. Sixteen antigenic virus subtypes by HA and 9 NA subtypes circulate among them.[33–35]

All the viral proteins are evolutionally stable in primary hosts, although intense exchange with the elements of segmented genome often takes place due to reassortment. This vast "pot" gives origin to numerous evolutionary branches of viruses circulating in secondary hosts—that is, in humans, other mammals, and poultry birds. Evolution speed increases drastically in new hosts.[36]

The most important element of virus adaptation to a new host is adjustment to new receptors of the same cell targets or (in some cases) to new targets. It would be interesting to trace the changes in receptor specificity during the transition from the previous host to the new one and its further evolution. Systematic study of influenza virus receptor specificity with the aid of synthetic sialooligosaccharides for 15 years demonstrated that all evolutionary branches of human influenza viruses acquire a high affinity to the same receptor, Neu5Acα2-6Galβ1-4GlcNAc (6′SLN), that is, that GlcNAc residue is important for recognition. At the same time, all the studied avian viruses of eight subtypes recognized disaccharide fragment Neu5Acα2–3Gal in composition of *various* oligosaccharides (fucosylated, sulfated, etc.).

Interestingly, different subtypes of avian influenza viruses were demonstrated to have the same molecular mechanism of Neu5Acα2–3Gal recognition. Their evolutionary stable CBS contains 10 conservative amino acids, six of which can be changed during the transfer to another host. Affinity of duck viruses to Neu5Acα2–3Gal is higher than to monosaccharide Neu5Ac, thus evidencing energetically advantageous interaction of CBS with galactose moiety.[37]

The mechanism of receptor specificity rebuilding during influenza viruses transfer to humans has been studied the best for H3N2 viruses. The very first isolates of human H3N2 differed from relative avian viruses by replacements Gln226→Leu and Gly228→Ser, resulting in increased affinity to 2–6 and decreased affinity to 2–3 sialylgalactose fragments.[5,10,38] An analogous mechanism has been realized during H2N2 virus subtype transfer to humans, where amino acids 226 and 228 have been replaced primarily. Interestingly, the same replacements Gln226→Leu and Gly228→Ser have been observed in H4N6 virus isolated form pigs. Receptor specificity of this isolate coincided with that of early H3N2 virus A/Aichi/2/68.[39]

Independent appearance of two identical replacements in three evolutionary branches demonstrates the efficiency of this mechanism for acquirement of the ability to recognize 6′SLN. In all three cases, viral HA in a new host is, from an evolutionary standpoint, very close to hemagglutinin of wild duck viruses of the given subtype. Indeed, two replacements, Gln226→Lcu and Gly228→Ser, are sufficient for readjustment of receptor specificity from recognizing of wild duck receptor to recognition of human receptor 6′SLN.[40,41]

Other amino acid replacements assisting the appearance of the ability to recognize 2–6 receptor during transfer from birds to humans have been observed in the case of B and H1N1 viruses.[11,42] Replacement Glu190→Asp was observed in all five sequenced human viruses H1N1 from year 1918. Viruses with single replacement demonstrated shared 2–6/2–3 receptor specificity and, additionally, high affinity to 6-Su-3′SLN and related sulfated OS. At the same time, the viruses with additional replacements Gly225→Asp do not bind Neu5Ac2–3Gal receptors and possess maximum affinity to human receptor 6′SLN.[43–46] Mutation amino acid 190 has been observed in all pig viruses H1N1 and H9N2 and in one of evolutionary branches of poultry viruses H9N2.[47] Study of pig viruses with this mutation demonstrated the optimal receptor to be Su-SiaLe^x, and these viruses also acquired the ability to recognize 6′SLN.[48–50] Additional replacement Glu190→Asp in the viruses with Asp225 provides preferential binding with 6′SLN compared to 6′SL.[11]

X-ray crystallography data of HA from human and pig H1N1 viruses revealed hydrogen bonds between Asp225 and galactose residue in composition of Neu5Ac2–6Gal and between Asp190 and amino group nitrogen of glucosamine in composition of 6′SLN.[51]

After 1992 the replacement Asp190→Glu was also observed in human H3N2 viruses, accompanied by the change of receptor properties: first, reduced agglutination of chicken erythrocytes[52,53]; second, loss of affinity to fetuin; and, finally, acquisition of the ability to differentiate 6′SL and 6′SLN.[54] After 2003, H3N2 viruses acquired Asp225 instead of Gly, thus leading to dramatic decrease of affinity to 6′SL and retaining affinity to 6′SLN. Most probably, bulky hydrophilic residue Asp225 prevents hydrophobic interactions of the oligosaccharide with amino acid 226. Thus, human viruses H3N2 acquired the ability to recognize trisaccharide 6′SLN, similarly to H1N1 viruses.[54]

Viruses B also display much stronger binding to trisaccharides SL and SLN than to monosaccharide Neu5Ac, thus indicating energetically favorite interactions with the asialo part of the receptor.[42] Notable discrimination between Neu5Ac2–3Gal and Neu5Ac2–6Gal was observed only for polyvalent receptors[9,11] but not for free oligosaccharides. During adaptation to human receptor, avian B viruses retain intact the residues 226 and 228 in the sequence Gln–Ser–Gly–Arg typical for avian viruses, but acquired replacements Tyr98→Phe and Glu190→Gln and insertion in the 225 amino acid region. Additionally, carbohydrate residue at amino acid 187, localized practically inside CBS in the left upper fissure of HA, plays an important role in retraining of receptor specificity. Loss of this residue and correspondingly the carbohydrate chain restores the virus ability to bind Neu5Ac2–3Gal.[9,11,55] A typical feature of viruses B is inability, in contrast to viruses H1 and H3, to differentiate Neu5Acα2–6Galβ1–4GlcNAc and Neu5Acα2–6Galβ1–4Glc.

Thus, adaptation of hemagglutinin CBS to a new receptor during the transfer of avian viruses to humans can proceed by various pathways though with the same result, namely, attainment of high affinity to trisaccharide 6′SLN.

2. Structure of Natural Cell Receptors and Fine Carbohydrate Specificity of HA: Too Much Discrepancies

It is well known that receptor specificity of influenza virus is host-dependent. Change of specificity also takes place at the cell culture level. Thus, growing of a human isolate on chicken embryos can lead to attainment of avian specificity even after a couple of passages; change of MDCK cells as host to closely related (both of kidney origin) Vero cells sometimes leads to tuning of receptor specificity. Two mechanisms of receptor specificity adaptation have been revealed. The first one is amino acid replacement in the CBS region; the second one is change of peptide chain glycosylation in proximity to CBS. Why the virus easily changes specificity and adapts to a new host in one case but not in other cases (e.g., during the transfer of viruses H5N1 from birds to humans) is not known for certain yet. Most probably, there are also two reasons for inducing the change of specificity in a new host. The first one is receptor differences in primary target cell. The second reason is dramatically different: The whole physiological cycle *virus/host* is exemplified by the pair duck (virus environment is stomach) versus pig (respiratory tract is infected).

Until recently it has been considered that, human viruses as a result of evolution, acquired Neu5Acα2–6Gal specificity because these carbohydrate chains are characteristic for human respiratory tract cells, whereas Neu5Acα2–3Gal specificity of avian viruses is the result of predomination of the corresponding structures on avian intestinal epithelium cells. However, more detailed analysis of avian viruses receptor specificity as well as composition of target cell carbohydrate chains demonstrated that this hypothesis is at least simplified.

Recently, studies with the aid of specific lectins have demonstrated that 2–3 but not 2–6 sialosides are exposed on cells of chicken embryo chorio-allantoic membrane and duck intestinal epithelial cells,[35,56,57] but *both* variants of chains have been observed on chicken embryo endothelial cells,[58] on intestine, and on tracheal epithelial cells of adult chicken[59]; moreover, these cells were capable of binding both human and avian viruses.[59,60] In addition, it has been shown that intestine and trachea epithelium of quail also carry both variants of sialylated chains and were capable of binding human viruses.[61] Analogous observations were made for a number of other bird species.[62]

Study of fine receptor specificity using a wide range of synthetic OS revealed principal importance of fucose substituent at GlcNAc residue of sialoreceptor for virus reception. Thus, duck viruses displayed high preference to non-fucosylated receptor Neu5Acα2–3Galβ1–4GlcNAc (3′SLN) and displayed low preference to its fucosylated variant—that is, SiaLe^x. Remarkably, mentioned viruses bind well only duck intestinal epithelium cells. At the same time, several chicken viruses possessed high specificity toward SiaLe^x; these viruses bound chicken cells well, thus allowing us to speculate about the presence of SiaLe^x on chicken epithelium cells.[62]

The distribution of influenza virus receptors on the human airway epithelium was investigated using lectins and well-characterized viruses. The results showed that both α2–3- and α2–6-linked sialosides were expressed on the surface of airway epithelial cells.[63–66]

Thus, influenza virus tropism cannot be abridged to the following simple formula: "The Neu5Ac2-3Gal receptor is presented on avian cells, so 2–3-specific viruses bind them; the Neu5Ac2–6Gal receptor is presented on human cells, so 2–6-specific viruses bind them." Obviously, it is important (possibly, even more important) what the virus *must not* bind during its way to a target cell—in particular intercellular matrix mucins and sialylated non-target cells, incapable of being infected. Furthermore, the choice of target cells in new hosts must support not only successful infection, but also effective transmissibility of virus.[67]

3. Mimetics?

In spite of great progress in glyco-biotechnology and chemical synthesis, scale oligosaccharide production remains a risky area for pharma investors. So, why can't an OS be substituted by cheap mimetics? We believe that in contrast to many other areas, glycomimetics are bad candidates for substitution of natural oligosaccharides in design of anti-adhesion therapeutics, because mimetic is unable to bind all the variety of virus strains. Indeed, the existing influenza virus (sub)types have acquired a different mechanism (specific set of amino acids in composition of CBS) of 6'SLN recognition (see above); moreover, the trisaccharide is recognized in two conformations[68,69]; thus, the search for such a complicated mimetic is believed to be a practically impossible task. Moreover, a mimetic should bind not only existing but also new strains. Thus, only the natural oligosaccharide itself is capable of binding all the evolutionary or drug-promoted variants of the lectin, and an optimum strategy for anti-adhesion drug design is a minimal strategy—not to make any changes at all, that is, to use the natural ligand as is.

One more expected advantage of a natural ligand compared to a mimetic is the expected low risk of side effects because a therapeutic will be, in fact, a variant of a molecule presented onto human cells or mucins—that is, a motif tolerant to its environment. Natural ligand instead of mimetics means the absence of lead candidates sorting out due to their side effects and, therefore, shortening of the drug development process.

Finally, here's the most obvious reasoning: We already know the structure of the receptor for human influenza viruses, so why invent a mimetic?

4. Other Anti-Influenza Therapeutics, Brief Overview

Antiviral Peptide. A 20 amino-acid peptide derived from the signal sequence of fibroblast growth factor exhibits antiviral including H5N1 strain activity. The peptide binds to HA and inhibits in 5–30 μM concentration the attachment to the cell receptor preventing infection. The binding is expected to change the conformation of HA, thereby decreasing the affinity for sialoreceptor on the cell surface. Another possibility is that the peptide interacts at or near the CBS of HA, thereby blocking binding pocket or causing steric hindrance during receptor docking.[70] Thus, this approach mechanistically seems to be similar to our anti-adhesion approach. Exact amino acid sequence of an HA molecule responsible for specific binding remains unknown, so it is impossible to anticipate evolutionary drift of this site and thus resistance potency of influenza viruses to this new therapeutic candidate.

Neuraminidase Inhibitors. Tamiflu (Oseltamivir) is a 312-Da systemic drug that is an oral inhibitor of viral NA. Tamiflu is developed by Gilead Biosciences and is licensed for manufacturing and sales to Roche. If started within 48 hr of symptoms' onset, Tamiflu is reported to reduce influenza symptoms by 1 day over a 5-day treatment course compared with placebo.[71] No data on the mortality reduction exist. Nausea, vomiting, and a few serious central nervous system side effects were reported. Resistance to neuraminidase drugs is reported at <5% rate, although higher rates of resistance to Tamiflu in children (6–18%) and in H5N1-infected patients were reported.[72] In a 2004 report of 10 H5N1-infected patients in Vietnam with 80% mortality, four out of five patients treated with Tamiflu died.[73] Relenza (Zanamivir) is also a small-molecule inhibitor of NA. Relenza is administered via inhalation of a powder, due to poor systemic availability. Relenza has been developed via rational drug design[74] by university research and company Biota Holdings and is marketed by GlaxoSmithKline. Relenza was the first worldwide neuraminidase inhibitor drug. Structurally, Relenza is more close to progenitor Neu5Ac molecule than Tamiflu, and this explains the very infrequent appearance of resistant strains.

Adamantane Derivatives. Amantadine (approved in 1976) and rimantadine are orally available agents for treatment of influenza A. The drugs interfere with viral protein M2 resulting in blocking of viral uncoating and replication. Their effectiveness against influenza A is similar to NA inhibitors and results in a 1-day reduction of symptoms if taken within 48 hr of onset. Most of their side effects concern gastro-intestinal and central nervous systems; amantadine is teratogenic in animals. The CDC reports progressive enhancement of drug-resistant strains, both H1 and H3.

Monoclonal Antibodies. In 2005, Gemini Science announced the development of a novel, fully human monoclonal antibody to the influenza A M2 protein for protection against and treatment of influenza infection. In preliminary studies using *in vitro* and *in vivo* systems, the antibody demonstrated broad activity against a wide range of human and avian influenza strains, including the recently emerging avian influenza strain, H5N1. Based upon these data, Gemini Science is initiating pre-clinical studies of the monoclonal antibody. This therapeutic is expected to have all the typical drawbacks of protein-based drugs, namely, high molecular weight, low stability, high production cost, high risk of allergy reactions, and, finally, high risk of resistant strains formation.

Vaccines. A person has to undergo regular vaccinations because new epidemic strains usually appear every 1–2 years. There is a stable unwillingness of the population to be vaccinated against the influenza. Shortage of modern vaccine due to production problems is not an unusual situation. Another general problem of all influenza vaccine preparation is storage instability. Probably, the most prospective modern vaccine series (H1, H3, H5) has been developed by GreenHills Biotechnology (Vienna). Vaccine virus lacks NS protein responsible for viral resistance to interferon; therefore live vaccine is capable only to a single infection cycle.

Recombinant Neuraminidase. NexBio (San Diego) announced[75] the start of clinical trials of anti-influenza preparation (*fludase*) based on recombinant NA from *V. cholerae*. The concept of this approach is to destroy human cell receptors for influenza virus. The approach is believed to have no chance for approval, because, first, incomplete removal of cell sialic acid may give the opposite result, that is, facilitated infection; and, second, sialooligosaccharides play a crucial role in many important cell processes; thus, removal of sialic acid ultimately causes numerous side effects.

This brief overview demonstrates that all conventional and modern preparations against influenza virus do not solve the problem of treatment this disease and prevention of expected avian pandemic. No doubt, principally new approaches are required. We believe that anti-adhesion paradigm itself or in combination with existing strategies are capable of solving influenza problem.

5. Synthesis of Self-Assembling Glycopeptides

The tetraantennary oligoglycine-based peptides and glycopeptides were synthesized by a conventional peptide chemistry using tetra(aminomethyl)methane as the starting material. Glycine residues were inserted individually or *en block* as hydroxysuccinimide-activated Boc-derivatives.[31] Carbohydrate residues were coupled to peptide backbone through acylation of amino groups of terminal glycyl residues by corresponding COO-nitrophenyl dervatives in two different ways: (i) $NaHCO_3$ was added to aqueous $[HCl \cdot Gly_7\text{-}NHCH_2]_4C$ (which exists as a monomer), resulting in the assembled $[Gly_7\text{-}NHCH_2]_4C$ followed by acylation of the formed peptide tectomer; (ii) alternatively, the glycopeptide was obtained by acylation of monomeric $[Gly_7\text{-}NHCH_2]_4C$ in the presence of LiBr. The degree of "glycosylation" by first method was ~75%, whereas the synthesis by second method allowed achievement of 100% substitution. Aqueous tectomers are stable at room temperature in the presence of salts at physiological concentrations, while a reversible disintegration occurs in the presence of concentrated solutions of lithium bromide or trifluoroacetic acid or upon heating.

ACKNOWLEDGMENTS

This study was support in part by research grants 05-04-48934, 01-04-49300, and 04-03-032683 from the Russian Foundation for Basic Research, RAS program "Molecular and Cell Biology," and ISTC grant No. 2464.

REFERENCES

1. Zopf, D.; Roth, S. Oligosaccharide anti-infective agents. *The Lancet* **1996**, *347*, 1017–1021.
2. Irvin, R. T.; Bautista, D. L. Hope for the post-antibiotic era? *Nature Biotechnol.* **1999**, *17*, 20–20.

3. Khorlin, A. Ya.; Privalova, I. M.; Bystrova, I. B. The synthesis of *N*-acetyl-neuraminyl-(2→3)- and -(2→6)-hexoses. *Carb. Res.* **1971**, *19*, 272–275.

4. Matrosovich, M. N. Towards the development of antimicrobial drugs acting by inhibition of pathogen attachment to host cells: A need for polyvalency. *FEBS Let.* **1989**, *252*, 1–4.

5. Paulson, J. C. Interaction of animal viruses with cell surface receptors. In *The Receptors*, vol. 2; Conn, M., Ed., Academic Press, Orlando, FL, **1985**, pp. 131–219.

6. Wiley, D. C.; Skehel, J. J. The structure and function of the hemagglutinin membrane glycoprotein of influenza virus. *Annu. Rev. Biochem.* **1987**, *56*, 365–394.

7. Herrler, G.; Hausmann, J.; Klenk, H. D. Sialic acid as receptor determinant of ortho- and paramyxoviruses. In *Biology of the Sialic Acids*, Rosenberg, A., Ed., Plenum Press, New York, **1995**, pp. 315–336.

8. Suzuki, Y. Gangliosides as influenza virus receptors. Variation of influenza viruses and their recognition of the receptor sialo-sugar chains. *Prog. Lipid Res.* **1994**, *33*, 429–457.

9. Gambaryan, A. S.; Tuzikov, A. B.; Piskarev, V. E.; Yamnikova, S. S.; L'vov, D. K.; Robertson, J. C.; Bovin, N. V.; Matrosovich, M. N. Specification of receptor-binding phenotypes of influenza virus isolates from different hosts using synthetic sialylglycopolymers: Non-egg-adapted human H1 and H3 influenza A, and influenza B viruses share a common high binding affinity for 6′-sialyl(*N*-acetllactosamine). *Virology* **1997**, *232*, 345–350.

10. Rogers, G. N.; D'Souza, B. L. Receptor-binding properties of human and animal H1 influenza virus isolates. *Virology* **1989**, *173*, 317–322.

11. Gambaryan, A. S.; Robertson, J. S.; Matrosovich, M. N. Effects of eggs—Adaptation on the receptor-binding properties of human influenza A and B viruses. *Virology* **1999**, *258*, 232–239.

12. Matrosovich, M. N.; Klenk, H.-D.; Kawaoka, Y. Receptor specificity, host-range, and pathogenicity of influenza viruses. In *Influenza Virology: Current Topics*, Kawaoka, Y., Ed., Caister Academic Press, Wymondham, England, **2006**, pp. 95–137.

13. Gambaryan, A. S.; Matrosovich, M. N. A solid-phase enzyme-linked assay for influenza virus receptor-binding activity. *J. Virol. Methods* **1992**, *39*, 111–123.

14. Gambaryan, A. S.; Boravleva, E. Y.; Matrosovich, T. Y.; Matrosovich, M. N.; Klenk, H. D.; Moiseeva, E. V.; Tuzikov, A. B.; Chinarev, A. A.; Pazynina, G. V.; Bovin, N. V. Polymer-bound 6′ sialyl-*N*-acetyllactosamine protects mice infected by influenza virus. *Antiviral Res.* **2005**, *68*, 116–123.

15. Tuzikov, A. B.; Chinarev, A. A.; Gambaryan, A. S.; Oleinikov, V. A.; Klinov, D. V.; Matsko, N. B.; Kadykov, V. A.; Ermishov, M. A.; Demin, I. V.; Demin, V. V.; Rye, P. D.; Bovin, N. V. Polyglycine II nanosheets: supramolecular antivirals? *ChemBioChem* **2003**, *4*, 147–154.

16. Lehn, J.-M. Perspectives in supramolecular chemistry—From molecular recognition towards molecular information processing and self-organization. *Angew. Chem. Int. Ed. Engl.* **1990**, *29*, 1304–1319.

17. Whitesides, G. M.; Mathias, J. P.; Seto, C. T. Molecular self-assembly and nanochemistry: A chemical strategy for the synthesis of nanostructures. *Science* **1991**, *254*, 1312–1319.

18. Lindsey, J. S. Self-assembly in synthetic routes to molecular devices. Biological principles and chemical perspectives: A review. *New J. Chem.* **1991**, *15*, 153–180.

19. Lawrence, D. S.; Jiang, T.; Levett, M. Self-assembling supramolecular complexes. *Chem. Rev.* **1995**, *95*, 2229–2260.

20. Bamford, C. H.; Brown, L.; Cant, E. M.; Elliott, A.; Hanby, W. E.; Malcolm, B. R. Structure of polyglycine. *Nature* **1955**, *176*, 396.

21. Shimizu, T.; Kogiso, M.; Masuda, M. Noncovalent formation of polyglycine II-type structure by hexagonal self-assembly of linear polymolecular chains. *J. Amer. Chem. Soc.* **1997**, *119*, 6209–6210.

22. Bella, J.; Puiggali, J.; Subirana, J. A. Glycine residues induce a helical structure in polyamides. *Polymer* **1994**, *35*, 1291–1297.

23. Gorokhova, I. V.; Chinarev, A. A.; Tuzikov, A. B.; Tsygankova, S. V.; Bovin, N. V. Spontaneous and promoted association of linear oligoglycines Russ. *J. Bioorg. Chem.* **2006**, *32*, 420–428.

24. Glick, G. D.; Knowles, J. R. Molecular recognition of bivalent sialosides by influenza virus. *J. Am. Chem. Soc.* **1991**, *113*, 4701–4703.

25. Sabesan, S.; Duus, J. F.; Neira S.; Domaille, P.; Kelm, S.; Paulson, J. C.; Bock, K. Cluster sialoside inhibitors for influenza virus: Synthesis, NMR, and biological studies. *J. Am. Chem. Soc.* **1992**, *114*, 8363–8375.

26. Unverzagt, C.; Kelm, S.; Paulson, J. C. Chemical and enzymatic synthesis of multivalent sialoglycopeptides. *Carbohydr. Res.* **1994**, *251*, 285–301.

27. Roy, R. Recent developments in the rational design of multivalent glyco-conjugates. *Topics Curr. Chem.* **1997**, *187*, 241–274.

28. Weis, W.; Brown, J. H.; Cusack, S.; Paulson, J. C.; Skehel, J. J.; Wiley, D. C. *Nature* **1988**, *333*, 426–431.

29. Watowich, S. J.; Skehel, J. J.; Wiley, D. C. Crystal structures of influenza virus hemagglutinin in complex with high-affinity receptor analogs. *Structure* **1994**, *2*, 719–731.

30. Cusack, S.; Ruigrok, R. W. H.; Krygsman P. C. J.; Mellema J. E. Structure and composition of influenza virus. A small-angle neutron scattering study. *J. Mol. Biol.* **1985**, *186*, 565–582.

31. Chinarev, A. A.; Tuzikov, A. B.; Gambaryan, A. S.; Matrosovich, M. N.; Imberty, A.; Bovin, N. V. Tetravalent blockers for influenza virus hemagglutinin. In *Sialobiology and Other Novel Forms of Glycosylation*, Ynoue, Y., Lee, Y. C., Troy, F. A., II, Eds., Gakushin Publishing Co, Osaka, **1999**; pp 135–143.

32. Mochalova, L. V.; Kurova, V. S.; Shtyrya, Y. A.; Korchagina, E. Y.; Gambaryan, A.S. Bovin N. V. Fluorescence assay for evaluation of the substrate specificity kinetics of influenza virus neuraminidase. *Arch. Virol.* **2007**, accepted for publication.

33. Webster, R. G.; Bean, W. J.; Gorman, O. T.; Chambers, T. M.; Kawaoka, Y. Evolution and ecology of influenza A viruses. *Microbiol. Rev.* **1992**, *56*, 152–179.

34. Alexander, D. J. A review of avian influenza in different bird species. *Vet. Microbiol.* **2000**, *74*, 3–13.

35. Horimoto, T.; Kawaoka, Y. Pandemic threat posed by avian influenza A viruses. *Clin. Microbiol. Rev.* **2001**, *14*, 129–149.

36. Suarez, D. L. Evolution of avian influenza viruses. *Vet. Microbiol.* **2000**, *74*, 15–27.

37. Matrosovich, M. N.; Gambaryan, A. S.; Teneberg, S.; Piskarev, V. E.; Yamnikova, S. S.; Lvov, D. K.; Robertson, J. S.; Karlsson, K. A. Avian influenza A viruses differ from human viruses by recognition of sialyloligosaccharides and gangliosides and by a higher conservation of the HA receptor-binding site. *Virology* **1997**, *233*, 224–234.

38. Connor, R. J.; Kawaoka, Y.; Webster, R. G.; Paulson, J. C. Receptor specificity in human, avian, and equine H2 and H3 influenza virus isolates. *Virology* **1994**, *205*, 17–23.

39. Karasin, A. I.; Brown, I. H.; Carman, S.; Olsen, C. W. Isolation and characterization of H4N6 avian influenza viruses from pigs with pneumonia in Canada. *J. Virol.* **2000**, *74*, 9322–9327.

40. Vines, A.; Wells, K.; Matrosovich, M.; Castrucci, M. R.; Ito, T.; Kawaoka, Y. The role of influenza A virus hemagglutinin residues 226 and 228 in receptor specificity and host range restriction. *J.Virol.* **1998**, *72*, 7626–7631.

41. Matrosovich, M.; Tuzikov, A.; Bovin, N.; Gambaryan, A.; Klimov, A.; Castrucci, M. R.; Donatelli, I.; Kawaoka, Y. Early alterations of the receptor-binding properties of H1, H2, and H3 avian influenza virus hemagglutinins after their introduction into mammals. *J. Virol.* **2000**, *74*, 8502–8512.

42. Gambaryan, A. S.; Piskarev, V. E.; Yamskov, I. A.; Tuzikov, A. B.; Bovin, N. V. Nifant`ev, N. E.; Matrosovich, M. N. Human influenza virus recognition of sialyloligosaccharides. *FEBS Lett.* **1995**, *366*, 57–60.

43. Reid, A. H.; Fanning, T. G.; Hultin, J. V.; Taubenberger, J. K. Origin and evolution of the 1918 "Spanish" influenza virus hemagglutinin gene. *Proc. Natl. Acad. Sci. USA* **1999**, *96*, 1651–1656.

44. Reid, A. H. 1918 influenza pandemic caused by highly conserved viruses with two receptor-binding variants. *Emerg. Infect. Dis.* **2003**, *9*, 1249–1253.

45. Glaser, L.; Stevens, J.; Zamarin, D.; Wilson, I. A. García-Sastre, A.; Tumpey, T. M.; Basler, C. F.; Taubenberger, J. K.; Palese, P. A Single amino acid substitution in 1918 influenza virus hemagglutinin changes receptor binding specificity. *J. Virol.* **2005**, *79*, 11533–11536.

46. Stevens, J.; Blixt, O.; Glaser, L.; Taubenberger, J. K.; Palese, P.; Paulson, J. C.; Wilson, I. A. Glycan microarray analysis of the hemagglutinins from modern and pandemic influenza viruses reveals different receptor specificities. *J. Mol. Biol.* **2006**, *355*, 1143–1155.

47. Matrosovich, M.; Krauss, S.; Webster, R. H9N2 influenza A viruses from poultry in Asia have human-virus-like receptor specificity. *Virology* **2001**, *281*, 156–162.

48. Gambaryan, A.; Yamnikova, S.; Lvov, D.; Tuzikov, A.; Chinarev, A.; Pazynina, G.; Webster, R.; Matrosovich, M.; Bovin, N. Receptor specificity of influenza viruses from birds and mammals: New data on involvement of the inner fragments of the carbohydrate chain. *Virology* **2005**, *334*, 276–283.

49. Gambaryan, A. S.; Karasin, A. I.; Tuzikov, A. B.; Chinarev, A. A.; Pazynina, G. V.; Bovin, N. V.; Matrosovich, M. N.; Olsen, C. W.; Klimov, A. I. Receptor-binding properties of swine influenza viruses isolated and propagated in MDCK cells. *Virus Res.* **2005**, *114*, 15–22.

50. Marinina, V. P.; Gambaryan, A. S.; Tuzikov, A. B.; Bovin, N. V.; Fedyakina, I. T.; Yamnikova, S. S.; Lvov, D. K.; Matrosovich, M. N. Evolution of receptor specificity of influenza H1 hemagglutinin during the transmission of duck virus to swine and human. *Vopr. Virusol.* **2004**, *4*, 25–30 (Moscow; in Russian).

51. Gamblin, S. J.; Haire, L. F.; Russell, R. J.; Stevens, D. J.; Xiao, B.; Ha, Y.; Vasisht, N.; Steinhauer, D. A.; Daniels, R. S.; Elliot, A.; Wiley, D. C.; Skehel, J. J. The structure and receptor-binding properties of the 1918 influenza hemagglutinin. *Science.* **2004**, *303*, 1838–1842.

52. Nobusawa, E.; Ishihara, H.; Morishita, T.; Sato, K.; Nakajima, K. Change in receptor-binding specificity of recent human influenza A viruses (H3N2): A single amino acid change in hemagglutinin altered its recognition of sialyloligosaccharides. *Virology* **2000**, *278*, 587–596.

53. Medeiros, R.; Escriou, N.; Naffakh, N.; Manuguerra, J.-C.; van der Werf, S. Hemagglutinin residues of recent human A (H3N2) influenza viruses that contribute to the inability to agglutinate chicken erythrocytes. *Virology* **2001**, *289*, 74–85.

54. Mochalova, L.; Gambaryan, A.; Romanova, J.; Tuzikov, A.; Chinarev, A.; Katinger, D.; Katinger, H.; Egorov, A.; Bovin N. Receptor-binding properties of modern human influenza viruses primarily isolated in Vero and MDCK cells and chicken embryonated eggs. *Virology* **2003**, *313*, 473–480.

55. Saito, T.; Nakaya, Y.; Suzuki, T.; Ito, R.; Saito, T.; Saito, H.; Takao, S.; Sahara, K.; Odagiri, T.; Murata, T.; Usui, T.; Suzuki, Y.; Tashiro, M. Antigenic alteration of influenza B virus associated with loss of a glycosylation site due to host-cell adaptation. *J. Med. Virol.* **2004**, *74*, 336–343.

56. Ito, T.; Suzuki, Y.; Takada, A.; Kawamoto, A.; Otsuki, K.; Masuda, H.; Yamada, M.; Suzuki, T.; Kida, H.; Kawaoka, Y. Differences in sialic acid-

galactose linkages in the chicken egg amnion and allantois influence human influenza virus receptor specificity and variant selection. *J. Virol.* **1997**, *71*, 3357–3362.

57. Ito, T.; Kawaoka, Y. Avian influenza. In *Textbook of Influenza*, Nicholson, K. G., Webster, R. G., Hay, A. J. Eds., Blackwell Science, London, **1998**, pp 126–136.

58. Feldmann, A.; Schafer, M. K.; Garten, W.; Klenk, H.-D. Targeted infection of endothelial cells by avian influenza virus A/FPV/Rostock/34 (H7N1) in chicken embryos. *J. Virol.* **2000**, *74*, 8018–8027.

59. Gambaryan, A. S.; Tuzikov, A. B.; Bovin, N. V.; Yamnikova, S. S.; Lvov, D. K.; Webster, R. G.; Matrosovich, M. N. Differences between influenza virus receptors on target cells of duck and chicken and receptor specificity of the 1997 H5N1 chicken and human influenza viruses from Hong Kong. *Avian Dis.* **2003**, *47* (3 Suppl.), 1154–1160.

60. Gambaryan, A.; Webster, R.; Matrosovich, M. Differences between influenza virus receptors on target cells of duck and chicken. *Arch. Virol.* **2002**, *147*, 1197–1208.

61. Wan, H.; Perez, D. R. Quail carry sialic acid receptors compatible with binding of avian and human influenza viruses. *Virology* **2006**, *346*, 278–286.

62. Gambaryan, A.; Marinina, V.; Solodar, T.; Tuzikov, A.; Pazynina, G.; Bovin, N.; Yamnikova, S.; Lvov, D.; Klimov, A.; Matrosovich, M. Different receptor specificity of influenza viruses from duck and chicken correspond to distinctions in composition of sialosugars on hosts' cells and mucins. *Vopr. Virusol.* **2006**, *4*, 24–32 (Moscow; in Russian).

63. Matrosovich, M. N.; Matrosovich, T. Y.; Gray, T.; Roberts, N. A.; Klenk, H. D. Human and avian influenza viruses target different cell types in cultures of human airway epithelium. *Proc. Natl. Acad. Sci. USA* **2004**, *101*, 4620–4624.

64. Kogure, T.; Suzuki, T.; Takahashi, T.; Miyamoto, D.; Hidari, K. I.; Guo, C. T.; Ito, T.; Kawaoka, Y.; Suzuki, Y. Human trachea primary epithelial cells express both sialyl(alpha2–3)Gal receptor for human parainfluenza virus type 1 and avian influenza viruses, and sialyl(alpha2–6)Gal receptor for human influenza viruses. *Glycoconj. J.* **2006**, *23*, 101–106.

65. Thompson, C. I.; Barclay, W. S.; Zambon, M. C.; Pickles, R. J. Infection of human airway epithelium by human and avian strains of influenza a virus. *J. Virol.* **2006**, *80*, 8060–8068.

66. Shinya, K.; Ebina, M.; Yamada, S.; Ono, M.; Kasai, N.; Kawaoka, Y. Influenza virus receptors in the human airway. *Nature* **2006**, *440*, 435.

67. Maines, T. R.; Chen, L. M.; Matsuoka, Y.; Chen, H.; Rowe, T.; Ortin, J.; Falcon, A.; Hien, N. T.; Mai, L. Q.; Sedyaningsih, E. R.; Harun, S.; Tumpey, T. M.; Donis, R. O.; Cox, N. J.; Subbarao, K.; Katz, J. M. Lack of transmission of H5N1 avian–human reassortant influenza viruses in a ferret model. *Proc. Natl. Acad. Sci. USA* **2006**, *103*, 12121–12126.

68. Eisen, M. B.; Sabesan, S.; Skehel, J. J.; Wiley, D. C. Binding of the influenza A virus to cell-surface receptors: Structures of five hemagglutinin–sialyloligosaccharide complexes determined by X-ray crystallography. *Virology* **1997**, *232*, 19–31.

69. Ha, Y.; Stevens, D. I.; Skehel, J. J.; Wiley, D. C. X-ray structures of H5 Avian and H9 swine hemagglutinins biund to avian and human receptor analogs. *Proc. Natl. Acad. Sci. USA* **2001**, *98*, 11181–11186.

70. Jones, J.C.; Turpin, E.A.; Bultmann, H.; Brandt, C.R.; Schultz-Cherry, S. Inhibition of influenza virus infection by a novel antiviral peptide that targets viral attachment to cells. *J. Virol.* **2006**, *80*, 11960–11967.

71. http://www.cdc.gov/flu/professionals/antiviralback.htm

72. Le, Q. M.; Kiso, M.; Someya, K.; Sakai, Y. T.; Nguyen, T. H.; Nguyen, K. H.; Pham, N. D.; Ngyen, H. H.; Yamada, S.; Muramoto, Y.; Horimoto, T.; Takada, A.; Goto, H.; Suzuki, T.; Suzuki, Y.; Kawaoka, Y. Avian flu: Isolation of drug-resistant H5N1 virus. *Nature* **2005**, *437*, 1108.

73. Hien, T. T.; Liem, N. T.; Dung, N. T.; San, L. T.; Mai, P. P.; Chau, N. v. V.; Suu, P. T.; Dong, V. C.; Mai, L. T. Q.; Thi, N. T.; Khoa, D. B.; Phat, L. P.; Truong, N. T.; Long, H. T.; Tung, C. V.; Giang, L. T.; Tho, N. D.; Nga, L. H.; Tien, N. T. K.; San, L. H.; Tuan, L. V.; Dolecek, C.; Thanh, T. T.; de Jong, M.; Schultsz, C.; Cheng, P.; Lim, W.; Horby, P.; the World Health Organization International Avian influenza Investigative Team; Farrar, J. Avian influenza A (H5N1) in 10 patients in Vietnam. *N. Engl. J. Med.* **2004**, *350*, 1179–1188.

74. von Itzstein, M.; Wu, W.-Y.; Kok, G. B.; Pegg, M. S.; Dyason, J. C.; Jin, B.; Phan, T. V.; Smythe, M. L.; White, H. F.; Oliver, S. W.; Colman, P. M.; Varghese, J. N.; Ryan, D. M.; Woods, J. M.; Bethell, R. C.; Hotham, V. J.; Cameron, J. M.; Penn, C. R. Rational design of potent sialidase-based inhibitors of influenza virus replication. *Nature* **1993**, *363*, 418–423.

75. Potera, C. NexBio takes novel approach to influenza prevention by disrupting receptors in airways. Fludase treatment touted as possible flu stopper. *Genet. Eng. News* **2005**, 25.

9

UNDERSTANDING INFLUENZA NEURAMINIDASE INHIBITORS USING QUANTITATIVE STRUCTURE–ACTIVITY RELATIONSHIP (QSAR) MODELS

RAJESHWAR P. VERMA AND CORWIN HANSCH
Department of Chemistry, Pomona College, Claremont, CA 91711

INTRODUCTION

Influenza is a highly contagious, acute viral respiratory disease that occurs seasonally in most parts of the world. This virus continues to be a major cause of morbidity and mortality worldwide despite the availability of vaccines and antiviral agents. It is responsible for an average of 140,000 hospitalizations and 36,000 deaths annually in the United States alone, and the problem is increasing due to the aging population and the susceptibility of the elderly. Thus, influenza is regarded as a virus of enormous public health importance.[1,2] Vaccination remains the primary method for prevention of influenza, but vaccine strains must be continually updated and also their protective efficacy is limited in patients over 65 years of age, who are the major target group.[3] The alternative to the vaccination lies in antiviral drugs.

The unique replication mechanism of influenza virus has allowed investigators to identify a number of potential molecular targets for

Combating the Threat of Pandemic Influenza: Drug Discovery Approaches,
Edited by Paul F. Torrence

drug design; these include hemagglutinin, neuraminidase, M2 protein, and endonuclease. Hemagglutinin (HA) and neuraminidase (NA) are the two major surface glycoproteins of influenza A and B viruses. HA is known to mediate binding of viruses to target cells via terminal sialic acid residue in glycoconjugates. In contrast to HA activity, NA cleaves terminal sialic acids from glycoproteins and glycolipids and it is critical for viral replication.[4] Thus, the discovery of NA inhibitors for the treatment of influenza infection has been an active area of research.

Four drugs are available to treat and/or prevent influenza. They are amantadine, rimantadine, zanamivir, and oseltamivir. Amantadine and rimantadine were the first anti-influenza drugs and block the ion channel of virus protein M2. They are effective only against type A influenza viruses and cause many side effects.[5] Two other drugs (zanamivir and oseltamivir) that inhibit both influenza A and B viruses are neuraminidase inhibitors and have recently been approved by FDA for the treatment and prevention of influenza.[6] Zanamivir is administered by oral inhalation due to high polar compounds, and oseltamivir is a prodrug that is converted (after oral intake) to its active form of the carboxylic acid (GS 4071) (Fig. 9.1). None of the four drugs has been shown to effectively prevent serious influenza-related complications such as bacterial or viral pneumonia. When either amantadine or rimantadine is used for therapy, drug-resistant flu viruses may appear in about one-third of patients. Laboratory studies have shown that influenza A and B viruses can develop resistance to zanamivir and oseltamivir. Thus, there is an urgent need for the development of newer NA inhibitors as anti-influenza drugs. More recently, we developed and published 17 QSAR models on various compound series for the inhibition of influenza A and B neuraminidase. Results from that study suggest that the

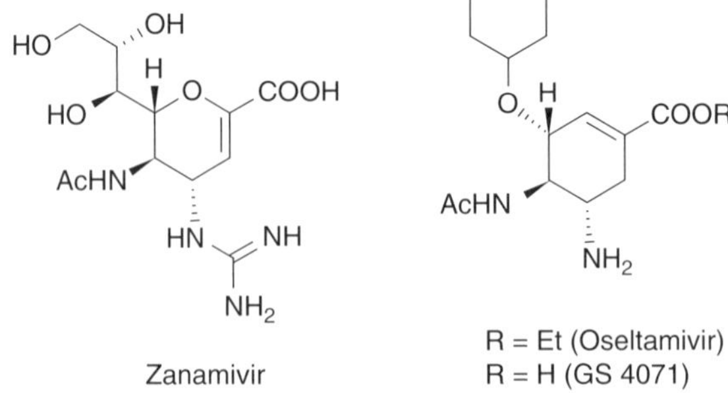

Fig. 9.1. Inhibitors of influenza A and B virus neuraminidase.

inhibitory activity of the neuraminidase inhibitors is mainly dependent on their hydrophobicity, which is one of the most important determinants of the activity.[7] In the present chapter, we describe the QSAR studies on carbocyclic compounds as influenza neuraminidase inhibitors to understand the chemical–biological interactions.

In the past 44 years, the use of QSAR, since the advent of this methodology,[8] has become increasingly helpful to understand many aspects of chemical–biological interactions in drug-design process and pesticide research as well as in the areas of toxicology. It is useful in elucidating the mechanisms of chemical–biological interactions in various biomolecules, particularly enzymes, membranes, organelles, cells, and human.[9–11] It has also been utilized for the evaluation of absorption, distribution, metabolism, and excretion (ADME) phenomena in many organisms and whole-animal studies.[12] The QSAR approach employs extra-thermodynamically derived and computational-based descriptors to correlate biological activity in isolated receptors, in cellular systems, and *in vivo*. Four standard molecular descriptors are routinely used in QSAR analysis: electronic, hydrophobic, steric, and topological indices. These descriptors are invaluable in helping to delineate a large number of receptor–ligand interactions that are critical to biological processes.[9] The quality of a QSAR model depends strictly on the type and quality of the data, and not on the hypotheses, and is valid only for the compound structure analogues to those used to build the model. QSAR models can stand alone, augment other computational approaches, or be examined in tandem with equations of a similar mechanistic genre to establish the authenticity and reliability.[13] Potential use of QSAR models for screening of chemical databases or virtual libraries before their synthesis appears equally attractive to chemical manufacturers, pharmaceutical companies, and government agencies.

MATERIALS AND METHODS

All the data used in this chapter have been collected from the literature (see individual QSAR for respective references). C is the molar concentration of a compound and $\log 1/C$ is the dependent variable that defines the biological parameter for QSAR equations. Physicochemical descriptors are auto-loaded, and multi-regression analyses (MRA) used to derive the QSAR are executed with the C-QSAR program.[14] The parameters used in this chapter have already been discussed in detail along with their application.[9] Briefly, $C \log P$ is the calculated partition coefficient in n-octanol/water and is a measure of hydrophobicity, and π is the hydrophobic parameter for the substituents. CMR is the calculated molar refractivity for the whole molecule. MR is calculated from the Lorentz–Lorenz equation and is described as follows: $(n^2 - 1/n^2 + 2)(\text{MW}/\rho)$, where n is the refractive index, MW is the molecular weight, and ρ is the density of a substance. MR is dependent on volume and polarizability. It can be used for a substituent or for the whole molecule. MR is thus a means of characterizing the bulk and polarizability of a substituent/compound. Although it contains no information about the shape, it has found considerable usage in biological QSAR where intermolecular effects predominate. MR is usually scaled at 0.1 to make it equiscalar with π. The indicator variable I is assigned the value of 1 or 0 for special features with special effects that cannot be parameterized and has been explained wherever used. Each regression equation includes 95% confidence limits for each term in parentheses.

In QSAR equations, n is the number of data points, r is the correlation coefficient between observed values of the dependent and the values calculated from the equation, r^2 is the square of the correlation coefficient represents the goodness of fit, q^2 is the cross-validated r^2 (a measure of the quality of the QSAR model), and s is the standard deviation. The cross-validated r^2 (q^2) is obtained by using the leave-one-out (LOO) procedure.[15] Q is the quality factor (quality ratio), where $Q = r/s$. Chance correlation, due to the excessive number of parameter (which increases the r and s values also), can, thus, be detected by the examination of Q value. F is the Fischer statistics (Fischer ratio), $F = fr^2/[(1 - r^2)m]$, where f is the number of degree of freedom, $f = n - (m + 1)$, n = number of data points, and m = number of variables. The modeling was taken to be optimal when Q reached a maximum together with F, even if slightly nonoptimal F values have normally been accepted. A significant decrease in F with the introduction of one additional variable (with increasing Q and decreasing s) could mean that the new descriptor is not as good as expected; that is, its introduction has endangered the statistical quality of the combination. However, the statistical quality could be improved by the introduction of a more convincing descriptor.[16–18] Compounds were assigned to be outliers on the basis of their deviation between observed and calculated activities from the equation ($>2s$).[19–21] Each regression equation includes 95% confidence limits for each term in parentheses. For a list of outliers in both data sets, refer to Table 9.1. Both the QSAR (**1** and **2**) reported here are derived by us and were not formulated by the original authors.

TABLE 9.1. Biological , Physicochemical, and Structural Parameters Used to Derive QSAR Eqs. (1) and (2) for the Inhibition of Carbocyclic Derivatives (I) to Influenza A Neuraminidase and Influenza B Neuraminidase

No.	R	$\log 1/C$ [Eq. (1)]			$\log 1/C$ [Eq. (2)]			$C\pi$-R	CMR-R	I_1	I_2
		Observed	Predicted	Δ	Observed	Predicted	Δ				
1		6.00	6.07	−0.07	7.00	6.62	0.38	0.21	1.67	0	0
2		6.51	6.50	0.01	7.52	7.21	0.31	0.77	2.14	0	0
3		7.60	6.84	0.76	8.40	7.56	0.84	1.32	2.60	0	0
4		7.46	7.08	0.38	8.15	7.68	0.47	1.88	3.06	0	0
5		7.59	7.24	0.35	7.85	7.57	0.28	2.44	3.53	0	0
6		7.12	7.31	−0.19	7.39	7.23	0.16	3.00	3.99	0	0
7[a]		6.58	7.28	−0.70	6.05	7.66	−1.61	2.17	3.53	0	0

TABLE 9.1. (*Continued*)

No.	R	log 1/C [Eq. (1)]			log 1/C [Eq. (2)]			Cπ-R	CMR-R	I_1	I_2
		Observed	Predicted	Δ	Observed	Predicted	Δ				
8[a]		6.59	6.32	0.27	7.52	6.50	1.02	0.11	2.29	0	0
9		5.72	6.11	−0.39	4.64	5.02	−0.38	−0.78	2.97	0	0
10		7.29	7.09	0.20	7.19	7.67	−0.48	1.71	3.06	0	0
11		7.28	7.27	0.01	7.21	7.64	−0.43	2.24	3.53	0	0
12		7.40	7.38	0.02	7.06	7.40	−0.34	2.77	3.99	0	0
13		7.49	7.22	0.27	7.52	7.66	−0.14	1.64	3.35	0	0
14		8.10	7.35	0.75	7.85	7.55	0.30	1.30	3.68	0	0

No.	R	log 1/C [Eq. (1)]			log 1/C [Eq. (2)]			Cπ-R	CMR-R	I_1	I_2
		Observed	Predicted	Δ	Observed	Predicted	Δ				
15	OH	5.20	5.44	−0.24	ND	6.79	ND	0.35	0.24	0	0
16	OCH$_3$	5.43	5.73	−0.30	ND	6.97	ND	0.51	0.71	0	0
17	OCH$_2$CH$_3$	5.70	6.07	−0.37	6.73	7.32	−0.59	0.90	1.17	0	0
18	OCH$_2$CH$_2$CH$_3$	6.74	6.38	0.36	ND	7.60	ND	1.43	1.63	0	0
19[a]	O(CH$_2$)$_3$CH$_3$	6.52	6.62	−0.10	6.67	7.68	−1.01	1.96	2.10	0	0
20	O(CH$_2$)$_4$CH$_3$	6.70	6.77	−0.07	ND	7.55	ND	2.49	2.56	0	0
21[a]	O(CH$_2$)$_5$CH$_3$	6.82	6.84	−0.02	5.84	7.22	−1.38	3.02	3.02	0	0
22	O(CH$_2$)$_6$CH$_3$	6.57	6.83	−0.26	ND	6.67	ND	3.55	3.49	0	0
23	O(CH$_2$)$_7$CH$_3$	6.74	6.74	0.00	5.46	5.92	−0.46	4.07	3.95	0	0
24	O(CH$_2$)$_8$CH$_3$	6.68	6.57	0.11	ND	4.96	ND	4.60	4.42	0	0
25	O(CH$_2$)$_9$CH$_3$	6.22	6.31	−0.09	ND	3.79	ND	5.13	4.88	0	0
26[b]	OCH$_2$CH(CH$_3$)$_2$	6.70	8.35	−1.65	ND	8.28	ND	1.83	2.10	0	1
27	OCH(CH$_3$)CH$_2$CH$_3$[R]	8.00	8.36	−0.36	8.15	8.27	−0.12	1.74	2.10	0	1
28	OCH(CH$_3$)CH$_2$CH$_3$[S]	8.05	8.36	−0.31	8.70	8.27	0.43	1.74	2.10	0	1
29	OCH(CH$_2$CH$_3$)$_2$	9.00	8.54	0.46	8.52	8.23	0.29	2.27	2.56	0	1
30		9.00	8.74	0.26	8.52	8.22	0.30	2.31	3.00	0	1
31		8.52	8.74	−0.22	7.62	8.22	−0.60	2.31	3.00	0	1
32[a]		9.00	8.25	0.75	8.40	4.90	3.50	4.91	4.88	0	1

TABLE 9.1. (*Continued*)

No.	R	log 1/C [Eq. (1)]			log 1/C [Eq. (2)]			Cπ-R	CMR-R	I_1	I_2
		Observed	Predicted	Δ	Observed	Predicted	Δ				
33		7.22	6.92	0.30	6.92	7.59	−0.67	2.40	2.85	0	0
34		7.80	8.61	−0.81	5.19	5.97	−0.78	4.39	4.70	0	1
35		9.00	8.39	0.61	5.67	4.89	0.78	4.92	5.17	0	1
36		6.28	6.92	−0.64	ND	7.67	ND	2.06	2.75	0	0
37		6.21	7.14	−0.93	ND	7.66	ND	2.17	3.22	0	0
38		9.52	9.25	0.27	7.15	7.09	0.06	3.69	5.07	0	1
39[b]		7.92	9.25	−1.33	7.46	7.09	0.37	3.69	5.07	0	1

TABLE 9.1. (*Continued*)

No.	R	log 1/C [Eq. (1)]			log 1/C [Eq. (2)]			Cπ-R	CMR-R	I_1	I_2
		Observed	Predicted	Δ	Observed	Predicted	Δ				
40		7.05	7.53	−0.48	ND	4.69	ND	4.74	6.66	0	0
41	N(CH$_3$)CH$_2$CH$_2$CH$_3$	7.19	7.11	0.08	7.19	7.16	0.03	1.89	2.31	1	1
42	N(CH$_3$)CH$_2$CH$_2$CH$_2$CH$_3$	6.74	7.27	−0.53	ND	7.06	ND	2.42	2.78	1	1
43	N(CH$_3$)CH(CH$_2$CH$_3$)$_2$	8.22	7.42	0.80	7.22	6.91	0.31	2.73	3.24	1	1
44	N(CH$_3$)CH$_2$CH$_2$C$_6$H$_5$	7.00	7.90	−0.90	6.25	6.77	−0.52	2.93	4.36	1	1
45	N(CH$_3$)-cy-C$_6$H$_{11}$	6.70	7.52	−0.82	ND	6.82	ND	2.86	3.53	1	1
46	N(CH$_2$CH$_3$)CH$_2$CH$_2$CH$_3$	7.05	7.27	−0.22	ND	7.06	ND	2.42	2.78	1	1
47	N(CH$_2$CH$_3$)CH$_2$CH$_2$CH$_2$CH$_3$	7.07	7.35	−0.28	6.76	6.75	0.01	2.95	3.24	1	1
48	N(CH$_2$CH$_2$CH$_3$)CH$_2$CH$_2$CH$_3$	7.92	7.35	0.57	7.22	6.75	0.47	2.95	3.24	1	1
49[b]	NHCH$_2$CH$_2$CH$_3$	6.70	5.12	1.58	6.62	6.41	0.21	1.25	1.85	1	0
50	NHCH(CH$_2$CH$_3$)$_2$	7.96	7.32	0.64	7.00	7.15	−0.15	2.09	2.78	1	1
51	NHCOCH$_2$CH$_3$	5.57	4.91	0.66	6.30	5.76	0.54	0.42	1.88	1	0
52[b]	NHCOCH(CH$_3$)$_2$	5.19	6.97	−1.78	5.77	6.66	−0.89	0.73	2.35	1	1
53[a,b]	NHCOCH(CH$_2$CH$_3$)$_2$	5.40	7.57	−2.17	5.49	7.16	−1.67	1.79	3.28	1	1
54	OCH$_2$OCH$_3$	5.70	5.93	−0.23	ND	6.70	ND	0.27	1.32	0	0
55	OCH$_2$CH$_2$CF$_3$	6.65	6.37	0.28	ND	7.47	ND	1.14	1.68	0	0
56	OCH$_2$CH=CH$_2$	5.66	6.33	−0.67	ND	7.48	ND	1.15	1.61	0	0
57	O-cy-C$_5$H$_9$	7.66	6.76	0.90	ND	7.68	ND	1.84	2.38	0	1
58	SCH$_2$CH$_2$CH$_3$	6.67	6.71	−0.04	ND	7.68	ND	1.99	2.29	0	0
59	(CH$_2$)$_3$CH$_3$	6.66	6.50	0.16	ND	7.61	ND	2.33	1.94	0	0

[b] Not used to derive Eq. (1).
[a] Not used to derive Eq. (2).
ND, Not determined.

RESULTS AND DISCUSSION

Inhibition of Influenza A Neuraminidase by Carbocyclic Derivatives (I)

Combined data of Lew et al. (Table 9.1)[22–26]:

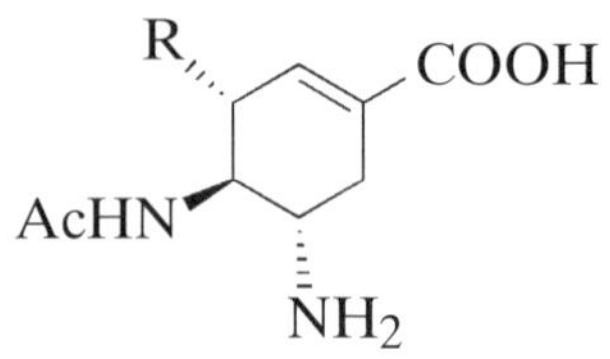

I

From the combined data in Table 9.1, we developed Eq. (1):

$$\log 1/C = 0.51(\pm 0.32)\text{C}\pi\text{-R} - 0.15(\pm 0.06)(\text{C}\pi\text{-R})^2 + 0.48(\pm 0.21)\,\text{CMR-R} - 1.35(\pm 0.44)I_1 + 1.73(\pm 0.38)I_2 + 5.17(\pm 0.50) \quad (1)$$

$n = 54$, $r^2 = 0.777$, $s = 0.494$, $q^2 = 0.709$, $Q = 1.785$, $F_{5,48} = 33.449$ optimum $\text{C}\pi\text{-R} = 1.76(0.95\text{–}2.43)$

This is a parabolic correlation in terms of Cπ-R (calculated hydrophobicity of R-groups) followed by linearly related to CMR-R (calculated molar refractivity of R-groups) and two indicator variables, which suggests that the inhibitory activity of carbocyclic derivatives (**I**) to influenza A neuraminidase first increases with an increase in hydrophobicity of the R-groups up to an optimum Cπ-R of 1.76 and then decreases. The positive coefficient of CMR-R (+0.48) suggests that the R-substituents having high molar refractivity/polarizability may improve the activity. Indicator variable $I_1 = 1$ and 0 is for the presence and absence of substituted amine groups at the R-position. Similarly, $I_2 = 1$ and 0 is for the presence and absence of branched alkoxy groups at the R-position. The negative coefficient of I_1 (−1.35) suggests that the absence of substituted amine groups at the R-position will enhance the inhibitory activity of carbocyclic derivatives (**I**) to influenza A neuraminidase. In contrast, the positive coefficient of I_2 (+1.73) suggests that the presence of the branched alkoxy groups at the R-position will increase the inhibitory activity. Thus, one should increase the inhibitory activity of carbocyclic derivatives (**I**) to influenza A neuraminidase by boosting the molar refractivity of R-groups and preserving R = branched alkoxy groups with Cπ-R ≈ 1.76.

Inhibition of Influenza B Neuraminidase by Carbocyclic Derivatives (I)

From the combined data of Lew et al. (Table 9.1)[22–24], we developed Eq. (2):

$$\log 1/C = 1.41(\pm 0.40)C\pi\text{-}R - 0.37(\pm 0.09)(C\pi\text{-}R)^2 - 1.12(\pm 0.45)I_1$$
$$+ 0.60(\pm 0.44)I_2 + 6.35(\pm 0.46) \tag{2}$$

$$n = 33, \qquad r^2 = 0.776, \qquad s = 0.496, \qquad q^2 = 0.638, \qquad Q = 1.776,$$
$$F_{4,28} = 24.250 \qquad \text{optimum } C\pi\text{-}R = 1.90(1.64-2.13)$$

All parameters used in this equation have the same meanings as described for Eq. (1). Equation (2) is very similar to the Eq. (1) and their optimum value for $C\pi$-R is also very close. This result is supported by the well-established fact that the neuraminidase inhibitors inhibit both influenza A and B viruses. The absence of the CMR-R term is not very clear. It may be due to the presence of the smaller data set (20 less compounds) than that of Eq. (1).

QSAR MODEL VALIDATION

QSAR model validation is an essential task to develop a statistically valid and predictive model, because the real utility of a QSAR model is in its ability to predict accurately the modeled property for new compounds. The following approaches have been used for the validation of QSAR (1) and (2):

- *Fraction of the Variance*: It is important to note that a QSAR model must have to explain a sufficiently high fraction of the variance for any data set. The fraction of the variance of an MRA model is expressed by r^2 (measure of the goodness of fit between model-predicted and experimental values). It is believed that the closer the value of r^2 to unity, the better the QSAR model. The values of r^2 for QSAR models (1) and (2) are 0.777 and 0.776, which suggests that these two QSAR models explain more than 77% of the variance of the data. According to the literature, the predictive QSAR model must have $r^2 > 0.6$.[27,28]
- *Cross-Validation Test*: The values of q^2 for QSAR models (1) and (2) are 0.709 and 0.638. The high values of q^2 validate these QSAR models. In the literature, it must be greater than 0.50.[27,28]

- *Standard Deviation (s)*: s is the standard deviation about the regression line. This is a measure of how well the function derived by the QSAR analysis predicts the observed biological activity. The smaller the value of s, the better the QSAR model. The value of s for QSAR models (1) and (2) are 0.494 and 0.496.

- *Quality Factor or Quality Ratio (Q)*: Chance correlation, due to the excessive number of parameter (which increases also the r and s values), is detected by the examination of Q value.[16–18] The high values of Q (1.785 and 1.776) for QSAR models (1) and (2) suggest that the high predictive powers of these QSAR models and also no overfitting.

- *Fischer Statistics (F)*: Fischer statistics (F) is a value derived from the F-test indicating the probability of a true relationship, or the significance level of the MLR model. The F-value is the ratio between explained and unexplained variance for a given number of degree of freedom. The larger the F-value, the greater the probability that the QSAR equation is significant. The F-values obtained for QSAR models (1) and (2) are 33.449 and 24.250, which are statistically significant at the 95% level.

- Both the QSAR models also fulfill the thumb rule condition, which is (number of data points)/(number of descriptors)≥ 4.

NEW MOLECULE PREDICTION

Both Eq. (1) and (2) are parabolic correlations in term of hydrophobic parameter of the R-substituents, where the optimum hydrophobicity of the R-substituents (1.76 and 1.90) is well-defined. We believe that these equations may be the predictive models to narrow the synthetic challenges in order to yield very specific neuraminidase inhibitors. On the basis of these models and keeping R = branched alkoxy groups having $C\pi$-R = 1.76–1.90, we can predict at least one compound (**II**) that may be the next synthetic target.

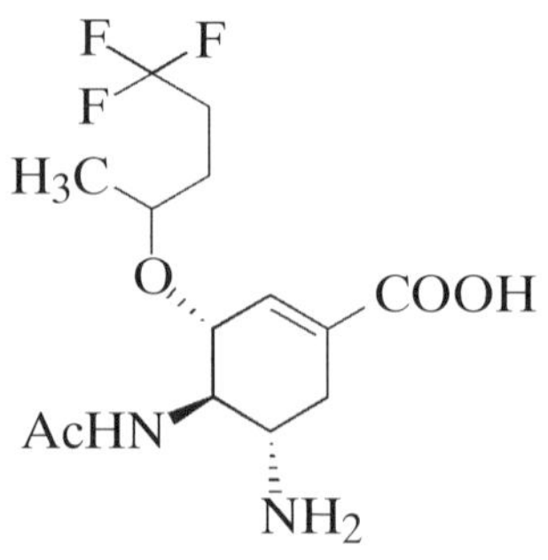

II

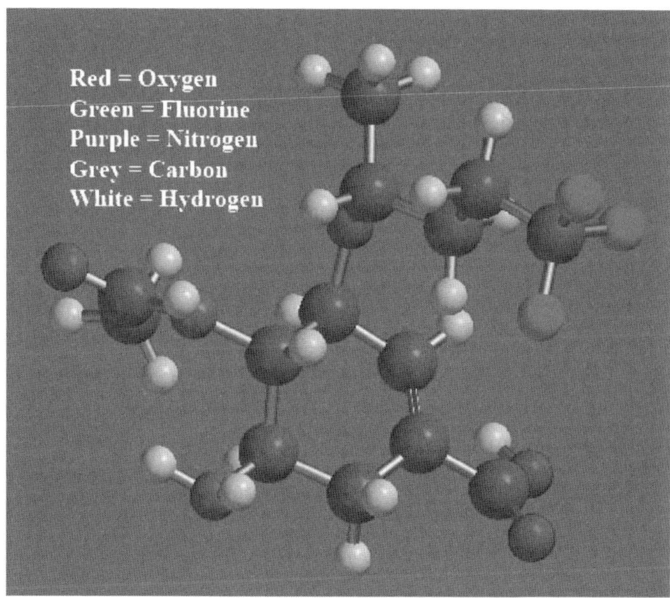

Fig. 9.2. The minimized energy geometry of compound (**II**) obtained from Spartan '06. See color insert.

The predicted log $1/C$ of compound (**II**) for the inhibition of influenza A neuraminidase and influenza B neuraminidase are 8.60 and 8.27, respectively, which are obtained from QSAR models **1** and **2**. The other parameters for this compound (**II**) are $C \log P = -1.72$, $C\pi$-$R = 1.78$, and CMR-$R = 2.61$. The minimized energy geometry of the compound (**II**) is shown in Fig. 9.2, which is obtained from the Spartan '06 program,[29] and used to calculate the following: minimized energy = 100.8982 kJ/mol, area = 343.14 Å^2, polar surface area (PSA) = 89.234 Å^2, volume = 312.35 Å^3, and molecular weight = 338.326 amu. It is interesting to note that the proposed molecule (**II**) fulfills all conditions of the "rule of five."

In the process of drug discovery and development, the estimation of molecular transport properties, particularly intestinal absorption and blood–brain barrier penetration, is one of the important key factors. Traditionally, calculated values of n-octanol/water partition coefficient have been used for this purpose.[30] A set of rules, which imposes the limitations on $\log P$, molecular weight, and the number of hydrogen bond donors and acceptors, is known as "rule of five" and was introduced by Lipinski et al.[31] According to Lipinski's "rule of five," drug-like molecules should have $\log P \leq 5$, molecular weight ≤ 500, number of hydrogen bond acceptors (expressed as the sum of Ns and Os) ≤ 10, and number of hydrogen bond donors (expressed as the sum of OHs and NHs) $\leq$ 5. Molecules violating more than one of these rules may have problems with bioavailability. As an alternative to Lipinski rules, polar surface area or VolSurf parameters can be used to predict oral absorption and blood–brain barrier penetration.[32] The polar surface area (PSA) of a molecule is a good parameter to predict compound (passive) absorption into the body. It is defined as the surface area of nitrogen and oxygen atoms in a molecule plus the surface of the hydrogen attached to these hetero-atoms. This has been established that a PSA value of over $140\,\text{Å}^2$ generally yields molecules that are poorly absorbed from the stomach and gastrointestinal tract.[33] Thus, the robust method of computationally screening large numbers of compounds prior to synthesis is to always keep the value of PSA $< 140\,\text{Å}^2$. Our predicted compound (**II**) has the PSA value $89.234\,\text{Å}^2$.

CONCLUSION

In this chapter, we developed two QSAR models [Eqs. (**1**) and (**2**)] on carbocyclic derivatives (**I**) for their inhibitory activities to influenza A and influenza B neuraminidase and found the importance of R-substituents. The data were collected from the five publications of Lew et al.[22–26] Both QSAR models are parabolic correlations in terms of the hydrophobic parameter of the R-substituents and very encouraging examples, where the optimum hydrophobicity of the R-substituents (1.76 and 1.90) is well-defined. We believe that these equations may be the predictive models to narrow the synthetic challenges in order to yield very specific neuraminidase inhibitors. On the basis of these models, we can predict at least one compound (**II**) that may be the next synthetic target. It is interesting to note that the proposed molecule (**II**) fulfills all the conditions of Lipinski's "rule of five." The PSA value of this compound (PSA $= 89.234\,\text{Å}^2$) is less than $140\,\text{Å}^2$, suggesting its ability to absorbed easily from the stomach and the gastrointestinal tract.

REFERENCES

1. Thompson, W. W.; Shay, D. K.; Weintraub, E.; Brammer, L.; Cox, N.; Anderson, L. J.; Fukuda, K. Mortality associated with influenza and respiratory syncytial virus in the United States. *J. Am. Med. Assoc.* **2003**, *289*, 179–186.

2. Carey, M. A.; Bradbury, J. A.; Seubert, J. M.; Langenbach, R.; Zeldin, D. C.; Germolec, D. R. Contrasting effects of cyclooxygenase-1 (COX-1) and COX-2 deficiency on the host response to influenza A viral infection. *J. Immunol.* **2005**, *175*, 6878–6884.

3. Nicholson, K. G.; Wood, J. M.; Zambon, M. Influenza. *Lancet* **2003**, *362*, 1733–1745.

4. Kim, C. U.; Lew, W.; Williams, M. A.; Zhang, L.; Liu, H.; Swaminathan, S.; Bischofberger, N.; Chen, M. S.; Tai, C. Y.; Mendel, D. B.; Laver, W. G.; Stevens, R. C. Influenza neuraminidase inhibitors possessing a novel hydrophobic interaction in the enzyme active site: design, synthesis, and structural analysis of carbocyclic sialic acid analogs with potent anti-influenza activity. *J. Am. Chem. Soc.* **1997**, *119*, 681–690.

5. Smith, P. W.; Sollis, S. L.; Howes, P. D.; Cherry, P. C.; Starkey, I. D.; Cobley, K. N.; Weston, H.; Scicinski, J.; Merritt, A.; Whittington, A.; Wyatt, P.; Taylor, N.; Green, D.; Bethell, R.; Madar, S.; Fenton, R. J.; Morley, P. J.; Pateman, T.; Beresford, A. Dihydropyrancarboxamides related to zanamivir: a new series of inhibitors of influenza virus sialidases. 1. Discovery, synthesis, biological activity, and structure–activity relationships of 4-guanidino- and 4-amino-4*H*-pyran-6-carboxamides. *J. Med. Chem.* **1998**, *41*, 787–797.

6. Chand, P.; Babu, Y. S.; Bantia, S.; Rowland, S.; Dehghani, A.; Kotian, P. L.; Hutchison, T. L.; Ali, S.; Brouillette, W.; El-Kattan, Y.; Lin, T.-H. Syntheses and neuraminidase inhibitory activity of multisubstituted cyclopentane amide derivatives. *J. Med. Chem.* **2004**, *47*, 1919–1929.

7. Verma, R. P.; Hansch, C. A QSAR study on influenza neuraminidase inhibitors. *Bioorg. Med. Chem.* **2006**, *14*, 982–996.

8. Hansch, C.; Maloney, P. P.; Fujita, T.; Muir, R. M. Correlation of biological activity of phenoxyacetic acids with Hammett substituent constants and partition coefficients. *Nature* **1962**, *194*, 178–180.

9. Hansch, C.; Leo, A. In *Exploring QSAR: Fundamentals and Applications in Chemistry and Biology, American Chemical Society*, Washington, D.C., 1995.

10. Selassie, C. D.; Garg, R.; Kapur, S.; Kurup, A.; Verma, R. P.; Mekapati, S. B.; Hansch, C. Comparative QSAR and the radical toxicity of various functional groups. *Chem. Rev.* **2002**, *102*, 2585–2605.

11. Verma, R. P.; Kurup, A.; Mekapati, S. B.; Hansch, C. Chemical–biological interactions in human. *Bioorg. Med. Chem.* **2005**, *13*, 933–948.

12. Hansch, C.; Leo, A.; Mekapati, S. B.; Kurup, A. QSAR and ADME. *Bioorg. Med. Chem.* **2004**, *12*, 3391–3400.

13. Selassie, C. D.; Mekapati, S. B.; Verma, R. P. QSAR: Then and now. *Curr. Top. Med. Chem.* **2002**, 2, 1357–1379.

14. C-QSAR Program, BioByte Corp., 201 W. 4th Street, Suite 204, Claremont, CA 91711, USA, www.biobyte.com.

15. Cramer, R. D., III; Bunce, J. D.; Patterson, D. E.; Frank, I. E. Cross validation, Bootstrapping and partial least squares compared with multiple regression in conventional QSAR studies. *Quant. Struct. –Act. Relat.* **1988**, *7*, 18–25.

16. Pogliani, L. Modeling with special descriptors derived from a medium-sized set of connectivity indices. *J. Phys. Chem.* **1996**, *100*, 18065–18077.

17. Pogliani, L. From molecular connectivity indices to semiempirical connectivity terms: Recent trends in graph theoretical descriptors. *Chem. Rev.* **2000**, *100*, 3827–3858.

18. Agrawal, V.; Singh, J.; Khadikar, P. V.; Supuran, C. T. QSAR study on topically acting sulfonamides incorporating GABA moieties: A molecular connectivity approach. *Bioorg. Med. Chem. Lett.* **2006**, *16*, 2044–2051.

19. Selassie, C. D.; Kapur, S.; Verma, R. P.; Rosario, M. Cellular apoptosis and cytotoxicity of phenolic compounds: a quantitative structure–activity relationship study. *J. Med. Chem.* **2005**, *48*, 7234–7242.

20. Verma, R. P.; Hansch, C. Cytotoxicity of organic compounds against ovarian cancer cells: A quantitative structure–activity relationship study. *Mol. Pharm.* **2006**, *3*, 441–450.

21. Verma, R. P.; Hansch, C. Understanding human rhinovirus infections in terms of QSAR. *Virology* **2007**, *359*, 152–161.

22. Lew, W.; Wu, H.; Chen, X.; Graves, B. J.; Escarpe, P. A.; MacArthur, H. L.; Mendel, D. B.; Kim, C. U. Carbocyclic influenza neuraminidase inhibitors possessing a C_3-cyclic amine side chain: Synthesis and inhibitory activity. *Bioorg. Med. Chem. Lett.* **2000**, *10*, 1257–1260.

23. Kim, C. U.; Lew, W.; Williams, M. A.; Wu, H.; Zhang, L.; Chen, X.; Escarpe, P. A.; Mendel, D. B.; Laver, W. G.; Stevens, R. C. Structure–activity relationship studies of novel carbocyclic influenza neuraminidase inhibitors. *J. Med. Chem.* **1998**, *41*, 2451–2460.

24. Lew, W.; Wu, H.; Mendel, D. B.; Escarpe, P. A.; Chen, X.; Laver, W. G.; Graves, B. J.; Kim, C. U. A new series of C_3-aza carbocyclic influenza neuraminidase inhibitors: Synthesis and inhibitory activity. *Bioorg. Med. Chem. Lett.* **1998**, *8*, 3321–3324.

25. Williams, M. A.; Lew, W.; Mendel, D. B.; Tai, C. Y.; Escarpe, P. A.; Laver, W. G.; Stevens, R. C.; Kim, C. U. Structure–activity relationships of carbocyclic influenza neuraminidase inhibitors. *Bioorg. Med. Chem. Lett.* **1997**, *7*, 1837–1842.

26. Lew, W; Williams, M. A.; Mendel, D. B.; Escarpe, P. A., Kim, C. U. C_3-thia and C_3-carba isosteres of a carbocyclic influenza neuraminidase inhibitor, (3*R*, 4*R*, 5*S*)-4-acetamido-5-amino-3-propoxy-1-cyclohexene-1-carboxylic acid. *Bioorg. Med. Chem. Lett.* **1997**, *7*, 1843–1846.

27. Golbraikh, A.; Tropsha, A. Beware of q^2! *J. Mol. Graph. Modl.* **2002**, *20*, 269–276.

28. Tropsha, A.; Gramatica, P.; Gombar, V. K. The importance of being earnest: Validation is the absolute essential for successful application and interpretation of QSPR models. *QSAR Comb. Sci.* **2003**, *22*, 69–77.

29. Spartan'06 Program, Wavefunction, Inc., 18401 Von Karman Avenue, Suite 370, Irvine, CA 92612, USA. www.wavefun.com.

30. Freitas, M. P. MIA-QSAR modelling of anti-HIV-1 acvtivities of some 2-amino-6-arylsulfonylbenzonitriles and their thio and sulfinyl congeners. *Org. Biomol. Chem.* **2006**, *4*, 1154–1159.

31. Lipinski, C. A.; Lombardo, F.; Dominy, B. W.; Feeney, P. J. Experimental and computational approaches to estimate solubility and permeability in drug discovery and development settings. *Adv. Drug. Delivery Rev.* **1997**, *23*, 3–25.

32. Kubinyi, H. Drug research: Myths, hype and reality. *Nature Rev.* **2003**, *2*, 665–668.

33. Clark, D. E. Rapid calculation of polar molecular surface area and its application to the prediction of transport phenomena. 1. Prediction of intestinal absorption. *J. Pharm. Sci.* **1999**, *88*, 807–814.

10

PEPTIDE INHIBITORS TARGETING VIRUS-CELL FUSION IN CLASS I ENVELOPED VIRUSES

GEORGE F. GAO

Center for Molecular Immunology and Center for Molecular Virology, Institute of Microbiology, Chinese Academy of Sciences, Datunlu, Beijing 100101, The People's Republic of China

INTRODUCTION

Viruses can be divided into two groups in terms of their surface architectures: (a) enveloped viruses that have an envelope derived from the double-layered lipid cell membrane with virus envelope proteins protruding into it and (b) non-enveloped viruses that do not have a envelope, with only a viral protein core.[1] Infection of virus starts from virus entry into the host cells to deliver its genome for replication and new virus assembly.[1] In enveloped viruses, the virus entry works by virus-cell membrane fusion, which takes place either in the cell-surface membrane (e.g., human immunodeficiency virus, HIV, takes this way)[1,2] or in the endosome inside the cell after the virus is taken into the cells through endocytosis (e.g., influenza virus goes through this way).[3,4]

Virus-cell fusion is mediated by protein–protein or protein–ligand (non-protein molecules) interaction in the interface of virus and cell.[4,5]

Combating the Threat of Pandemic Influenza: Drug Discovery Approaches,
Edited by Paul F. Torrence

On the virus surface there exist several surface proteins, named envelope proteins. The numbers of the envelope proteins on the virus surface depend on different kinds of viruses from different virus families (Table 10.1).[6] Their functions can be different, but at least one or two, in general, are involved in virus fusion.[1] Those proteins are usually named as fusion proteins—for example, gp160 in HIV or S protein in severe acute respiratory syndrome coronavirus (SARS-CoV).[7–10] Envelope proteins bind to their cell-surface receptors, either protein (e.g., CD4 as HIV virus receptor) or other molecules (e.g., sialic acid as influenza virus receptor). There is a prominent phenomenon, called binding-induced conformational changes, in the envelope protein during the virus fusion process.[4,11–13] This is referred to as the envelope protein conformational changes induced by its binding to the cellular receptors. This conformational change is the driving force to initiate the virus-cell fusion. Research on the envelope protein–receptor binding and the induced conformational change in the recent years on different enveloped viruses has led to some important discovery for us to understand the process of virus fusion and entry. This also leads to several concepts to elucidate the molecular mechanism involved and development for the new antiviral drugs, including some polypeptides.[5,8–10,14]

In this chapter, I will review recent progress in the development of anti-virus fusion peptides by addressing the important hepted repeat (HR) polypeptides in some notorious viruses, such as HIV, Newcastle disease virus (NDV), and influenza virus, which are all Class I enveloped viruses.

TWO CLASSES OF VIRAL ENVELOPE FUSION PROTEINS

Recent studies have shown that virus fusion proteins are classified at least into two groups: Class I and Class II (Table 10.1); these correlate well to virus surface structures, and each has its unique entry mechanism.[1,8,15,16] Under the electronic microscopy (EM), viruses with Class I fusion protein are seen having some protruding spikes. Sometimes it even has a "crown" appearance, thus being called "coronavirus" (members of Family *Coronaviridae*)[1], whereas viruses with Class II fusion protein shows a relative "flat" surface. HIV, SARS-CoV, and influenza virus have Class I envelope proteins. Flavivirus, instead, such as yellow fever virus, has Class II envelope proteins.

Class I envelope protein orients on the virus surface perpendicularly to the host membrane, forming a kind of "stick"; a number of them are

TABLE 10.1. Viral Envelope Fusion Proteins

Types of Virus Fusion	Families	Representatives	Fusion Proteins	With Known Structure	References
		Characteristics of Viruses			
Class I	*Orthomyxoviridae*	Influenza virus	HA	Yes	5, 54, 55
		Human immunodeficiency virus (HIV)	gp41	Yes	18
		Simian immunodeficiency virus (SIV)	gp41	Yes	56
	Retroviridae	Human T cell leukemia virus (HTLV)	gp21	Yes	57
		Murine leukemia virus	Env	Yes	58
		Avian sarcoma and leucosis virus	gA	No	59
	Filoviridae	Ebola virus	GP2	Yes	60
	Arenaviridae	Lymphocytic choriomeningitis virus (LCMV)	G2	No	61
	Coronaviridae	Severe acute respiratory syndrome cononavirus (SARS-CoV)	S	Yes	22
		Mouse hepatitis virus (MHV)	S	Yes	21
		Human parainfluenza virus	F	Yes	62
		Sendai virus	F	Yes	63, 64
		Simian virus 5	F	Yes	65
		Mumps	F	Yes	20
	Paramyxoviridae	Newcastle disease virus (NDV)	F	Yes	36, 66–68
		Measles virus	F	No	69
		Hendra virus	F	Yes	19
		Nipah virus	F	Yes	19
		Respiratory syncytial virus (RSV)	F	Yes	25
Class II	*Flaviviridae*	West Nile virus (WNV)	E	Yes	70,71
		Dengue virus	E	Yes	28
		Tick-borne encephalitis virus	E	Yes	72
	Togaviridae	Semiliki forest virus	E1	Yes	73
Undefined class	*Bunyaviridae*	Unkuniemi	G2	No	74
	Herpesviridae	Herpes simplex virus	gB	Yes	75
	Rhabdoviridae	Vesicular stomatitis virus	G	Yes	76
	Poxviridae	Vaccinia	Unknown	No	77

circled around the virus surface ("crown" structure), with the presence of amino-terminal or amino-proximal fusion peptides, which are short stretches of amino acids (usually hydrophobic) believed to interact directly with the target cell membrane by inserting their hydrophobic amino acids into the cellular lipid membrane after the envelope protein-cell receptor binding (exposure of the hydrophobic fusion peptide).[5] Through this way the cellular membrane and viral membrane starts to fuse together to form a single membrane. Though the detailed mechanism for the membrane fusion is largely unknown, however, research on HIV fusion core made an important breakthrough in 1997 by two American groups (worth mentioning my mentor at Harvard, the late Dr. Don C. Wiley) for the Class I virus fusion.[17,18] Most of the Class I envelope fusion proteins form homotrimers, with several known crystal structures to confirm this particular features.[19–25] The molecular mechanism of Class I fusion proteins has thoroughly reviewed by Skehel and Wiley[5] in 2000. Readers are encouraged to read it to get more background for the rational of the design of the peptide fusion inhibitors.

In contrast, Class II envelope fusion protein is quite different, at a glance, from Class I fusion protein. It lies down onto and parallels to the viral membrane, leading to an un-"crowned" appearance under the EM. There is also a stretch of hydrophobic amino acids acting as fusion peptide that will insert into the cellular membrane during the membrane fusion, similar to Class I envelope proteins.[15,16,26–28] This fusion peptide usually locates in the middle of the folded envelope fusion protein.[16,28] Flavivirus envelope protein, a member of Class II fusion protein, forms homodimer on the cell surface and has three domains: I, II, and III. Recent crystal structure work by Dr. Stephen C. Harrison's group (Dr. Harrison was my second mentor at Harvard) has shown that the homodimeric fusion protein E of dengue virus (a member of Family *Flaviviridae*) would irreversibly change into homotrimers under the endosomal low-pH condition.[15,16,26–28] The three domains in these two multimeric states are relatively "intact" but with large rearrangement to fulfill their changed conformations (a kind of rigid-body rearrangement).[26–28]

Research on the conformational changes of these two class viral fusion proteins, in general, contributes some important concepts of protein conformational changes for other systems. This, in part, explains why the open reading frames (ORFs) of human genome are much less than we have ever expected as some functions are carried out by the same protein with different conformations.

UNIQUE HEPTAD REPEAT (HR) SEQUENCES IN CLASS I ENVELOPE PROTEINS AND INHIBITORY EFFECTS OF HR POLYPETIDES TO VIRUS ENTRY

Current understanding of virus fusion process shows that there are some obvious structural domains/modules in viral envelope fusion proteins—for example, receptor binding domain, fusion peptide, transmembrane domain, and so on (Fig. 10.1).[1,6] These can even easily be recognized in the gene sequences by eye or by some computer programs—for example, the heptad repeat (HR) regions in Class I viral

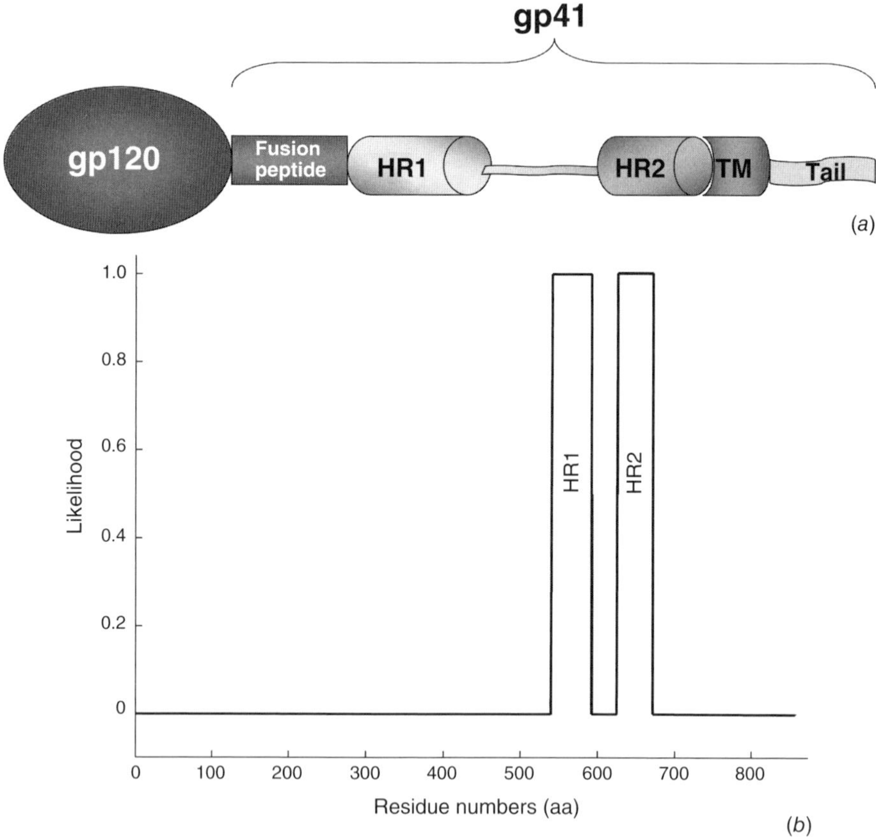

Fig. 10.1. Structural and functional domains of HIV envelope protein gp160. (a) Schematic representation of these domains: Receptor-binding subunit gp120 and fusion subunit gp41 are depicted. The positions of the HR1, HR2, fusion peptide, transmembrane (TM), and cytoplasmic tail (Tail) are shown in detail. (b) Typical HR1/2 prediction result of the HIV gp160 using LearnCoil-VMF program.

TABLE 10.2. Known Fusion Proteins with HR Inhibitory Activities in Class I Enveloped Viruses

Viruses	Characteristics of Fusion Protein			
	Fusion Proteins	Domain with Known Inhibitory Activity	With Known Structure	References
HIV	gp41	HR1/HR2	Yes	49, 50, 78–80
SARS-CoV	S	HR2	Yes	81
MHV	S	HR2	Yes	21, 82, 83
Murine leukemia virus	Env	HR2	Yes	24, 84, 85
Human parainfluenza virus	F	HR2	Yes	62
Sendai virus	F	HR2	Yes	86
Simian virus 5	F	HR1/HR2	Yes	65
NDV	F	HR1/HR2	Yes	31
Avian sarcoma and leucosis virus	E	HR2	No	59
Measles virus	F	HR1/HR2	Yes	69
Hendra virus	F	HR2	Yes	19
Nipah virus	F	HR2	Yes	19
RSV	F	HR1/HR2	Yes	25, 33, 35

fusion proteins (Fig. 10.1). HRs are amino acid repeats of 3–4 seven-amino-acid peptide, and each repeat starts with a characteristic leucine (L) or isoleucine (I) or sometimes other hydrophobic amino acids. This characteristic HR sequence has been found in many virus envelope proteins (Table 10.2).

HR sequences have a typical α-helix structure and can easily be predicted by some computer programs—for example, Dr. Peter Kim's LearnCoil-VMF (http://nightingale.lcs.mit.edu/cgi-bin/vmf)[29] (Fig. 10.1). HRs are usually found in pairs and they are referred to as HR1 (or HR-A or HR-N) and HR2 (or HR-B or HR-C). They are separated by different lengths of amino acids between them, dependent on virus families. Retrovirus envelope protein has a shorter-spaced sequence than that of paramyxovirus. Lu et al.[30] first showed, using HIV gp41 as a model, that HR1 and HR2 bind each other in an antiparallel manner by proteinase K digestion experiments. This pioneering biochemical analysis is the milestone for our understanding of the molecular and mechanistic mechanism of Class I virus fusion.

HRs can act as effective inhibitors for virus entry.[6,31–33] Initially, this phenomenon was discovered by chance in HIV studies by Jiang et al.[34] They first demonstrated that some peptides (HR2) derived from gp41 of HIV inhibited HIV fusion and realized that these peptides showed typical α-helix structure. This leads to an assumption that some polypeptides with α-helix sequences of the envelope protein can, in an unknown manner, inhibit virus fusion and entry. Later, a lot of fusion inhibitors have been tested based on this observation in HIV, and the concept was expanded to other viruses, including paramyxoviruses (Table 10.2).[31,33,35–38] However, the mechanism underlying this effect is unclear. It is a typical empirical observation.

In the early studies, HR2 has been found to consistently show the inhibition effect for all the tested viruses; however, the inhibition of HR1 was shown to be unstable, which was believed due to the hydrophobicity of the HR1 peptide. Our recent studies by using a paramyxovirus as a model have shown that inhibition of HR1 and HR2 are indeed different.[31,35]

Based on the structural data recently obtained (see below for detailed discussion), some *de novo* polypeptide inhibitors have been developed.[31,32,35,39,40] They are analogues or homologues of the HR1 and HR2. In 2001, the Kim group[40] first reported that a 5-helix HIV gp41 could act as a potent virus fusion inhibitor with a more stable character, which would help for clinical application. Later on, our group tested the concept in other viruses and further expanded the idea to develop some new polypeptides (e.g., HR121, HR212, etc.).

STRUCTURE OF CLASS I ENVELOPE PROTEIN FUSION CORE AND FUSION MECHANISM INVOLVED

Though the striking sequence characters are obviously conserved among Class I envelope proteins, it is more striking that the HR forms a characteristic 6-helix coiled coil bundle in an antiparallel manner of HR1 and HR2 (Fig. 10.2).[17–19,21–23,25,41] HR1 and HR2 bind to each other tightly, and the complex is very thermally stable.[5,7,8] This 6-helix coiled coil structure is believed to represent the post-fusion state of the part of envelope structure and is named as viral fusion core. It is assumed that HR1 and HR2 are apart in the pre-fusion state of the envelope protein. After the receptor binding the new conformation of the envelope is formed, notably the formation of the fusion core. In the fusion core, HR1 and HR2 bind each other after an intermediate conformational state, which is a short-lived state but is important for fusion inhibitor design because blocking the protein further folding into the fusion core and keeping them in the intermediate state offer us a good chance for drug dicovery.

In the fusion core structure, three HR1s form a trimeric coiled coil core surrounded by three HR-2s, which also have α-helix structures,

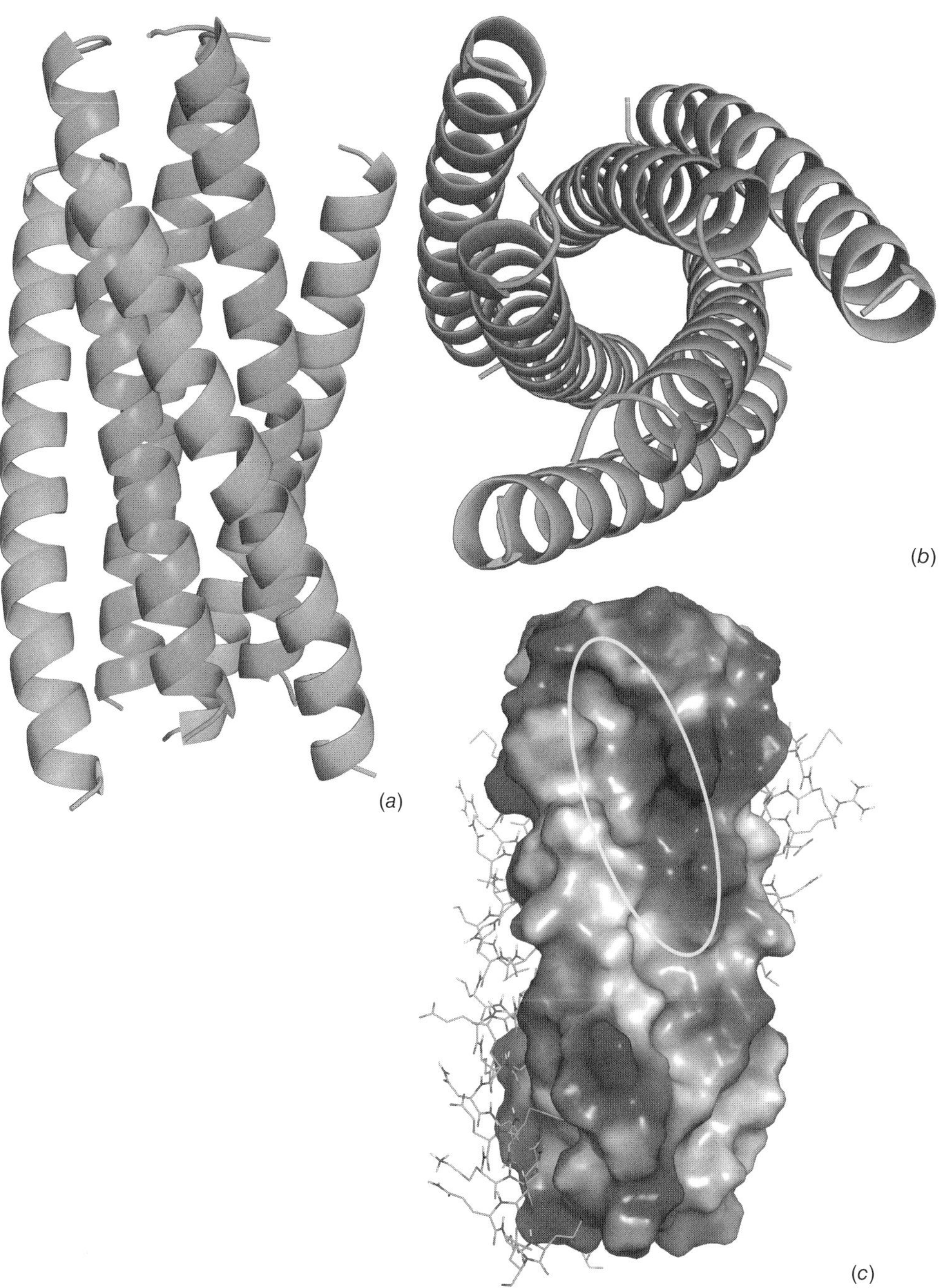

Fig. 10.2. Crystal structure of the fusion core of the HIV HR1/HR2 6-helix bundle. (a) Side view of the α-helix structure. HR1 (green) forms a tightly bound trimer surrounded by three HR2 (cyan). (Source of the structure: PDB code 1AIK.) (b) Top view of the fusion core. (c) Fusion structure (HR1 in space-filling form to show the surface potential and HR2 in stick form) with one HR2 removed to show the cavities (circled), which are targets for small-molecule design. See color insert.

thereby being called 6-helix bundle or "trimer-of-hairpins" (Fig. 10.2). The binding of HR1 and HR2 is in a head–tail form, or antiparallel manner; that is, the N-terminal amino acids of HR1 bind to C-terminal amino acids of the HR2. This is due to the folding process as the HR1 and HR2 are in a single sequential polypeptide sequence. After binding of the fusion peptide locating at the N-terminus of HR1 to the cell membrane, through an intermediate state, the HR1 and HR2 bend to bind each other, leading the virus membrane and cell membrane to the close proximity necessary for membrane fusion to occur, fulfilling the membrane fusion process. Just before the HR1 binds to HR2 during the folding process, the two HRs are exposed in this intermediate state, called prehairpin intermediate. Therefore if either the HR1 or HR2 is introduced, they will compete with the endogenous counterpart for binding, blocking the formation of the fusogenic 6-helix bundle fusion core, thereby working as an effective fusion inhibitor.

Detailed structural analysis of several fusion cores has shown that there are some clear cavities in the HR1 folded area for HR2 binding. These cavities are good targets for novel drug discovery of small molecules. These small molecules can be used to replace the HR2, thereby blocking the HR1/2 binding. This concept has been applied in the small-molecule search of human respiratory syncytial virus (hRSV)[42,43] and HIV.[44] However, to get these into clinical use, it will take some time. Current research focuses on this because small molecules are easy to deliver to the body and are more stable.

PEPTIDE INHIBITORS FOR HIV FUSION

HIV virus is a typical one with Class I envelope protein (named gp160 or two subunits, gp120 and gp41) protruding on the virion surface.[1,8,10,45] Early studies on its HR six-helix bundle structure[17,18,30,41] paved the road toward our understanding of the molecular and mechanistic mechanism of virus fusion in those viruses who have a Class I fusion proteins.

In fact the HR2 inhibitory effect of HIV was discovered by chance,[34] not based on the understanding of the 6-helix bundle formation of the HR1/HR2. Indeed it is the discovery of the HIV coiled coil structure that promotes the science of the classification of two classes of the fusion proteins.[6] This also leads to the establishment of a company named Trimeris Inc. for further development of HR inhibitors and their homologues or analogues (http://www.trimeris.com). The inhibitory activity of the HIV HR2 provides compelling evidence that the prehairpin intermediate indeed exists and is a useful target for anti-HIV therapy. This concept has extended to be applied to other Class I viruses.

With great efforts, peptide derived from the HR2 (T20, or brand name Fuzeon, or generic name Enfuvirtide) has been developed from the laboratory bench into a clinically-applicable drug, with an IC_{50} value in the low nanomolar range. This has been approved by the US Food and Drug Administration (FDA) and European Commission as an alternative for treatment of HIV-1 infection in adults and children who have failed to respond to the current antiretroviral drugs and proved to be very effective.[46]

Although it is a great success for the concept and in the laboratory, the use of T20 in patients has some disadvantages. First, large amounts of this peptidic drug (about 200 mg/day/patient) are required to maintain the *in vivo* antivirus efficacy in humans because of the short half-life of the drug *in vivo* due to its intrinsic degradation character of the peptide.[46–48] Second, the procedure to produce this peptide is tedious and time-consuming, and therefore the capacity to supply enough drugs for patients is very limited. We and other groups have attempted to develop some new polypeptides targeting the HR1 and HR2 with potent anti-HIV activity but with higher stability and lower cost of production. Based on the study that HR1 and HR2 can form stable 6-helix bundle if these two is linked by a short flexible amino acid linker and can be produced by recombinant *E. coli* expression system,[40,41] we and others made use of the fusogenic core (HR1-linker-HR2) as a scaffold to link another HR1 (denoted HR121, HR1-linker-HR2-linker-HR1) or HR2 (denoted HR212, HR2-linker-HR1-linker-HR2) or three HR1 and two HR2 (5-Helix, HR1-linker-HR2-linker-HR1-linker-HR2-linker-HR1) for the development of more stable polypeptide inhibitors. The results show that they are all potent HIV fusion inhibitors with IC_{50} in a range of nanomolar and improved solubility and stability. Because they are produced using recombinant techniques, they are low-cost with sufficient supplies. These are under clinical development.

Taking the current gene therapy into account, one would immediately think that these polypeptides, if produced inside the cells, might be used to block the envelope protein folding inside the cells as a gene therapy tool. This concept has been examined by Hildinger and Egelhofer and their colleagues and proved to be an alternate of HIV therapy.[49,50]

Currently, treatment with T-20 is priced about $20,000 and $25,000 per patient per year in the United States and Europe, respectively. A clinically feasible drug would be stable, easy-delivering, and cheap-producing; therefore, in addition to our approach to develop novel polypeptide inhibitors, some peptide analogues or small molecules are our ultimate goal for HIV therapeutic drugs in the future, which are vigorously pursued by scientists around the world.

PEPTIDE INHIBITORS FOR PARAMYXOVIRUS FUSION: TARGETING NEWCASTLE DISEASE VIRUS

Like other Class I enveloped virus, paramyxovirus envelope fusion protein also has heptad repeat sequences.[13,51] Studies on fusion mechanism or crystal structures of some important paramyxovirus HRs have led to the rational design of some fusion inhibitors.[31,33,35]

There are two separate envelope proteins in paramyxovirus involved in virus entry: attachment protein and fusion protein. The former is responsible for cell-receptor binding, whereas the latter is responsible for fusion. Following the rule of Class I envelope protein in the fusion process, typical coiled coil 6-helix HR bundle, or fusion core, is formed in the fusion protein F of all the studied paramyxoviruses,[19,20,25] after a series of conformational changes. Blocking the fusion core formation by using either HR1 or HR2 has been proved effective in paramyxovirus.

By using Newcastle disease virus (NDV) as a model,[31] we found that, though they are effective in fusion inhibition, the IC_{50} of HR1 and HR2 is in the range of micromolar, a magnitude lower than that of HIV HRs. Similar observations have been seen in other paramyxoviruses.[33,35–38] This implies that although they might follow the general rule of Class I virus fusion, papramyxovirus has some specific characters in the fusion process. In NDV, both attachment protein (HN) and fusion protein (F) are absolutely required for F-protein-mediated fusion. The conformational change of F protein is prompted by HN protein binding to cellular receptors. Therefore the interaction of HN and F is essential for virus to initiate the fusion. F protein is synthesized initially as a precursor, F_0, which is later cleaved into disulfide-bond-linked F_2 and F_1 by furin-like enzyme of the host cells.[11] This cleavage process is essential for NDV fusion and entry. Some NDV strains are not cleaved into the subunits and therefore the efficacy of fusion is very low, leading to some avirulent viruses.[11,12] Our studies[31,36] showed that peptides corresponding to both HR1 and HR2 of NDV F protein can inhibit virus-mediated cell fusion, but the inhibition of the two peptides probably occurs through a different mechanism, maybe at different stages during F protein conformational changes.

Based on the structural and functional analyses, we have developed several *de novo* polypeptides for NDV fusion inhibition, namely HR121, HR212, and 5-Helix as we discussed in HIV inhibitor section. Indeed we do show that the concept does work in the NDV system, and later the observation is expanded to hRSV inhibitor design.[35]

INFLUENZA VIRUS FUSION AND POTENTIAL PEPTIDE FUSION-INHIBITORS

There are also two envelope proteins for influenza virus, hemagglutinin (HA) and neuraminadase (NA),[1,5] but their functions are totally different. HA is a typical fusion protein and is responsible for binding to cellular receptors and membrane fusion,[1,5] whereas NA is responsible for virus release from the infected cells. HA is synthesized as an HA_0 precursor and processed later by cellular furin-like enzyme into two subunits, HA_1 (cellular receptor binding subunit) and HA_2 (the actual fusion subunit).[5] HA is also a typical Class I viral envelope protein with two HR structures in the HA_2 subunit, HR1 and HR2[5] (Fig. 10.3). Crystal structures of both pre-fusion and low-pH-induced post-fusion HA have been solved, and clear conformational changes and domain rearrangement have been revealed.[52,53] In the post-fusion state of the HA, the two HRs bind each other, forming a typical coiled-coil 6-helix bundle, or hairpin fusion core (Fig. 10.3). This clearly provides a good target for potential fusion inhibitors based on the HR sequences. Unfortunately, work in influenza virus has not yet been done so far, and the potential use of these polypeptides in the eve of a possible flu-pandemic is extremely welcomed.

Influenza virus fusion occurs inside the cells in the endosome after being taken up into the cell by endocytosis; therefore it is impossible to have the HRs to inhibit the virus entry on the cell membrane level. However, if the peptides can be delivered into the cells, they might function to inhibit the endosomal-viral membrane fusion. Our preliminary data on peptide-soaking into the cells show some inhibitory effects on virus titers in an *in vitro* infection system (Liu and Gao, unpublished data).

Based on the successful work in HIV studies,[49,50] we have introduced (by transfection) the influenza virus HA protein HRs (both HR1 and HR2) into the MDCK cells (a permissive cell line to support influenza virus growth) and have found that HR expression inside the cells affects virus titers, implying that they might block the virus fusion in the endosome (Liu and Gao, unpublished data). This gene therapy

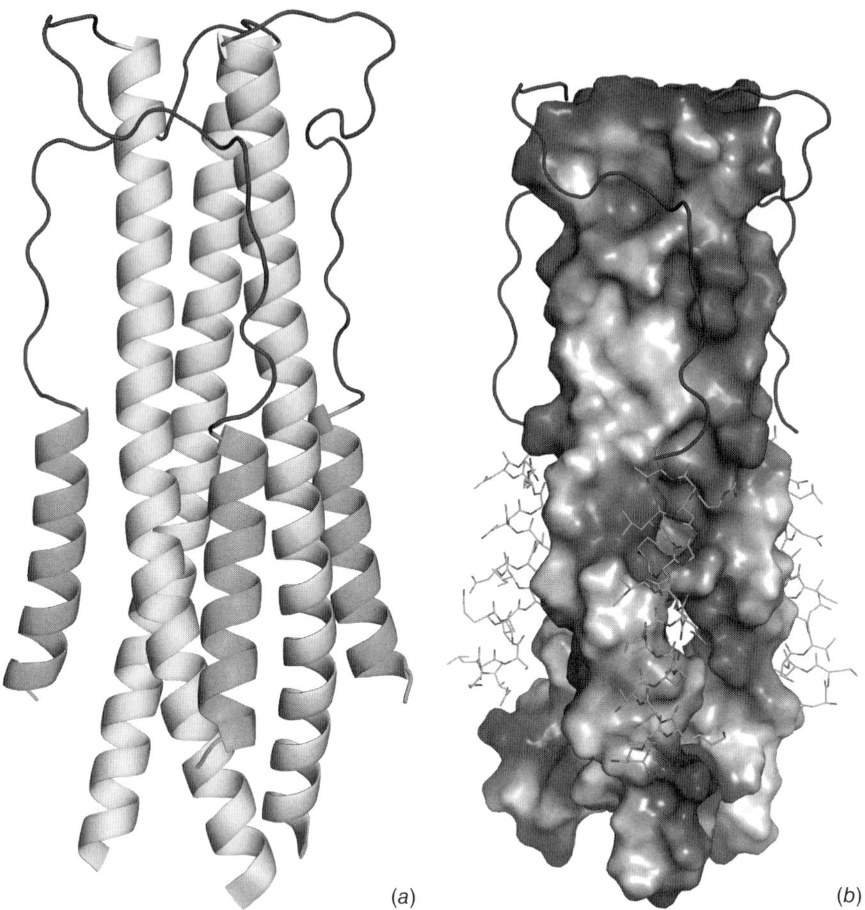

Fig. 10.3. Crystal structure of the HR1/HR2 complex of influenza virus HA. (a) Typical α-helix structure of the three long HR1 (yellow) surrounded by three shorter HR2 (cyan) with some flexible loops shown in blue. (Source of the structure: PDB code 2viu.) (b) Space-filling presentation of the structure in part a to show the HR1 surface potential and the bound HR2 in stick. See color insert.

approach provides us an alternative for drug stockpiling of a potential influenza pandemic.

CONCLUSIONS AND PERSPECTIVES

Our understanding of the molecular and mechanistic mechanism of virus fusion and entry is gradually clear. Preventing virus fusion or entry has become a new therapeutic strategy to prevent virus infection, and virus fusion inhibition is currently one of the most promising approaches. Binding-induced conformational changes of viral envelope protein have been shown to play an important role in envelope virus fusion and entry. Catching the intermediate state of a protein folding process duing the conformational changes can stop the protein from further folding, thereby blocking the virus membrane fusion. The successful use in clinics of the T20 (or Enfuvirtide or Fuzeon) in HIV-infected patient makes a promise for further development of other HR polypeptide inhibitors, including SARS-CoV and influenza virus, which might be used in the event of a potential pandemic of influenza worldwide. Work in either the soluble HR form or *in vivo* delivery of the HR genes into the cells as a gene therapy strategy needs to be rigorously further explored for influenza virus.

ACKNOWLEDGMENTS

George F. Gao is a Distinguished Young Investigator of the National Natural Science Foundation of China (NSFC, Grant No. 30525010). Work in GFG's lab is supported, in part, by Beijing Natural Science Foundation (Grant No. 5062028), NSFC (Grant No. 30599434), and the Ministry of Science and Technology (MOST) of P. R. China (Frontier Science Project 973, Grant No. 2005CB523001; The 10th and 11th 5-Year Plan National Key Technologies R&D Program, Grant Nos. 2004BA519A29 and 2006BAD06A01). I am grateful to Mr. Feng Gao, Ms. Yan Wu, Mr. Youjun Feng, Mr. Hao Peng, Ms. Jun-e Liu, and Mr. Fang (Francis) Yuan for help in the preparation of this manuscript.

REFERENCES

1. Knipe, D. M.; Howley, P. M.; Fields, B. N. *Fields' Virology*, 4th ed., Lippincott Williams & Wilkins, Philadelphia, **2001**, p. 2 v. (xix, 3087, 72 pp.).

2. Chazal, N.; Gerlier, D. Virus entry, assembly, budding, and membrane rafts. *Microbiol. Mol. Biol. Rev.* **2003**, *67*(2), 226–237, table of contents.

3. Mousavi, S. A.; Malerod, L.; Berg, T.; Kjeken, R. Clathrin-dependent endocytosis. *Biochem. J.* **2004**, *377*(Pt 1), 1–16.

4. Skehel, J. J.; Wiley, D. C. Coiled coils in both intracellular vesicle and viral membrane fusion. *Cell* **1998**, *95*(7), 871–874.

5. Skehel, J. J.; Wiley, D. C. Receptor binding and membrane fusion in virus entry: The influenza hemagglutinin. *Annu. Rev. Biochem.* **2000**, *69*, 531–569.

6. Wang, X. Z., G. W. H.; Wang, M.; Gao, G. F. The molecular mechanism of enveloped virus-cell membrane fusion. *Prog. Biochem. Biophys.* **2004**, *31*(6), 482–491.

7. Bentz, J. Membrane fusion mediated by coiled coils: A hypothesis. *Biophys. J.* **2000**, *78*(2), 886–900.

8. Eckert, D. M.; Kim, P. S. Mechanisms of viral membrane fusion and its inhibition. *Annu. Rev. Biochem.* **2001**, *70*, 777–810.

9. Colman, P. M.; Lawrence, M. C. The structural biology of type I viral membrane fusion. *Nat. Rev. Mol. Cell. Biol.* **2003**, *4*(4), 309–319.

10. Wyatt, R.; Sodroski, J. The HIV-1 envelope glycoproteins: fusogens, antigens, and immunogens. *Science* **1998**, *280*(5371), 1884–1888.

11. Nagai, Y.; Klenk, H. D.; Rott, R. Proteolytic cleavage of the viral glycoproteins and its significance for the virulence of Newcastle disease virus. *Virology* **1976**, *72*(2), 494–508.

12. Nagai, Y.; Inocencio, N. M.; Gotoh, B. Paramyxovirus tropism dependent on host proteases activating the viral fusion glycoprotein. *Behring Inst. Mitt.* **1991** (89), 35–45.

13. Lamb, R. A. Paramyxovirus fusion: A hypothesis for changes. *Virology* **1993**, *197*(1), 1–11.

14. Eckert, D. M.; Kim, P. S. Design of potent inhibitors of HIV-1 entry from the gp41 N-peptide region. *Proc. Natl. Acad. Sci. USA* **2001**, *98*(20), 11187–11192.

15. Heinz, F. X.; Allison, S. L. The machinery for flavivirus fusion with host cell membranes. *Curr. Opin. Microbiol.* **2001**, *4*(4), 450–455.

16. Heinz, F. X.; Allison, S. L. Structures and mechanisms in flavivirus fusion. *Adv. Virus. Res.* **2000**, *55*, 231–269.

17. Weissenhorn, W.; Dessen, A.; Harrison, S. C.; Skehel, J. J.; Wiley, D. C. Atomic structure of the ectodomain from HIV-1 gp41. *Nature* **1997**, *387*(6631), 426–430.

18. Chan, D. C.; Fass, D.; Berger, J. M.; Kim, P. S. Core structure of gp41 from the HIV envelope glycoprotein. *Cell* **1997**, *89*(2), 263–273.

19. Lou, Z.; Xu, Y.; Xiang, K.; Su, N.; Qin, L.; Li, X.; Gao, G. F.; Bartlam, M.; Rao, Z. Crystal structures of Nipah and Hendra virus fusion core proteins. *FEBS J.* **2006**, *273*(19), 4538–4547.

20. Liu, Y.; Xu, Y.; Lou, Z.; Zhu, J.; Hu, X.; Gao, G. F.; Qiu, B.; Rao, Z.; Tien, P. Structural characterization of mumps virus fusion protein core. *Biochem. Biophys. Res. Commun.* **2006**, *348*(3), 916–922.

21. Xu, Y.; Liu, Y.; Lou, Z.; Qin, L.; Li, X.; Bai, Z.; Pang, H.; Tien, P.; Gao, G. F.; Rao, Z. Structural basis for coronavirus-mediated membrane fusion. Crystal structure of mouse hepatitis virus spike protein fusion core. *J. Biol. Chem.* **2004**, *279*(29), 30514–30522.

22. Xu, Y.; Lou, Z.; Liu, Y.; Pang, H.; Tien, P.; Gao, G. F.; Rao, Z. Crystal structure of severe acute respiratory syndrome coronavirus spike protein fusion core. *J. Biol. Chem.* **2004**, *279*(47), 49414–49419.

23. Malashkevich, V. N.; Singh, M.; Kim, P. S. The trimer-of-hairpins motif in membrane fusion: Visna virus. *Proc. Natl. Acad. Sci. USA* **2001**, *98*(15), 8502–8506.

24. Fass, D.; Davey, R. A.; Hamson, C. A.; Kim, P. S.; Cunningham, J. M.; Berger, J. M. Structure of a murine leukemia virus receptor-binding glycoprotein at 2.0 angstrom resolution. *Science* **1997**, *277*(5332), 1662–1666.

25. Zhao, X.; Singh, M.; Malashkevich, V. N.; Kim, P. S. Structural characterization of the human respiratory syncytial virus fusion protein core. *Proc. Natl. Acad. Sci. USA* **2000**, *97*(26), 14172–14177.

26. Modis, Y.; Ogata, S.; Clements, D.; Harrison, S. C. Variable surface epitopes in the crystal structure of dengue virus type 3 envelope glycoprotein. *J. Virol.* **2005**, *79*(2), 1223–1231.

27. Modis, Y.; Ogata, S.; Clements, D.; Harrison, S. C. Structure of the dengue virus envelope protein after membrane fusion. *Nature* **2004**, *427*(6972), 313–319.

28. Modis, Y.; Ogata, S.; Clements, D.; Harrison, S. C. A ligand-binding pocket in the dengue virus envelope glycoprotein. *Proc. Natl. Acad. Sci. USA* **2003**, *100*(12), 6986–6991.

29. Singh, M.; Berger, B.; Kim, P. S. LearnCoil-VMF: Computational evidence for coiled-coil-like motifs in many viral membrane-fusion proteins. *J. Mol. Biol.* **1999**, *290*(5), 1031–1041.

30. Lu, M.; Blacklow, S. C.; Kim, P. S. A trimeric structural domain of the HIV-1 transmembrane glycoprotein. *Nat. Struct. Biol.* **1995**, *2*(12), 1075–1082.

31. Zhu, J.; Jiang, X.; Liu, Y.; Tien, P.; Gao, G. F. Design and characterization of viral polypeptide inhibitors targeting Newcastle disease virus fusion. *J. Mol. Biol.* **2005**, *354*(3), 601–613.

32. Ni, L.; Gao, G. F.; Tien, P. Rational design of highly potent HIV-1 fusion inhibitory proteins: Implication for developing antiviral therapeutics. *Biochem. Biophys. Res. Commun.* **2005**, *332*(3), 831–836.

33. Wang, E.; Sun, X.; Qian, Y.; Zhao, L.; Tien, P.; Gao, G. F. Both heptad repeats of human respiratory syncytial virus fusion protein are potent inhibitors of viral fusion. *Biochem. Biophys. Res. Commun.* **2003**, *302*(3), 469–475.

34. Jiang, S.; Lin, K.; Strick, N.; Neurath, A. R. HIV-1 inhibition by a peptide. *Nature* **1993**, *365*(6442), 113.

35. Ni, L.; Zhao, L.; Qian, Y.; Zhu, J.; Jin, Z.; Chen, Y. W.; Tien, P.; Gao, G. F. Design and characterization of human respiratory syncytial virus entry inhibitors. *Antivir. Ther.* **2005**, *10*(7), 833–840.

36. Yu, M.; Wang, E.; Liu, Y.; Cao, D.; Jin, N.; Zhang, C. W.; Bartlam, M.; Rao, Z.; Tien, P.; Gao, G. F. Six-helix bundle assembly and characterization of heptad repeat regions from the F protein of Newcastle disease virus. *J. Gen. Virol.* **2002**, *83*(Pt 3), 623–629.

37. Buckland, R.; Malvoisin, E.; Beauverger, P.; Wild, F. A leucine zipper structure present in the measles virus fusion protein is not required for its tet-

ramerization but is essential for fusion. *J. Gen. Virol.* **1992**, *73*(Pt 7), 1703–1707.

38. Rapaport, D.; Ovadia, M.; and Shai, Y. A synthetic peptide corresponding to a conserved heptad repeat domain is a potent inhibitor of Sendai virus–cell fusion: An emerging similarity with functional domains of other viruses. *EMBO J.* **1995**, *14*, 5524–5531.

39. Ni, L.; Zhu, J.; Zhang, J.; Yan, M.; Gao, G. F.; Tien, P. Design of recombinant protein-based SARS-CoV entry inhibitors targeting the heptad-repeat regions of the spike protein S2 domain. *Biochem. Biophys. Res. Commun.* **2005**, *330*(1), 39–45.

40. Root, M. J.; Kay, M. S.; Kim, P. S. Protein design of an HIV-1 entry inhibitor. *Science* **2001**, *291*(5505), 884–888.

41. Lu, M.; Kim, P. S. A trimeric structural subdomain of the HIV-1 transmembrane glycoprotein. *J. Biomol. Struct. Dyn.* **1997**, *15*(3), 465–471.

42. Gao, G. F. Filling the hole: Evidence of a small molecule binding to the fusion core pocket in human respiratory syncytial virus. *Expert Opin. Invest. Drugs* **2005**, *14*(2), 195–197.

43. Cianci, C.; Langley, D. R.; Dischino, D. D.; Sun, Y.; Yu, K. L.; Stanley, A.; Roach, J.; Li, Z.; Dalterio, R.; Colonno, R.; Meanwell, N. A.; Krystal, M. Targeting a binding pocket within the trimer-of-hairpins: Small-molecule inhibition of viral fusion. *Proc. Natl. Acad. Sci. USA* **2004**, *101*(42), 15046–15051.

44. Zhou, G.; Ferrer, M.; Chopra, R.; Kapoor, T. M.; Strassmaier, T.; Weissenhorn, W.; Skehel, J. J.; Oprian, D.; Schreiber, S. L.; Harrison, S. C.; Wiley, D. C. The structure of an HIV-1 specific cell entry inhibitor in complex with the HIV-1 gp41 trimeric core. *Bioorg. Med. Chem.* **2000**, *8*(9), 2219–2227.

45. Weissenhorn, W.; Dessen, A.; Calder, L. J.; Harrison, S. C.; Skehel, J. J.; Wiley, D. C. Structural basis for membrane fusion by enveloped viruses. *Mol. Membr. Biol.* **1999**, *16*(1), 3–9.

46. Cuzin, L.; Alvarez, M. Enfuvirtide for prophylaxis against HIV infection. *N. Engl. J. Med.* **2003**, *349*(22), 2169–2170; author reply 2169–2170.

47. Hicks, C. B.; Cahn, P.; Cooper, D. A.; Walmsley, S. L.; Katlama, C.; Clotet, B.; Lazzarin, A.; Johnson, M. A.; Neubacher, D.; Mayers, D.; Valdez, H. Durable efficacy of tipranavir–ritonavir in combination with an optimised background regimen of antiretroviral drugs for treatment-experienced HIV-1-infected patients at 48 weeks in the Randomized Evaluation of Strategic Intervention in multi-drug resistant patients with Tipranavir (RESIST) studies: An analysis of combined data from two randomised open-label trials. *Lancet* **2006**, *368*(9534), 466–475.

48. Fletcher, C. V. Enfuvirtide, a new drug for HIV infection. *Lancet* **2003**, *361*(9369), 1577–1578.

49. Hildinger, M.; Dittmar, M. T.; Schult-Dietrich, P.; Fehse, B.; Schnierle, B. S.; Thaler, S.; Stiegler, G.; Welker, R.; von Laer, D. Membrane-anchored

peptide inhibits human immunodeficiency virus entry. *J. Virol.* **2001**, *75*(6), 3038–3042.

50. Egelhofer, M.; Brandenburg, G.; Martinius, H.; Schult-Dietrich, P.; Melikyan, G.; Kunert, R.; Baum, C.; Choi, I.; Alexandrov, A.; von Laer, D. Inhibition of human immunodeficiency virus type 1 entry in cells expressing gp41-derived peptides. *J. Virol.* **2004**, *78*(2), 568–575.

51. Lamb, R. A.; Joshi, S. B.; Dutch, R. E. The paramyxovirus fusion protein forms an extremely stable core trimer: Structural parallels to influenza virus haemagglutinin and HIV-1 gp41. *Mol. Membr. Biol.* **1999**, *16*(1), 11–19.

52. Wilson, I. A.; Skehel, J. J.; Wiley, D. C. Structure of the haemagglutinin membrane glycoprotein of influenza virus at 3 A resolution. *Nature* **1981**, *289*(5796), 366–373.

53. Chen, J.; Lee, K. H.; Steinhauer, D. A.; Stevens, D. J.; Skehel, J. J.; Wiley, D. C. Structure of the hemagglutinin precursor cleavage site, a determinant of influenza pathogenicity and the origin of the labile conformation. *Cell* **1998**, *95*(3), 409–417.

54. Gamblin, S. J.; Haire, L. F.; Russell, R. J.; Stevens, D. J.; Xiao, B.; Ha, Y.; Vasisht, N.; Steinhauer, D. A.; Daniels, R. S.; Elliot, A.; Wiley, D. C.; Skehel, J. J. The structure and receptor binding properties of the 1918 influenza hemagglutinin. *Science* **2004**, *303*(5665), 1838–1842.

55. Bullough, P. A.; Hughson, F. M.; Skehel, J. J.; Wiley, D. C. Structure of influenza haemagglutinin at the pH of membrane fusion. *Nature* **1994**, *371*(6492), 37–43.

56. Yang, Z. N.; Mueser, T. C.; Kaufman, J.; Stahl, S. J.; Wingfield, P. T.; Hyde, C. C. The crystal structure of the SIV gp41 ectodomain at 1.47 Å resolution. *J. Struct. Biol.* **1999**, *126*(2), 131–144.

57. Kobe, B.; Center, R. J.; Kemp, B. E.; Poumbourios, P. Crystal structure of human T cell leukemia virus type 1 gp21 ectodomain crystallized as a maltose-binding protein chimera reveals structural evolution of retroviral transmembrane proteins. *Proc. Natl. Acad. Sci. USA* **1999**, *96*(8), 4319–4324.

58. Fass, D.; Harrison, S. C.; Kim, P. S. Retrovirus envelope domain at 1.7 angstrom resolution. *Nat. Struct. Biol.* **1996**, *3*(5), 465–469.

59. Netter, R. C.; Amberg, S. M.; Balliet, J. W.; Biscone, M. J.; Vermeulen, A.; Earp, L. J.; White, J. M.; Bates, P. Heptad repeat 2-based peptides inhibit avian sarcoma and leukosis virus subgroup a infection and identify a fusion intermediate. *J. Virol.* **2004**, *78*(24), 13430–13439.

60. Weissenhorn, W.; Carfi, A.; Lee, K. H.; Skehel, J. J.; Wiley, D. C. Crystal structure of the Ebola virus membrane fusion subunit, GP2, from the envelope glycoprotein ectodomain. *Mol. Cell* **1998**, *2*(5), 605–616.

61. Eschli, B.; Quirin, K.; Wepf, A.; Weber, J.; Zinkernagel, R.; Hengartner, H. Identification of an N-terminal trimeric coiled-coil core within arenavirus

glycoprotein 2 permits assignment to class I viral fusion proteins. *J. Virol.* **2006**, *80*(12), 5897–5907.

62. Yin, H. S.; Paterson, R. G.; Wen, X.; Lamb, R. A.; Jardetzky, T. S. Structure of the uncleaved ectodomain of the paramyxovirus (hPIV3) fusion protein. *Proc. Natl. Acad. Sci. USA* **2005**, *102*(26), 9288–9293.

63. Wang, X.; Xu, Y.; Cole, D. K.; Lou, Z.; Liu, Y.; Rao, Z.; Wang, M.; Gao, G. F. Biochemical, biophysical and preliminary X-ray crystallographic analyses of the fusion core of Sendai virus F protein. *Acta Crystallogr. D Biol. Crystallogr.* **2004**, *60*(Pt 9), 1632–1635.

64. Ludwig, K.; Baljinnyam, B.; Herrmann, A.; Bottcher, C. The 3D structure of the fusion primed Sendai F-protein determined by electron cryomicroscopy. *EMBO J.* **2003**, *22*(15), 3761–3771.

65. Baker, K. A.; Dutch, R. E.; Lamb, R. A.; Jardetzky, T. S. Structural basis for paramyxovirus-mediated membrane fusion. *Mol. Cell* **1999**, *3*(3), 309–319.

66. Lalezari, J. P.; Henry, K.; O'Hearn, M.; Montaner, J. S.; Piliero, P. J.; Trottier, B.; Walmsley, S.; Cohen, C.; Kuritzkes, D. R.; Eron, J. J., Jr.; Chung, J.; DeMasi, R.; Donatacci, L.; Drobnes, C.; Delehanty, J.; Salgo, M. Enfuvirtide, an HIV-1 fusion inhibitor, for drug-resistant HIV infection in North and South America. *N. Engl. J. Med.* **2003**, *348*(22), 2175–2185.

67. Zhu, J.; Li, P.; Wu, T.; Gao, F.; Ding, Y.; Zhang, C. W.; Rao, Z.; Gao, G. F.; Tien, P. Design and analysis of post-fusion 6-helix bundle of heptad repeat regions from Newcastle disease virus F protein. *Protein Eng.* **2003**, *16*(5), 373–379.

68. Chen, L.; Gorman, J. J.; McKimm-Breschkin, J.; Lawrence, L. J.; Tulloch, P. A.; Smith, B. J.; Colman, P. M.; Lawrence, M. C. The structure of the fusion glycoprotein of Newcastle disease virus suggests a novel paradigm for the molecular mechanism of membrane fusion. *Structure* **2001**, *9*(3), 255–266.

69. Zhu, J.; Zhang, C. W.; Qi, Y.; Tien, P.; Gao, G. F. The fusion protein core of measles virus forms stable coiled-coil trimer. *Biochem. Biophys. Res. Commun.* **2002**, *299*(5), 897–902.

70. Kanai, R.; Kar, K.; Anthony, K.; Gould, L. H.; Ledizet, M.; Fikrig, E.; Marasco, W. A.; Koski, R. A.; Modis, Y. Crystal structure of West Nile virus envelope glycoprotein reveals viral surface epitopes. *J. Virol.* **2006**, *80*(22), 11000–11008.

71. Nybakken, G. E.; Nelson, C. A.; Chen, B. R.; Diamond, M. S.; Fremont, D. H. Crystal structure of the West Nile virus envelope glycoprotein. *J. Virol.* **2006**, *80*(23), 11467–11474.

72. Rey, F. A.; Heinz, F. X.; Mandl, C.; Kunz, C.; Harrison, S. C. The envelope glycoprotein from tick-borne encephalitis virus at 2 Å resolution. *Nature* **1995**, *375*(6529), 291–298.

73. Lescar, J.; Roussel, A.; Wien, M. W.; Navaza, J.; Fuller, S. D.; Wengler, G.; Wengler, G.; Rey, F. A. The Fusion glycoprotein shell of Semliki forest virus: An icosahedral assembly primed for fusogenic activation at endosomal pH. *Cell* **2001**, *105*(1), 137–148.

74. Pobjecky, N.; Smith, J.; Gonzalez-Scarano, F. Biological studies of the fusion function of California serogroup Bunyaviruses. *Microb. Pathog.* **1986**, *1*(5), 491–501.

75. Heldwein, E. E.; Lou, H.; Bender, F. C.; Cohen, G. H.; Eisenberg, R. J.; Harrison, S. C. Crystal structure of glycoprotein B from herpes simplex virus 1. *Science* **2006**, *313*(5784), 217–220.

76. Roche, S.; Bressanelli, S.; Rey, F. A.; Gaudin, Y. Crystal structure of the low-pH form of the vesicular stomatitis virus glycoprotein G. *Science* **2006**, *313*(5784), 187–191.

77. Moss, B. Poxvirus entry and membrane fusion. *Virology* **2006**, *344*(1), 48–54.

78. Chan, D. C.; Chutkowski, C. T.; Kim, P. S. Evidence that a prominent cavity in the coiled coil of HIV type 1 gp41 is an attractive drug target. *Proc. Natl. Acad. Sci. USA* **1998**, *95*(26), 15613–15617.

79. Ji, H.; Shu, W.; Burling, F. T.; Jiang, S.; Lu, M. Inhibition of human immunodeficiency virus type 1 infectivity by the gp41 core: Role of a conserved hydrophobic cavity in membrane fusion. *J. Virol.* **1999**, *73*(10), 8578–8586.

80. Judice, J. K.; Tom, J. Y.; Huang, W.; Wrin, T.; Vennari, J.; Petropoulos, C. J.; McDowell, R. S. Inhibition of HIV type 1 infectivity by constrained alpha-helical peptides: Implications for the viral fusion mechanism. *Proc. Natl. Acad. Sci. USA* **1997**, *94*(25), 13426–13430.

81. Bosch, B. J.; Martina, B. E.; Van Der Zee, R.; Lepault, J.; Haijema, B. J.; Versluis, C.; Heck, A. J.; De Groot, R.; Osterhaus, A. D.; Rottier, P. J. Severe acute respiratory syndrome coronavirus (SARS-CoV) infection inhibition using spike protein heptad repeat-derived peptides. *Proc. Natl. Acad. Sci. USA* **2004**, *101*(22), 8455–8460.

82. Xu, Y.; Cole, D. K.; Lou, Z.; Liu, Y.; Qin, L.; Li, X.; Bai, Z.; Yuan, F.; Rao, Z.; Gao, G. F. Construct design, biophysical, and biochemical characterization of the fusion core from mouse hepatitis virus (a coronavirus) spike protein. *Protein Expr. Purif.* **2004**, *38*(1), 116–122.

83. Xu, Y.; Zhu, J.; Liu, Y.; Lou, Z.; Yuan, F.; Liu, Y.; Cole, D. K.; Ni, L.; Su, N.; Qin, L.; Li, X.; Bai, Z.; Bell, J. I.; Pang, H.; Tien, P.; Gao, G. F.; Rao, Z. Characterization of the heptad repeat regions, HR1 and HR2, and design of a fusion core structure model of the spike protein from severe acute respiratory syndrome (SARS) coronavirus. *Biochemistry* **2004**, *43*(44), 14064–14071.

84. Ou, W.; Silver, J. Inhibition of murine leukemia virus envelope protein (env) processing by intracellular expression of the env N-terminal heptad repeat region. *J. Virol.* **2005**, *79*(8), 4782–4792.

85. Witte, O. N.; Wirth, D. F. Structure of the murine leukemia virus envelope glycoprotein precursor. *J. Virol.* **1979**, *29*(2), 735–743.

86. Ghosh, J. K.; Shai, Y. A peptide derived from a conserved domain of Sendai virus fusion protein inhibits virus-cell fusion. A plausible mode of action. *J. Biol. Chem.* **1998**, *273*(13), 7252–7259.

11

NOVEL INFLUENZA THERAPEUTICS

LAURA M. ASCHENBRENNER, NICOLE PELLETIER, MANG YU, AND FANG FANG

NexBio Inc., San Diego, CA 92121

Influenza is a highly infectious acute respiratory disease that has plagued the human race since ancient times. It is characterized by recurrent annual epidemics and periodic major worldwide pandemics. Due to high disease-related morbidity and mortality, the direct and indirect socioeconomic impacts of influenza (IFV) are enormous. In the United States alone, annual epidemics cause approximately 300,000 hospitalizations and 36,000 deaths. In the twentieth century, three influenza pandemics (1918, 1957, and 1968) were recorded and together they have taken an enormous toll of millions of lives and billions of dollars. The avian IFV, H5N1, which initially emerged in the late 1990s, has spread to hundreds of poultry farms in Asia, Europe, and Africa. As of March 12, 2007, 278 people have been confirmed to be infected by the virus in 10 countries and 168 of them have died. Accumulated epidemiological evidence has documented that since 1999, the H5N1 virus has evolved rapidly in ducks and has become increasingly virulent and pathogenic in both chickens and mice.[1] Recent molecular and genetic evidence has shown that the H5N1 virus isolated from the human outbreak of avian flu in Turkey has acquired mutations that are likely to

Combating the Threat of Pandemic Influenza: Drug Discovery Approaches,
Edited by Paul F. Torrence
Copyright © 2007 by John Wiley & Sons, Inc.

make the virus better adapted to infect humans.[2] These are serious warning signs that a pandemic could be imminent.

Currently, vaccination and antiviral chemical compounds are the only prophylaxis and therapeutic remedies to control epidemic influenza. Inactivated or attenuated live human influenza vaccines are now in worldwide use, especially in the high-risk groups; however, these vaccines need to be updated annually to maintain efficacy and require a substantial period of time for manufacture. The United States vaccine supply for the influenza season of 2004–2005 was abruptly cut in half due to manufacturing problems, highlighting potential issues of inconsistency and unreliability of future product supply. It is estimated that in facing a pandemic outbreak, it could take up to 8 months before the updated influenza vaccines are ready for distribution.[3] Historical record has shown that in the past, flu pandemics have spread to most continents within 6 months, and future pandemics are expected to spread even faster due to increased international travel.[4] At the present time, no vaccine exists against the potential pandemic strain H5N1. Furthermore, it has become increasingly clear that proper prediction of the pandemic virus strain will be difficult in light of the recent discovery that genetically and antigenically distinct sublineages of H5N1 virus have become established among poultry in different geographical regions of Southeast Asia.[5] It is inevitable that vaccines will be either unavailable or in short supply during the first wave of future pandemics.

Antiviral chemical compounds are becoming the mainstay for therapeutic treatment during inter-pandemic periods and are currently the only option for controlling pandemics during the initial period. Two classes of antiviral compounds are currently on the market: (a) the M2 inhibitors such as amantadine and rimantadine and (b) the viral neuraminidase inhibitors (NAIs) oseltamivir (Tamiflu®) and zanamivir (Relenza®). The first class only works for influenza A and is commonly associated with side effects and drug resistance. In addition, they are generally considered useless against the potential IFV pandemic of the H5N1 subtype.[6] In January 2006, the Centers for Disease Control and Prevention (CDC) advised physicians to stop prescribing rimantadine and amantadine because 91% of influenza viruses have become resistant to this class of drug, underscoring the importance of developing new classes of influenza therapeutics.

The NA inhibitors entered the marketplace in recent years and are effective against both influenza A and B viruses. However, oseltamivir, which now dominates the NA inhibitor market, was linked to a surprisingly high frequency (18%) of drug-resistant viruses in children.[7] A mutant IFV strain (H274Y) that is highly resistant to oseltamivir has been isolated from two patients who had been treated with the drug, and both patients died from the infection.[8] The community emergence and spread of viruses resistant to oseltamivir, if it were to occur, would have significant implications for influenza A/H5N1 prevention and control. Furthermore, it has been repeatedly observed that some of the oseltamivir resistant viral strains also exhibit cross-resistance against other NAIs.[9–11] The introduction of new NAIs to the market may not provide the solution to oseltamivir resistance. Therapeutics with a novel mechanism of action are urgently needed for influenza treatment.

Targeting distinct steps in the influenza virus life cycle is a strategy for developing novel influenza therapeutics (Fig. 11.1). Influenza initiates infection by binding to the sialic acid receptors on the surface of the airway epithelium and is then internalized with the host cells' machinery. As the endosomal vesicle containing the newly internalized virion matures, the pH of the vesicle becomes more acidic, thereby initiating HA-dependent fusion between the vesicle and the virion. Once

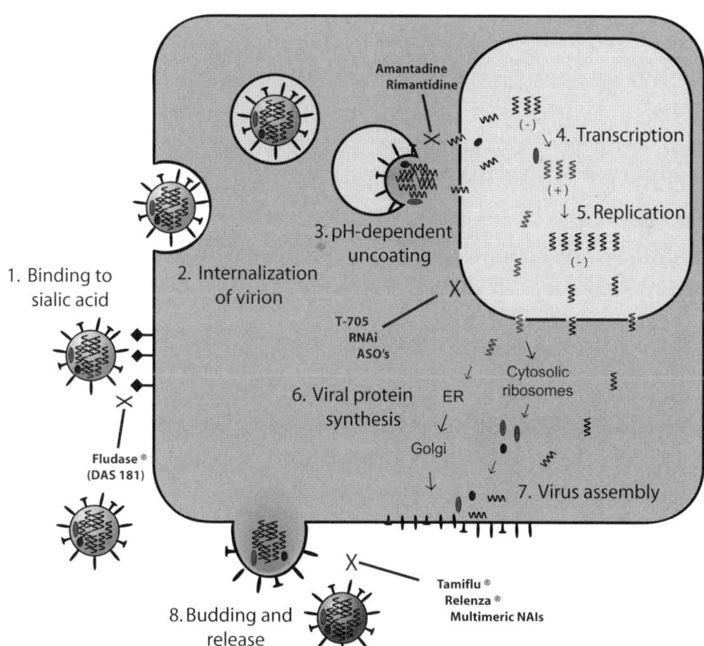

Fig. 11.1. Influenza virus life cycle. Fludase® (DAS181) prevents viral binding and entry; amantadine and rimantadine inhibit pH-dependent uncoating of the virion; ASOs, siRNA, and T-705 target viral replication, transcription, and subsequent translation; Tamiflu®, Relenza®, and long-lasting multimeric forms of NAIs target the budding and release stage of the influenza virus life cycle.

TABLE 11.1. Novel Therapeutic Candidates and Strategies Against Influenza

Candidates or Strategy	Mechanism of Action	Current Development Stage	Developed By
DAS181 (Fludase®)	Inhibition of host cell receptor binding	Phase 1 clinical trial	NexBio Inc.
T-705	Inhibition of RNA replication	Phase 1 clinical trial	Toyama Chemical Co.
Antisense oligonucleotides and siRNA	Inhibition of RNA replication and translation	Preclinical	AVI Biopharma Alnylam Pharmaceuticals
Multimeric zanamivir	Inhibition of viral release	Preclinical	Biota

the fusion has occurred, the contents are released into the cytoplasm and the viral RNA along with replication components are translocated to the nucleus. Here, both transcription and replication take place. Viral proteins are synthesized and assembled on the apical surface of the cell. The assembled virions are then released and spread to the neighboring cells.

Novel therapeutic candidates have been designed to target various steps of the virus life cycle including host receptor binding, viral RNA replication, viral RNA translation, and viral release. They are summarized in Table 11.1, and discussed in more detail in this review.

DAS181 (FLUDASE®): A NOVEL INFLUENZA VIRUS RECEPTOR INACTIVATOR

An investigation into the life cycle of influenza viruses revealed that binding to the host cell receptor is the key event to initiate infection, and this holds true for every subtype and strain of influenza virus. If viral attachment to its cellular receptor is blocked by a specific antibody, infection does not take place.[12] Neutralizing anti-influenza antibodies isolated from individuals exposed to influenza virus work by inhibiting viral infection by blocking the viral HA protein from binding to the host cell receptor, sialic acid. The vaccines that have been proven effective typically work by inducing the formation of the receptor blocking neutralizing antibodies.[13] These facts clearly demonstrated that blocking the first step (i.e., viral binding to host cell receptors) in the viral life cycle is potentially the most effective approach to prevent influenza viral infection.

However, since most viral surface antigens are mutation prone, neutralizing antibodies against influenza viruses are only effective toward the strains to which they are raised and cannot provide broad-based protection to the mutant strains. To create a broad-spectrum influenza therapeutic agent, NexBio Inc., a San Diego-based biopharmaceutical company, undertook a novel approach to block the specific binding between all types of influenza viruses to their host cell receptors. NexBio's strategy is to render the target cells inaccessible to influenza viruses by inactivating the influenza virus receptor, sialic acids, on the cell surface. To this end, NexBio invented and produced DAS181, a novel recombinant fusion protein consisting of a sialidase catalytic domain fused with a human respiratory epithelium-anchoring domain for blocking viral infection.

The host cell receptors for influenza A and B viruses are cell-surface sialic acids.[14] Sialic acids are α-keto acids with 9-carbon backbones that are usually found at the outermost positions of oligosaccharide chains that are attached to glycoproteins and glycolipids. The predominant type of sialic acid is N-acetylneuraminic acid (Neu5Ac), which is the biosynthetic precursor for most other types. Two major linkages between Neu5Ac and the penultimate galactose residues of the carbohydrate side chains are found in nature, Neu5Ac α(2,3)-Gal (α2,3-linked sialic acids) and Neu5Ac α(2,6)-Gal (α2,6-linked sialic acids). Both α2,3- and α2,6-linked sialic acids can be recognized as receptors by influenza viruses.[15] Human viruses recognize α2,6-linked sialic acids while avian and equine viruses recognize α2,3-linked sialic acids.[14,16]

The human tracheal epithelium expresses both forms of sialic acids, but α(2,6)-linked sialic acids are more abundant and present on both the ciliated and nonciliated cells, while the α(2,3)-linked sialic acids are less abundant and restricted to only some ciliated cells.[17] This explains why the avian virus can infect humans, but the virus transmission is very inefficient. The relatively low abundance of α(2,3)-linked sialic acid in the human airway epithelium underlies the species barrier for avian viruses. This also indicates that merely reducing the sialic acid level on the airway surface would have a significant impact on IFV infectivity.

Sialidases, also referred to as neuraminidases, are a family of exoglycosidases that catalyze the removal of terminal sialic acid residues from various glycoconjugates, such as glycoproteins and glycolipids. Sialic acids on the cell surface can be removed by treating the cells with a sialidase. The respiratory epithelium-anchoring domain is a high-affinity heparin-binding peptide domain that attaches the enzyme onto heparin-like molecules such as heparan sulfate, or other negatively charged polysaccharides that are ubiquitously present on the epithelial cell surface. The anchoring domain enhances the potency of the sialidase by juxtaposing the molecule to the target sialic acid functional groups and thus increases retention time on the respiratory epithelium. In fact, the epithelial anchoring domain increases the potency of sialic acid removal on MDCK cells by over 10 times.[18]

Sialidases have been shown to be effective inhibitors of influenza virus infection in a number of *in vitro* experimental models. Even before sialic acids were proven to be the receptor for influenza viruses, it was observed that when sialic acids were enzymatically removed from cell surfaces, the cells were less susceptible to infection by influenza viruses. [19–22] These findings, however, had not been translated into a practical approach for clinically treatment of influenza until the creation of DAS181.

Sialidase activities are normally present in many human tissues, including the salivary glands and the lungs.[23] In fact, sialidase treatment of guinea pig respiratory tract significantly reduced substance P-induced bronchoconstriction[24] and inhibited tracheal contraction induced by an antigen (ovalbumin) or compound 48/80.[25] Furthermore, sialidase treatment did not change the rheological properties of mucus, nor did it affect the normal mucus transport activity on ciliated epithelium.[26,27] These features suggest that a sialidase like DAS181 is unlikely to be overtly toxic to the airway or produce airway hyper-responsiveness and hyper-reactivity.

Studies have shown that DAS181 has potent broad-spectrum anti-influenza activity in cell culture and animal models. Using the conventional MDCK cell culture model, the antiviral activity of DAS181 and its analogue has been demonstrated against over 20 laboratory strains and clinical isolates of IFV of the H1N1, H2N2, H3N2, H5N1, H9N2, and H7N7 subtypes. DAS181 was shown to be active against all of the tested IFV strains in this model system. The 50% and 90% inhibitory concentrations (EC_{50} and EC_{90}) in cell protection and viral inhibition assays were in the range of 0.04 to 15.6 nM and 0.4 to 51.6 nM, respectively. The *in vitro* anti-IFV activity of DAS181 appears to be stronger than Tamiflu® and Relenza® by several orders of magnitude; the reported cell protection EC_{50} values of Tamiflu® and Relenza® ranged from <10 nM to 3.4 μM.[10]

DAS181 maintained similar potency even when the infectious dose of virus was increased by 100- to 1000-fold. By contrast, the activity of many antiviral compounds is influenced by the infectious viral dose; they are often more active in cell culture at low MOI and thus less active (or inactive) at higher virus-to-cell ratio. For the NAIs, oseltamivir and RWJ-270201, every fivefold increase in MOI, in the MOI range of 0.0002 to 0.02 raised EC_{50} of both compounds by 7- to 10-fold (from 10 nM at MOI 0.0002 to >10 μM at MOI 0.02).[10] DAS181 potency remained undiminished even when the cell treatment was performed 24 hr prior to the virus challenge.[18] By targeting the host cells rather than the virus, DAS181 has shown distinct anti-IFV properties from the virus-targeting compounds, such as the NAIs. In MDCK cell cultures, the state of cell surface desialylation was sustained for over 3 days after a single DAS181 treatment.[18]

In the model system of the well-differentiated human airway epithelium (HAE), which closely mimic the human airway epithelium morphologically and functionally,[28,29] DAS181 demonstrated similarly potent activity against influenza A and B virus strains. In this model system, the treatment effect of a single dose of DAS181 lasted for over one week (unpublished results).

In a murine model of influenza infection, DAS181 displayed potent anti-influenza activity. Twice daily dosing of 30 U (approximately 1 mg/kg/day) demonstrated 100% survival protection and over 5 logs of reduction in viral titer using the lethal A/NWS/33 (H1N1) strain of influenza. Doses as low as 0.3 U (approximately 10 μg/kg) still yielded 100% survival protection and gave rise to 4 logs of reduction in viral lung titer. In the same murine model, once every other day DAS181 treatment could be delayed to as late as 48 hrs post infection and still result in 100% survival.[18] Studies testing a DAS181 analogue in a ferret model of influenza infection gave similar results; viral titers in nasal washes were reduced and there were less signs of inflammation in the nasal washes. When the treatment was initiated at two days prior to the virus challenge, about 30% of the ferrets were completely protected from infection as demonstrated by negative seraconversion by the treated animals.[18] DAS181 has also demonstrated unprecedented activity against the highly pathogenic H5N1 virus (A/Vietnam/1203/04) in a lethal mouse model. In a series of studies, DAS181 administered once a day starting from one day prior to the virus challenge achieved 100% animal survival, and 70% of the animals were completely protected from the virus infection as demonstrated by the lack of seroconversion. The viral titer in the lungs was reduced by 4 to 6 $\log_{10}$ units, and the virus infection of the brains was completely prevented. When the DAS181 treatment was initiated at up to 72 hr after the virus infection, significant animal survival and virus inhibition was achieved.[30]

Based on its design, DAS181 has the following features that constitute an ideal therapeutic candidate against influenza: (1) By containing a sialidase that can effectively degrade both receptor sialic acids, Neu5Ac α(2,6)-Gal and Neu5Ac α(2,3)-Gal, DAS181 confers protection against the broadest range of influenza viruses, including both human and animal viruses. It also remains effective as the virus continuously mutates and evolves. As a result, DAS181 may overcome the shortcomings of influenza vaccines, which require annual updates due to antigenic drifts and antigenic shifts of the virus. (2) DAS181 targets the host cells rather than the virus. It simply prevents the virus from finding host receptors on the mucosal surface without selective killing of a large segment of the wild-type viral gene pool. Therefore, the likelihood of selecting resistant viral strains may be greatly reduced in comparison to therapeutics that target viral components.

Based on previous studies, it is expected that influenza strains resistant to DAS181 will be difficult to establish. A previous attempt to establish a stable sialidase-resistant influenza viral variant was only successful by using a combination of a bacterial sialidase with a polyclonal antibody directed toward the IFV NA.[31–34] The virus isolated under such conditions carried a large internal truncation in the NA gene and displayed a much reduced virulence both *in vitro* and *in vivo*.[33,35] It was revealed that the IFV mutants compensated for the lack of NA activity by having mutations around the HA receptor-binding pocket to reduce the virus's affinity for cellular receptors.[35] These studies demonstrated that the survival of the IFV mutants that were established by sialidase/anti-NA antibody double selection was only made possible by sacrificing the ability of the virus to infect host cells.

NexBio Inc. has submitted an IND application on DAS181 with the United States FDA.

T-705: AN INHIBITOR OF INFLUENZA VIRUS REPLICATION

Influenza viruses carry their genetic information as negative strands of RNA. Human host cells use DNA, rather than RNA templates for replication and transcription of their genetic information; they do not contain enzymes necessary to transcribe or replicate the RNA-based viral genome. Therefore the virus must supply its own RNA-dependent polymerases, making this unique enzyme an ideal target for the inhibition of influenza viral replication. Influenza nucleocapsids contain active viral RNA polymerase which bears signals that direct its entry into the nucleus of infected cells. During infection, each segment of the viral RNA genome is transcribed and replicated by viral polymerase in the host cell nucleus.

T-705 is a nonpeptide small-molecule influenza drug candidate that targets the viral gene replication process. Toyama Chemical Co. of Japan has developed the pyrazine derivative, T-705 (6-fluoro-3-hydroxy-2-pyrazinecarboxamide), which is reported to inhibit viral reproduction through inhibition of viral RNA polymerase.[36] Additional investigation showed that T-705 could function as a prodrug that can be phosphorylated into the nucleotide analogue drug T-705–4-ribofuranosyl-5′-triphosphate (T-705RTP) for viral RNA polymerase inhibition. Its mode of action is similar to that proposed for ribavirin which is a guanosine analogue antiviral compound. Ribavirin has demonstrated efficacy against RNA and DNA viruses, including influenza.

Studies demonstrating reversal of T-705's anti-influenza activity by the addition of purines and purine nucleosides suggest that T-705 inhibits viral polymerase through a competitive mechanism. In addition, a specific cellular metabolite of T-705 (T-705RTP) was shown to inhibit isolated influenza RNA polymerase in a pattern consistent with GTP competition. The inhibition appears to be specific because *in vitro* cellular DNA and RNA synthesis was unaffected.[36] It remains to be demonstrated whether T-705 and its metabolites exclusively affect polymerase activity or if they also competitively interfere with purine uptake and intracellular conversion.[37]

T-705 has shown selective inhibition of activity of a wide array of influenza A, B, and C viruses *in vitro*. Cell culture-based assays demonstrate efficacy against several strains of influenza A in the subtypes H1N1, H2N2, and H3N2 with EC_{50} ranging from 80 nM to 3 μM (0.013 to 0.5 μg/mL).[37,38] In addition, the therapeutic efficacy of T-705 was evaluated in a survival study of virus-infected mice. Orally administered T-705 (100 or 200 mg/kg/day, four times per day, beginning 1 hr post-infection) was shown to increase survival rates and decrease viral titer in lungs of virus-infected mice in a dose-dependent manner.[37] In recent studies at Utah State University, T-705 demonstrated efficacy against four strains of avian H5N1 influenza in cell culture with EC_{90} ranging from 1.3 to 7.7 μM. T-705 at 300 mg/kg/day administered up to 96 hr post-infection also prevented death in mice infected with lethal dose of a low pathogenic H5N1 influenza strain (A/Duck/MN/1525/81).[39] Studies demonstrated that T-705 had a better safety profile than amantadine and ribavirin; it displays no cytotoxicity in immortal mammalian cell lines at concentrations up to 10 times higher than levels where 50% cytotoxicity is observed for amantadine and ribavirin.[36]

Another nucleic acid analogue in this class of anti-influenza medicines that has demonstrated anti-influenza activity is LY217896 (1, 3,

4-thiadiazol-2-ylcyanamide). *In vitro* this compound provided protection against a broad range of influenza A and influenza B viruses with EC_{50} ranging from 2.8 to 11 μM (0.4 to 1.5 μg/mL). It also exhibited activity *in vivo* by preventing death in a lethal mouse model of influenza infection as well as in the ferret model.[40] Unfortunately, this molecule later failed to show efficacy in human clinical trials.[38,41] Since the viral RNA polymerase is a critical protein for inhibition of viral replication and potentially offers a high degree of drug target selectivity, it remains an attractive target for anti-influenza drug discovery. With superior potency and a better safety profile than LY217896, T-705 continues to be a promising new candidate for an influenza medicine. Toyama Chemical began Phase I clinical studies with T-705 in January 2007 under a Japanese IND and has also submitted an IND application with the United States FDA.

INHIBITING VIRAL REPLICATION AND TRANSCRIPTION: ANTISENSE OLIGONUCLEOTIDE AND SMALL INTERFERING RNA STRATEGIES

Because of their innate specificity toward the targeted viral RNA (vRNA) sequence and the critical role of influenza vRNA for replication and transcription, both antisense oligonucleotides (ASOs) and small interfering RNA (siRNA) are attractive technology platforms for viral-genome-based drug discovery. ASO and siRNA technologies employ either single-stranded or double-stranded short oligonucleotide sequences, respectively, that are complementary to mRNA, vRNA, or cRNA, to exert their inhibitory or gene silencing activities through different mechanisms. Second- and third-generation ASOs (2′-*O*-methoxy-substituted (MES) oligonucleotides and morpholino oligonucleotides) bind to their complementary RNA targets and primarily disrupt translation by steric hindrance[42] as well as the RNase H-mediated target cleavage activity.[42,43] The more pharmacokinetically favored, second-generation ASOs with a modified backbone to confer nuclease resistance have tremendously enhanced the therapeutic potency for either systemic, aerosol, or topical routes of delivery. Both of these ASOs rely on stoichiometric occupation and binding to the intended sequence of RNA target. In addition to the target binding, therapeutic siRNA technology employs the cellular RNA-induced silencing complex (RISC), which hones in on the target RNA sequence and mediates the cleavage of the target RNA.[44] Unlike inhibition by ASOs, the active RISC complex can be recycled for cleavage of additional target strands of

RNA. In comparison to the single-stranded morpholino or the MES ASOs, the RISC mechanism may require less siRNA to achieve the same therapeutic effect. Still, the second-generation ASOs are considered pharmaceutically more stable and pharmacokinetically superior to the siRNAs and could prove to be a more effective means for anti-influenza therapy.

Several groups have demonstrated the effectiveness of these potential anti-influenza therapies *in vitro* and *in vivo*. These strategies are covered in more detail in two separate contributions within this volume. Two promising ASOs targeted against either the AUG translation site of PB1 or the 3′-terminal region of the vRNA genome displayed broad-spectrum anti-influenza activity against H1N1, H3N2, H3N8, H7N7, and H5N1 *in vitro*. These top performing ASOs reduced viral titer by 2–$3\log_{10}$ units at $20\,\mu M$.[45] Similarly, siRNAs targeting either the influenza NP, PA, or PB1 have been shown to be active against H1N1, H5N1, and H7N7 in a cell culture model as well as in a mouse model of influenza infection using an intravenous route of administration. The top-performing siRNA candidates reduced viral titer in mouse lungs by 1–$2\log_{10}$ units at $3\,mg/kg$.[46–48]

Both ASO and siRNA therapeutics can be designed to bind to the highly conserved regions of viral RNA and offer broad-spectrum activity against all strains and subtypes of influenza A and B. However, because of sequence divergence, no single siRNA or ASO candidate therapeutic has yet been shown to display activity against both influenza A and B viruses. This issue could be addressed by using combinations of antisense oligonucleotides. Since influenza is an infection that is limited to the respiratory tract and the lungs, local administration of the drug candidates is possible to enhance target organ/tissue delivery and to limit the potential systemic side effects and toxicity. Both naked oligonucleotides as well as polycationic complexed oligonucleotides have been delivered successfully to the lungs of mice in a nebulized aerosol as an aqueous solution and can certainly be a viable option for human delivery. Both ASO and siRNA technologies utilize a 20- to 22-mer short nucleotide sequence to precisely target a specific viral gene. Yet similar anti-influenza activity is maintained with as many as two nucleotide changes in the influenza sequence.[38]

Thus far, AVI Biopharma has advanced one of the third-generation ASOs with NeuGene® chemistry into preclinical development (AVI-6001). Alnylam Pharmaceuticals has advanced the siRNA lead, ALN-RSVO1, for another respiratory virus, RSV, through phase I clinical trials and has phase II clinical efficacy studies planned. Through a partnership with Novartis, Alnylam Pharmaceuticals is developing an siRNA for pandemic H5N1 influenza virus. Although both companies have good lead compounds, the efficacy of the Neugene and Alnylam anti-influenza therapeutics has yet to be clearly demonstrated in clinical development.

INHIBITION OF VIRAL RELEASE: MULTIMERIC NEURAMINIDASE INHIBITORS

For the past several years the neuraminidase inhibitors (NAIs), oseltamivir and zanamivir, have been the mainstay of anti-influenza therapy. They have proven to be safe and effective for treatment of human influenza A and influenza B viruses. Recently, several studies have demonstrated their effectiveness against the potentially pandemic H5N1 strains in mouse and ferret challenge models[49–52] demonstrating their potential for use as a pandemic influenza drug.

The influenza viral envelope is covered with spikes that are composed of three types of protein: hemagglutinin (HA), which binds to host cell receptors and mediates fusion of viral and cellular membranes; neuraminidase (NA), which facilitates release of the new viruses from host cells; and a small number of M2 proteins which serve as ion channels. Specifically, the NA tetramer is thought to prevent self-aggregation of influenza virions during the budding and release stage of the virus life cycle as well as facilitate cell spreading through the mucus.[33] NAIs specifically inhibit viral neuraminidase, thereby preventing the efficient spreading of new viruses through the respiratory tract.

Building upon an already reliable class of influenza therapeutics, multimeric neuraminidase inhibitors are yet another novel approach to treat influenza. Because multivalent interactions can dramatically increase the affinity of ligands to receptors,[53,54] multimeric forms of the neuraminidase inhibitors are being investigated as a way to increase the potency of the NAIs. In both cell-based CPE (cytopathic effect) assays and plaque reduction assays, as well as *in vivo* mouse studies, dimeric forms of zanamivir can be up to 1000-fold more active than the monomeric form with an optimal linker length of 16–18 Å.[55] Dimeric forms of zanamavir could result in three types of multivalent interactions: binding between two sites on an NA tetramer (intratetramer), binding between two sites on different NA tetramers within the same virion (intravirion), and binding between two sites on NA tetramers on different virions (intervirion). Based on the molecular spacing of the NA tetramers on the surface of the virion, it was proposed that most of the interactions are either intratetramer or intervirion, and this potentially leads to the formation of large matrices of influenza virions resulting in further aggregation of virus and better prevention of viral spreading. An added benefit to the use of zanamavir dimers as a therapeutic agent is that the clearance rate is greatly diminished and lung retention of the therapeutic molecule is increased. This could potentially decrease the number of doses needed for effective prophylaxis and treatment. Similar improvements were observed with the use trimeric and tetrameric forms of zanamivir in anti-influenza assays. These compounds reduced viral titer by up to $4\log_{10}$ units when administered at a dose of 1 mg/kg/day. In comparison to the monomeric zanamivir, they were at least 40-fold more active. A single dose of the dimeric or tetrameric form could be administered 10 days prior to infection compared to two days prior to infection for the monomeric form and still exert significant anti-influenza effects in a mouse model of infection.[56]

In summary, broad-spectrum novel anti-influenza agents with different modes of action are urgently needed to address the unmet therapeutic needs and imminent pandemics, because the current supply of anti-influenza drugs is rapidly becoming inadequate. As more novel classes of anti-influenza therapeutics become available, the potential for combination therapy also becomes more feasible. Potential benefits of combination therapy include reduced drug resistance[57] and superior efficacy and potency.[58–62] Despite the overwhelming challenges of developing the ideal influenza medicine, DAS181, a sialidase fusion protein, viral polymerase inhibitors such as T-705, antisense oligonucleotides, siRNA, and long-lasting multimeric neuraminidase inhibitors represent some of the most promising upcoming anti-influenza therapeutics in development.

REFERENCES

1. Chen, H.; Deng, G.; Li, Z.; Tian, G.; Li, Y.; Jiao, P.; Zhang, L.; Liu, Z.; Webster, R. G.; Yu, K. The evolution of H5N1 influenza viruses in ducks in southern China. *Proc. Natl. Acad. Sci. USA* **2004**, *101*, 10452–10457.

2. Butler, D. Alarms ring over bird flu mutations. *Nature* **2006**, *439*, 248–249.

3. Wood, J. M. Developing vaccines against pandemic influenza. *Philos. Trans. R. Soc. Lond. B. Biol. Sci.* **2001**, *356*, 1953–1960.

4. Gust, I. D.; Hampson, A. W.; Lavanchy, D. Planning for the next pandemic of influenza. *Rev. Med. Virol.* **2001**, *11*, 59–70.

5. Chen, H.; et al. Establishment of multiple sublineages of H5N1 influenza virus in Asia: implications for pandemic control. *Proc. Natl. Acad. Sci USA* **2006**, *103*, 2845–2850.

6. Moscona, A. Neuraminidase inhibitors for influenza. *N. Engl. J. Med.* **2005**, *353*, 1363–1373.

7. Kiso, M.; Sakai-Tagawa, Y.; Shiraishi, K.; Kawakami, C.; Kimura, K.; Hayden, F. G.; Sugaya, N.; Kawaoka, Y. Resistant influenza A viruses in children treated with oseltamivir: Descriptive study. *Lancet* **2004**, *364*, 759–765.

8. de Jong, M. D.; Tran, T. T.; Truong, H. K.; Vo, M. H.; Smith, G. J.; Nguyen, V. C.; Bach, V. C.; Phan, T. Q.; Do, Q. H.; Guan, Y.; Peiris, J. S.; Tran, T. H.; Farrar, J. Oseltamivir resistance during treatment of influenza A (H5N1) infection. *N. Engl. J Med.* **2005**, *353*, 2667–2672.

9. Gubareva, L. V.; Bethell, R.; Hart, G. J.; Murti, K. G.; Penn, C. R.; Webster, R. G. Characterization of mutants of influenza A virus selected with the neuraminidase inhibitor 4-guanidino-Neu5Ac2en. *J. Virol.* **1996**, *70*, 1818–1827.

10. Smee, D. F.; Huffman, J. H.; Morrison, A. C.; Barnard, D. L.; Sidwell, R. W. Cyclopentane neuraminidase inhibitors with potent *in vitro* anti-influenza virus activities. *Antimicrob. Agents. Chemother.* **2001**, *45*, 743–748.

11. McKimm-Breschkin, J. L. Resistance of influenza viruses to neuraminidase inhibitors—a review. *Antiviral Res.* **2000**, *47*, 1–17.

12. Bender, B. S.; Small, P. A., Jr. Influenza: pathogenesis and host defense. *Semin. Respir. Infect.* **1992**, *7*, 38–45.

13. Ghendon, Y. The immune response to influenza vaccines. *Acta Virol.* **1990**, *34*, 295–304.

14. Ito, T. Interspecies transmission and receptor recognition of influenza A viruses. *Microbiol. Immunol.* **2000**, *44*, 423–430.

15. Schauer, R. Chemistry, metabolism, and biological functions of sialic acids. *Adv. Carbohydr. Chem. Biochem.* **1982**, *40*, 131–234.

16. Stevens, J.; Blixt, O.; Glaser, L.; Taubenberger, J. K.; Palese, P.; Paulson, J. C.; Wilson, I. A. Glycan microarray analysis of the hemagglutinins from modern and pandemic influenza viruses reveals different receptor specificities. *J. Mol. Biol.* **2006**, *355*, 1143–1155.

17. Matrosovich, M. N.; Matrosovich, T. Y.; Gray, T.; Roberts, N. A.; Klenk, H. D. Human and avian influenza viruses target different cell types in cultures of human airway epithelium. *Proc. Natl. Acad. Sci. USA* **2004**, *101*, 4620–4624.

18. Malakhov, M. P.; Aschenbrenner, L. M.; Smee, D. F.; Wandersee, M. K.; Sidwell, R. W.; Gubareva, L. V.; Mishin, V. P.; Hayden, F. G.; Kim, D. H.; Ing, A.; Campbell, E. R.; Yu, M.; Fang, F. Sialidase fusion protein as a novel broad-spectrum inhibitor of influenza virus infection. *Antimicrob. Agents Chemother.* **2006**, *50*, 1470–1479.

19. Gottschalk, A. *The Viruses*, Academic Press, New York, **1959**, pp. 51–61.
20. Bergelson, L. D.; Bukrinskaya, A. G.; Prokazova, N. V.; Shaposhnikova, G. I.; Kocharov, S. L.; Shevchenko, V. P.; Kornilaeva, G. V.; Fomina-Ageeva, E. V. Role of gangliosides in reception of influenza virus. *Eur. J. Biochem.* **1982**, *128*, 467–474.
21. Griffin, J. A.; Basak, S.; Compans, R. W. Effects of hexose starvation and the role of sialic acid in influenza virus release. *Virology* **1983**, *125*, 324–334.
22. Els, M. C.; Laver, W. G.; Air, G. M. Sialic acid is cleaved from glycoconjugates at the cell surface when influenza virus neuraminidases are expressed from recombinant vaccinia viruses. *Virology* **1989**, *170*, 346–351.
23. Achyuthan, K. E.; Achyuthan, A. M. Comparative enzymology, biochemistry and pathophysiology of human exo-alpha-sialidases (neuraminidases). *Comp. Biochem. Physiol. B Biochem. Mol. Biol.* **2001**, *129*, 29–64.
24. Jarreau, P. H.; Harf, A.; Levame, M.; Lambre, C. R.; Lorino, H.; Macquin-Mavier, I. Effects of neuraminidase on airway reactivity in the guinea pig. *Am. Rev. Respir. Dis.* **1992**, *145*, 906–910.
25. Kai, H.; Makise, K.; Matsumoto, S.; Ishii, T.; Takahama, K.; Isohama, Y.; Miyata, T. The influence of neuraminidase treatment on tracheal smooth muscle contraction. *Eur. J. Pharmacol.* **1992**, *220*, 181–185.
26. King, M.; Gilboa, A.; Meyer, F. A.; Silberberg, A. On the transport of mucus and its rheologic simulants in ciliated systems. *Am. Rev. Respir. Dis.* **1974**, *110*, 740–745.
27. Meyer, F. A.; King, M.; Gelman, R. A. On the role of sialic acid in the rheological properties of mucus. *Biochim. Biophys. Acta* **1975**, *392*, 223–232.
28. Zhang, L.; Peeples, M. E.; Boucher, R. C.; Collins, P. L.; Pickles, R. J. Respiratory syncytial virus infection of human airway epithelial cells is polarized, specific to ciliated cells, and without obvious cytopathology. *J Virol.* **2002**, *76*, 5654–5666.
29. Sinn, P. L.; Williams, G.; Vongpunsawad, S.; Cattaneo, R.; McCray, P. B., Jr. Measles virus preferentially transduces the basolateral surface of well-differentiated human airway epithelia. *J. Virol.* **2002**, *76*, 2403–2409.
30. Belser, J.; Lu, X.; Szretter, K.; Jin, X.; Aschenbrenner, L.; Lee, A.; Hawley, S.; Kim, D.; Malakhov, M.; Yu, M.; Fang, F.; Katz, J. A novel sialidase fusion protein DAS181 (Fludase®) protects mice against lethal H5N1 avian influenza infection. Unpublished work, **2007**.
31. Yang, P.; Bansal, A.; Liu, C.; Air, G. M. Hemagglutinin specificity and neuraminidase coding capacity of neuraminidase-deficient influenza viruses. *Virology* **1997**, *229*, 155–165.
32. Liu, C.; Air, G. M. Selection and characterization of a neuraminidase-minus mutant of influenza virus and its rescue by cloned neuraminidase genes. *Virology* **1993**, *194*, 403–407.

33. Liu, C.; Eichelberger, M. C.; Compans, R. W.; Air, G. M. Influenza type A virus neuraminidase does not play a role in viral entry, replication, assembly, or budding. *J. Virol.* **1995**, *69*, 1099–1106.

34. Hughes, M. T.; Matrosovich, M.; Rodgers, M. E.; McGregor, M.; Kawaoka, Y. Influenza A viruses lacking sialidase activity can undergo multiple cycles of replication in cell culture, eggs, or mice. *J. Virol.* **2000**, *74*, 5206–5212.

35. Hughes, M. T.; Matrosovich, M.; Rodgers, M. E.; McGregor, M.; Kawaoka, Y. Influenza A viruses lacking sialidase activity can undergo multiple cycles of replication in cell culture, eggs, or mice. *J. Virol.* **2000**, *74*, 5206–5212.

36. Furuta, Y.; Takahashi, K.; Kuno-Maekawa, M.; Sangawa, H.; Uehara, S.; Kozaki, K.; Nomura, N.; Egawa, H.; Shiraki, K. Mechanism of action of T-705 against influenza virus. *Antimicrob. Agents Chemother.* **2005**, *49*, 981–986.

37. Furuta, Y.; Takahashi, K.; Fukuda, Y.; Kuno, M.; Kamiyama, T.; Kozaki, K.; Nomura, N.; Egawa, H.; Minami, S.; Watanabe, Y.; Narita, H.; Shiraki, K. *In vitro* and *in vivo* activities of anti-influenza virus compound T-705. *Antimicrob. Agents Chemother.* **2002**, *46*, 977–981.

38. Ge, Q.; Pastey, M.; Kobasa, D.; Puthavathana, P.; Lupfer, C.; Bestwick, R. K.; Iversen, P. L.; Chen, J.; Stein, D. A. Inhibition of multiple subtypes of influenza A virus in cell cultures with morpholino oligomers. *Antimicrob. Agents Chemother.* **2006**, *50*, 3724–3733.

39. Sidwell, R. W.; Barnard, D. L.; Day, C. W.; Smee, D. F.; Bailey, K. W.; Wong, M. H.; Morrey, J. D.; Furuta, Y. Efficacy of orally administered T-705 on lethal avian influenza A (H5N1) virus infections in mice. *Antimicrob. Agents Chemother.* **2007**, *51*, 845–851.

40. Colacino, J. M.; DeLong, D. C.; Nelson, J. R.; Spitzer, W. A.; Tang, J.; Victor, F.; Wu, C. Y. Evaluation of the anti-influenza virus activities of 1,3,4-thiadiazol-2-ylcyanamide (LY217896) and its sodium salt. *Antimicrob. Agents Chemother.* **1990**, *34*, 2156–2163.

41. Hayden, F. G.; Rollins, B. S.; Hay, A. J. Anti-influenza virus activity of the compound LY253963. *Antiviral Res.* **1990**, *14*, 25–38.

42. Dias, N.; Stein, C. A. Antisense oligonucleotides: Basic concepts and mechanisms. *Mol. Cancer Therapeutics* **2002**, *1*, 347–355.

43. Crooke, S. T. Molecular mechanisms of action of antisense drugs. *Biochim. Biophys. Acta-Gene Struct. Expr.* **1999**, *1489*, 31–44.

44. Dykxhoorn, D. M.; Lieberman, J. Running interference: Prospects and obstacles to using small interfering RNAs as small molecule drugs. *Annu. Rev. Biomed. Eng.* **2006**.

45. Ge, Q.; Pastey, M.; Kobasa, D.; Puthavathana, P.; Lupfer, C.; Bestwick, R. K.; Iversen, P. L.; Chen, J.; Stein, D. A. Inhibition of multiple subtypes of influenza A virus in cell cultures with morpholino oligomers. *Antimicrob. Agents Chemother.* **2006**, *50*, 3724–3733.

46. Tompkins, S. M.; Lo, C. Y.; Tumpey, T. M.; Epstein, S. L. Protection against lethal influenza virus challenge by RNA interference *in vivo*. *Proc. Natl. Acad. Sci. USA* **2004**, *101*, 8682–8686.

47. Ge, Q.; McManus, M. T.; Nguyen, T.; Shen, C. H.; Sharp, P. A.; Eisen, H. N.; Chen, J. RNA interference of influenza virus production by directly targeting mRNA for degradation and indirectly inhibiting all viral RNA transcription. *Proc. Natl. Acad. Sci. USA* **2003**, *100*, 2718–2723.

48. Ge, Q.; Filip, L.; Bai, A.; Nguyen, T.; Eisen, H. N.; Chen, J. Inhibition of influenza virus production in virus-infected mice by RNA interference. *Proc. Natl. Acad. Sci. USA* **2004**, *101*, 8676–8681.

49. Govorkova, E. A.; Ilyushina, N. A.; Boltz, D. A.; Douglas, A.; Yilmaz, N.; Webster, R. G. Efficacy of oseltamivir therapy in ferrets inoculated with different clades of H5N1 influenza virus. *Antimicrob. Agents Chemother.* **2007**.

50. Govorkova, E. A.; Leneva, I. A.; Goloubeva, O. G.; Bush, K.; Webster, R. G. Comparison of efficacies of RWJ-270201, zanamivir, and oseltamivir against H5N1, H9N2, and other avian influenza viruses. *Antimicrob. Agents Chemother.* **2001**, *45*, 2723–2732.

51. Leneva, I. A.; Goloubeva, O.; Fenton, R. J.; Tisdale, M.; Webster, R. G. Efficacy of zanamivir against avian influenza A viruses that possess genes encoding H5N1 internal proteins and are pathogenic in mammals. *Antimicrob. Agents Chemother.* **2001**, *45*, 1216–1224.

52. Gubareva, L. V.; McCullers, J. A.; Bethell, R. C.; Webster, R. G. Characterization of influenza A/HongKong/156/97 (H5N1) virus in a mouse model and protective effect of zanamivir on H5N1 infection in mice. *J. Infect. Dis.* **1998**, *178*, 1592–1596.

53. Bertozzi, C. R.; Kiessling, L. L. Chemical glycobiology. *Science* **2001**, *291*, 2357–2364.

54. Borman, S. Multivalency: Strength in numbers. *Chem. Eng. News* **2000**, *78*, 48–53.

55. Macdonald, S. J.; Watson, K. G.; Cameron, R.; Chalmers, D. K.; Demaine, D. A.; Fenton, R. J.; Gower, D.; Hamblin, J. N.; Hamilton, S.; Hart, G. J.; Inglis, G. G.; Jin, B.; Jones, H. T.; McConnell, D. B.; Mason, A. M.; Nguyen, V.; Owens, I. J.; Parry, N.; Reece, P. A.; Shanahan, S. E.; Smith, D.; Wu, W. Y.; Tucker, S. P. Potent and long-acting dimeric inhibitors of influenza virus neuraminidase are effective at a once-weekly dosing regimen. *Antimicrob. Agents Chemother.* **2004**, *48*, 4542–4549.

56. Watson, K. G.; Cameron, R.; Fenton, R. J.; Gower, D.; Hamilton, S.; Jin, B.; Krippner, G. Y.; Luttick, A.; McConnell, D.; Macdonald, S. J.; Mason, A. M.; Nguyen, V.; Tucker, S. P.; Wu, W. Y. Highly potent and long-acting trimeric and tetrameric inhibitors of influenza virus neuraminidase. *Bioorg. Med. Chem. Lett.* **2004**, *14*, 1589–1592.

57. Ilyushina, N. A.; Bovin, N. V.; Webster, R. G.; Govorkova, E. A. Combination chemotherapy, a potential strategy for reducing the emergence of drug-resistant influenza A variants. *Antiviral Res.* **2006**, *70*, 121–131.

58. Galabov, A. S.; Simeonova, L.; Gegova, G. Rimantadine and oseltamivir demonstrate synergistic combination effect in an experimental infection with type A (H3N2) influenza virus in mice. *Antivir. Chem. Chemother.* **2006**, *17*, 251–258.

59. Tsiodras, S.; Mooney, J. D.; Hatzakis, A. Role of combination antiviral therapy in pandemic influenza and stockpiling implications. *BMJ* **2007**, *334*, 293–294.

60. Govorkova, E. A.; Fang, H. B.; Tan, M.; Webster, R. G. Neuraminidase inhibitor-rimantadine combinations exert additive and synergistic anti-influenza virus effects in MDCK cells. *Antimicrob. Agents Chemother.* **2004**, *48*, 4855–4863.

61. Ghezzi, P.; Ungheri, D. Synergistic combination of *N*-acetylcysteine and ribavirin to protect from lethal influenza viral infection in a mouse model. *Int. J. Immunopathol. Pharmacol.* **2004**, *17*, 99–102.

62. Shigeta, S.; Mori, S.; Watanabe, J.; Soeda, S.; Takahashi, K.; Yamase, T. Synergistic anti-influenza virus A (H1N1) activities of PM-523 (polyoxometalate) and ribavirin *in vitro* and *in vivo*. *Antimicrob. Agents Chemother.* **1997**, *41*, 1423–1427.

INDEX